Rethinking Health Care

Rethinking Health Care

Innovation and Change
in America

Max Heirich

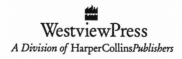

WestviewPress
A Division of HarperCollinsPublishers

Copyright © 1998 by Westview Press, A Division of HarperCollins Publishers, Inc.

Published in 1998 in the United States of America by Westview Press, 5500 Central Avenue, Boulder, Colorado 80301-2877, and in the United Kingdom by Westview Press, 12 Hid's Copse Road, Cumnor Hill, Oxford OX2 9JJ

A CIP catalog record for this book is available from the Library of Congress.
ISBN 0-8133-3454-3

The paper used in this publication meets the requirements of the American National Standard for Permanence of Paper for Printed Library Materials Z39.48-1984.

10   9   8   7   6   5   4   3   2   1

Contents

Acknowledgement

Many people have been part of the research venture which has culminated in this manuscript. In saying thank you it is hard to know where to begin.

Sources of institutional support have made it possible to study health from the many angles seen in this book. A University of Michigan sabbatical leave in 1974 helped me start a series of studies which have culminated in this book. A later sabbatical provided time for preparation of this manuscript which sets those kinds of developments in a larger socio-political context.

Both governmental and private sources funded research which deepened my understanding of various dimensions of American health care. Joint grants from the Heart, Lung, and Blood Institute of the National Institutes of Health and from the United Auto Workers-General Motors Health and Safety Innovation Fund, from 1984-1988 (to Andrea Foote, Jack Erfurt, and to me through the University of Michigan's Institute of Labor and Industrial Relations) sponsored experimental intervention research on worksite wellness programs, which deepened my understanding of some current health care dynamics. Judie LaRosa, Ted Miller, and Robert Wiencek, who oversaw these grants from NIH, the United Auto Workers, and General Motors, respectively, were quite helpful. I have appreciated, as well, access I have been given both to off-the-record meetings of business and labor health officials and to officers of health care philanthropies.

My thanks, also, to Rick J. Carlson and Ken Pelletier, who have been invaluable informants and consultants about health care policy and new developments for several years. The Ann Arbor and the Michigan Holistic Health Councils, the national Coalition of Holistic Health Organizations, and the advisory council for the NIH Office of Alternative Medicine gave me access to local, state, and national networks of holistic health participants who helped me better understand this particular health movement. Berkley Bedell, Brian Berman, Dan Butts, Barrie Cassileth, Ray Castellino, Brian Clements, Sally Collins, David Eisenberg, Steven Finando, Fred Goldberg, James S. Gordon, Phyllis Green, Gar Hildenbrand, Jennifer Jacobs, Gregory Kelley, Charlotte Kerr, Lao Lassiter, Ralph Moss, Sharon Scandrett-Hibdon, Tom Stiles, John Upledger, Nancy White, Frank Wiewel, and Richard Williams each taught me quite different things about the character and style of the holistic health movement, as did the staff of the NIH Office of Alternative Medicine.

The University of Michigan Residential College, Department of Sociology, and the University of Michigan Medical School's Inteflex program provided opportunity for me to teach about and to analyze the nature and character of American health care developments as the argument of this book was taking shape. My thanks to them, and to the approximately twelve hundred students who took these classes, helping me think through these issues as we interacted over a number of years.

A few colleagues have been especially helpful as I have wrestled with the problem of trying to understand the surprising and complex social phenomenon that emerged as American political and economic interest and our health care system interacted over time. Les Howard and William Norris stand out for their consistently thoughtful, challenging, provocative responses as I have struggled to understand these developments. Other friends and colleagues also have provided an important base of interest, support, and reaction as this project has gone forward. In addition to people already named I think with appreciation of Terry and Margaret Davies, Ruth Simmons and the late George Simmons, the late Jack Erfurt and the late Andrea Foote, Van Harrison, Jan Wright, and the late Raoul Betancourt, along with Doug, Dana, Alan, Julia and Debby Heirich, whose interest and feedback concerning various phases of this analysis have been quite helpful over the past few years. Rene Anspach, Charles Bright, James A. Bryant, Carola Burroughs, M. Linden Griffith, Joseph Jacobs, Clayton Koppock, Patricia Locke, Kristen Luker, Carolene Marks, Joyce Seltzer, Ellen Silverstone, and Tom Weisskopf provided helpful critiques of an earlier version of this manuscript from the vantage point of several intellectual disciplines, and Laurie Lehne, Rick Lempert, William Norris, and Deba Patnaik offered fine-grained critiques of that draft which were both challenging and extremely helpful. Their organizational suggestions, critiques of sometimes too facile arguments, and attention to clarity of wording have improved the quality of this account. The present argument has benefited, as well, from suggestions made by Barbara A. Anderson, Adam Bloomfield, Maaike Bouwmeister, Bruce Brock, Eugene Feingold, Maurice Gordon, Bridget Hamilton, Marianne Hillemeier, Nichelle Hughley, Carolyn Holmes, Nancy Kachel, Irit Kleinman, Hollie Malamud, Tricia Marine, Kim McNally, Sallyanne Payton, Erika Pennil, Brendon Riley, Stephanie Robert, Marilynn Rosenthal, Barbara Sloat, Kevin Stankiewiecz, Duujian Tsai, Cater Webb, Bethany White, and Christina Yadao, by anonymous reviewers of an earlier draft of this book and from Deba Patnaik's and Ruth Simmon's continuing interest and attention to detail. Gene Tanke has given editorial attention which has been quite helpful. I am quite grateful for all their suggestions.

Polly Coltman, Jean Chung, Kirsten Lietz, and Janelle Neroda, reference librarians for the University of Michigan School of Public Health Library, and Steven Jensen and his crew of research librarians at the Ann Arbor Public Library were constantly helpful as I pieced together the picture of contemporary health care trends that appears in this book. The reference help given during the period of time that I was working on this manuscript while recovering from a broken hip has left me deeply grateful for their assistance, which went beyond the limits of professional courtesy. I appreciate, as well, Tom Weisskopf's generosity in sharing data sources and helping me clarify confusing aspects of contemporary economic policy and Sy Berki's advice concerning health care financing literature and appropriate measures to use with some of the data.

The contributions of these colleagues, friends and sources of support have strengthened the analysis that you are about to read. Needless to say, the responsibility for any deficiencies that remain is mine.

Special thanks to Lindsay Custer, Claudia Dwass, Paula Espindola, Laura Ghiron, Daniel Kabira, Daxa Patel, Amy-Katrin St. Clair and Cater Webb for their help with endnote and manuscript preparation tasks. The University of Michigan's Department of Sociology and Institute of Labor and Industrial Relations provided computer support for manuscript preparation. Alan Heirich taught me computer programs and helped solve endless logistical problems in manuscript preparation in earlier stages of this project and was an ever-available "Man Friday" as I ran into various kinds of computer problems over a period of several years. Debby Heirich helped with manuscript preparation at critical stages of this project. My heartfelt thanks to both of them. Thanks also to Bryan Aupperle, Erna-Lynne Bogue, Dan DuRoss, Karis Gluski, Janis Michael, and Bennet Fauber for additional computer advice and help. Finally, a special vote of thanks to the staff of the Worker Health Program at the University of Michigan's Institute of Labor and Industrial Relations, including Cindy Sieck's very helpful research assistance, the late Patricia A. Strauch's copy editing, proofreading, formatting, and computerized manuscript preparation of earlier versions of this manuscript, and especially now to Carol L. Kent, who has acted as copy editor and has prepared the camera-ready copy of this book manuscript. Her knowledge, skill, commitment and dedication, and her careful attention to detail are deeply appreciated.

Introduction

The Deepening Crisis

It is time to rethink where we are trying to go with health care in America, and how we might begin to get there. Most agree that changes are needed, but efforts to reform health care as a whole have washed ashore, drowning in the whirlpools and eddies of special interest politics. This is all-too-familiar: from 1917 to the present, most political efforts to reform health care in the United States at a basic level have suffered similar fates. The plight of our most recent political expedition into these waters can be instructive, but only if understood as part of a larger saga. Meanwhile, over the past half-century, public and private efforts to introduce more limited reforms have often succeeded. They have changed the fundamental character of health care, but have not tamed its cost dynamic. Some of these more limited reforms have made the problems which remain more intense.

American health care has become dramatically different from that which developed elsewhere in the world. Its character has changed during the past 60 years, as health-care providers, business leaders, politicians, and various segments of the American public responded to new circumstances. Wars, evolving economic relations, population changes, and a variety of demands and pressures from social and political movements affected the organization of health-care services in the U.S. The end result has been ironic: on the one hand, American medicine has become the pace-setter for the rest of the world in terms of medical research and high-tech delivery of sophisticated medical services. Yet when the actual health status of the population is measured, the United States continues to fall short of what is being achieved in several other advanced industrial societies.[1] There is a growing consensus that American health care is in crisis, and that major changes are needed to make health services more affordable and more available to large segments of the public now being left out of the system.

Health care in America is far from static. For at least a half century a process of constant, incremental reform has reshaped the *organization* of health care as well as the actual services that are offered. As early as 1970, political analysts and public opinion polls agreed that the American health-care system was in trouble: costs were increasing at twice the rate of general inflation. Despite a variety of reforms, that dynamic has continued. As medical costs rise, each passing year finds fewer Americans protected by health insurance. High-tech medical innovation has produced a remarkable ability to affect life and death processes, so that the wealthy who are sick come to the United States from many parts of the world for care. However, before the collapse of the Soviet Union, the United States was the only industrialized nation other than South Africa that did not guarantee its own population access to health services, and in the U.S. the costs for health services have increased much more rapidly than anywhere else in the world. Medical care has become so expensive that few private households can afford to pay for it entirely out-of-pocket.

An important stream of health-care reform began about a century ago with the establishment of medical science as the basis for health-care delivery. It has been joined through time by organizational and funding innovations; these have worked much the way the joining of major tributaries sometimes influences the development of a larger river, changing both its size and its character. No longer is mainstream American health care adequately captured by the term, medical science. American health-care providers now describe themselves, with considerable accuracy, as part of "the health-care industry". Indeed, health care now is one of the most dynamic parts of the American economy, and its growth cannot be choked back without severe repercussions for the economy as a whole. Health care employs more Americans than any other economic area. For decades, now, hospitals, the pharmaceutical industry, medical equipment and the hospital construction industries have been major growth sectors in the economy; and as is well known, health care's share of the gross national product has quadrupled in the past 40 years. Heavily subsidized by federally funded research, by state and federal commitments to care for health costs of the elderly and those receiving public welfare payments, and by private employee health benefits guaranteed by many businesses, American health care sets the pace internationally for innovative treatment. It also sets the pace for cost: American health-care costs almost twice as much per person as that found in most other industrialized countries.

For several decades, however, U.S. standing on various international measures of the health of the population has been slipping. With the highest health-care spending in the world, one might expect the best health outcomes. Instead, the United States ranks twelfth to fifteenth on many measures of the health of the population, and ranks twenty-fourth for infant mortality. For some sectors of the population, infant mortality rates rival those found in the least economically developed countries.[2] Meanwhile state and federal governments find themselves hard-pressed to meet mandated, but constantly increasing medical costs, and more and more businesses either provide no health insurance coverage for their employees or decline responsibility for covering some of their more expensive ongoing medical problems. As a result, 40 million Americans currently have no health insurance, and over twice that many Americans have faced serious difficulty when health problems arise.[3] These double-trends, of constantly rising medical costs and the increasing refusal of public and private third-party payers to provide a blank check for this growth in cost, have torn the safety net available to Americans facing health-care problems. Formulas which were developed almost half a century ago for providing health care no longer work the way they did earlier. Nor—because of the complexity of earlier health-care innovations in America—can other nations' health-care systems, which produce better health outcomes for their populations, be simply transferred to the United States. The mix and distribution of physicians, and the vested interests in health care that must be accommodated, are sufficiently different in the U.S. so that formulas other nations use to get health care to the total population at a reasonable cost are only partially relevant to the American dilemma. Something more original will be needed.

We have been approaching health-care reform as if it is a simple problem in social engineering. Design a system, introduce it, and let the problems solve themselves. The process of health-care reform in the U.S., however, works rather differently than that, in practice. As American health care develops and flows forward through time, constantly changing, constantly in flux, it often sweeps new inputs away or sends them in unintended directions. There are, nonetheless, patterns to its flow, principles underlying the dynamic of its development. These can become part of our planning, if they are observed accurately. Innovations from the past show it is possible to affect the speed of its flow and sometimes its direction. Often, however, our efforts have increased the problematic dynamic at work. Only if we understand the variety of forces that affect it and how they work together are our innovations likely to have a more positive outcome.

Recent public debate about directions for health-care reform pitted three contending "solutions" to problems in health-care delivery against one another. Some advocated creating a Canadian-style health-care system in the U.S., a "single payer plan" where taxes finance health-care expenditures. Hospitals, whether publicly or privately owned, receive both annual budgets and payment from the provincial government, and they treat all who come without further charges. Private physicians are reimbursed by the provincial governments, which also regulate the prices that can be charged for physicians' services. There was little political support in the U.S. for such a solution, however: higher taxes and state regulation were ideological anathema, political poison, which also threatened the freedom of one of the most vibrant sectors of the American economy. The health-care industry's investment ties to other sectors of the economy and the insurance industry's investment in U.S. Treasury bonds guaranteed that developing a state-regulated health-care system was not politically feasible.[4] Nor was it clear that such a proposal would have solved U.S. health-care problems. These reforms would not address the geographic maldistribution of health services in the U.S., or the disproportionate ratio of specialists to primary care doctors. Moreover the Canadian system's cost is second only to that of the U.S., the world's most expensive health-care system. Like the U.S., Canada is having trouble paying for its health care, and several provinces are cutting back on the services they provide.[5]

At the opposite extreme, many conservatives argued that we should let "market forces" solve health-care problems, abandoning both government regulation and government subsidies for the health-care industry. If there were greater competition for the health-care dollar, they argued, prices would come down and the public would be better served. The voting block of elderly Americans dependent upon government-subsidized health insurance, the 40 million Americans without health insurance who cannot participate in the market because of the cost of services,[6] and the Medicaid population who find difficulty getting doctors to treat them for discounted payments, make it clear that the stakes are high for the American public. To ignore this can be politically dangerous. Market forces have not drawn physicians to the 2,000 communities where they are in short supply, nor to currently avoided population groups in U.S. metropolitan areas. Monopoly rights to practice medicine combine with "cooperative" organization of "health-care markets" to skew the way health-care market competition works. As federal health-care policy moved toward a more nearly market approach to health-care problems in the 1980s the number of Americans lacking basic health-care services rose sharply. American health care is both an economic commodity and a public necessity. Primarily economic solutions to problems of health care all too often ignore the human equation. However, when other proposals for health-care reform are stymied, market force approaches win by default. There is little evidence thus far, however, that the health needs of the public get better served.

"Managed competition," a "middle-way" between these two extremes, provided the conceptual base for proposals made in 1993 by President Clinton's Health Insurance Reform Task Force. This approach kept a role for government as definer of social problems that must be addressed, and as a regulator of market conditions: i.e., government-imposed rules for market competition in health care would guarantee that providers gave services to everyone and would define the price limits within which competition could be waged for the health-care dollar.[7] The Clinton Plan borrowed many details from the German health-care system; the proposal, however, added more government regulation than was palatable either to the health-care industry or the general American public. Congress began basically rewriting the Clinton health insurance reform proposals, before the venture bogged down in political partisanship. Eventually, public distrust of the Clinton health reform proposals helped conservative Republicans sweep control of Congress.

None of the directions for health-care reform proposed in 1994 carried the day. Equally important, it seems unlikely that any of them could have succeeded, had it been chosen.

This was the sixth round within the twentieth century of legislative efforts to make sure all Americans get the health-care services they need, at prices they (and various third parties that help pay for health care) can afford. Only twice have fundamental legislative reform efforts affecting access to health care or its financing succeeded. In 1965, Medicare and Medicaid were created. In 1972, legislation helped set up health maintenance organizations (HMOs) that would receive fixed annual payments to cover all health needs of their subscribers, rather than be paid fees for each service performed. These two reforms changed the structure of U.S. health care in important ways; one helped set in motion the cost escalation that has plagued the system ever since and the other, designed to counter this trend, challenged the traditional autonomy of physicians, while having only modest impact on the emerging cost dynamic.

Although most of the major reform efforts during the past 25 years have failed, policy makers introduced several innovations, which, if less sweeping in their impact, nonetheless were intended to improve the accessibility of health-care services and to control the costs and the quality of care given. Quite different approaches, reflecting rather different ideological strategies, have been tried in various decades. None, however, has worked. Health-care problems continue to escalate, independent of the various measures taken to improve the situation.

In the mid-1970s, off-the-record meetings of influential leaders—held first at Airlie House near Washington, D.C., and then at the Waldorf-Astoria in New York City—asked whether the health-care system had outlived its usefulness and needed to be replaced by something more attuned to the realities of contemporary health issues.[8] At the same time, the mass media were focusing attention on four problems: (1) the cost of health care was soaring dramatically; (2) despite major programs of government-sponsored health insurance for the elderly and those on welfare, health-care services remained inaccessible to millions of Americans; (3) a surge of malpractice cases against doctors and hospitals was bringing into the open issues of quality control in the practice of medicine; and (4) a lack of humaneness now confronted many Americans seeking health services, who found that bureaucratic regulations and a concern for their ability to pay for medical services all too often determined their access to health care.[9]

Dramatic public and private efforts to reform the American health-care system sought to address these problems. Health-care providers were subjected to cost control supervision by government, business, and insurance companies. Programs to reimburse health-care providers on an annual per-patient basis, rather than for each service performed, gained favor, as did fixed reimbursement costs per hospital illness. Business professionals now managed or advised many health facilities and introduced new management decision strategies into health-care administration. Private investment capital replaced public subsidies and introduced new kinds of market competition into many areas of health care.

Other reforms tackled problems of access to health services. New health professions (nurse-clinician, nurse-practitioner, nurse-midwife, and physicians' assistant) were created, expanding the number of professionals able to provide primary health-care services. Medical schools dramatically increased the number of doctors being trained, while recruiting greater numbers of women and members of ethnic minorities. For a time, debt forgiveness programs recruited young doctors for tours of duty in under-served communities. Health maintenance organizations (HMOs), offering a "managed care" approach to primary health care that provides services for a fixed per-person cost each year, enrolled 70 million Americans. Ninety million Americans get health service from Preferred Provider Organizations (PPOs) chosen by their employers because they offered a discounted rate for services.

Quality control issues also were addressed. New professional oversight committees were created to provide tighter review of the actual practice of medicine on a day-to-day basis, in the hope of lessening the need for malpractice suits while maintaining cost-efficient health care. Outcome-focused health care gained favor.

In short, between 1970 and 1995 an astonishing degree of innovation occurred in American health care. Yet by 1995 the American "health-care crisis" had grown far deeper and more complex. Each of the problems identified 25 years before had grown noticeably worse.

The increase in cost had been staggering. National health-care expenditures in 1970 already amounted to $74.4 billion (an almost 80 percent cost increase since Medicare and Medicaid had been established five years earlier). By 1995 the annual costs had grown to one trillion dollars.[10] Even after adjusting for inflation, health-care costs had increased more than three-fold since 1970, and health care's share of the gross national product (GNP) had almost doubled. The overall cost of the health-care system now was challenging the economic viability of federal and state budgets, and health costs to American businesses in 1989 were equal to 98 percent of their after-tax profits (i.e., had American businesses not paid for health care, their after-tax profits would have doubled).[11] Ironically, as costs for health care mounted, many hospitals also faced serious financial crises as they coped with new reimbursement formulas from governmental and private insurance sources.

Meanwhile, the number of Americans lacking access to basic health services increased sharply during the 1980s and 1990s. The working poor, ineligible for welfare and Medicaid, were especially hard hit, as were a few ethnic minorities. Estimates of the number of Americans who had no health insurance in 1990 ranged from 31.5 to 37 million, and by 1995 had increased to 40 million.[12] In addition, the U.S. Census found that 63.6 million people lacked health insurance coverage for at least part of the three-year period from 1986 through 1988.[13] In 1991 the *Journal of the American Medical Association (JAMA)* published a study showing that hospital patients who lacked health insurance were three times as likely to die in the hospital as were persons with insurance, and were much less likely to receive expensive medical procedures.[14] Infant mortality rates among urban low-income populations were three times as high as those for the rest of the population; and a resurgence of childhood epidemics was occurring as fewer children received immunizations.[15] While 18.6 percent of non-Hispanic white Americans lacked health insurance for all or part of 1987, 29.8 percent of African-Americans and 41.4 percent of Hispanic-Americans had no health insurance.[16] The problem of access to care, however, went beyond inability to pay: almost 2,000 rural American communities had inadequate (or no) primary care medical services, and few physicians were available to provide the primary health-care services needed by low-income and minority populations within major metropolitan areas. At the same time, a surplus of physicians who were specialists serving affluent areas of metropolitan communities added to the health costs of the nation.[17] Not surprisingly in light of these facts, the relative international standing of the U.S. on a variety of health indices continued to drop.[18]

A continuing increase in the number of malpractice suits underscored the quality control problems inherent in high-tech medicine. Between 1980 and 1985 alone, the ratio of malpractice suits to physicians tripled, rising to 10 law suits annually per 100 physicians. And the areas of medicine facing the largest increases in malpractice claims were those in which high-technology medicine had made the greatest inroads.[19] Finally, issues of humaneness took on a new intensity. The uninsured were being turned away from treatment centers. The elderly were sometimes released early from hospitals so that new Medicare payment formulas would maximize hospital income. Those dependent on Medicaid found that many hospitals and nursing homes would not accept them because of the program's low reimbursement formulas. And increasing numbers of doctors refused to handle health insurance claims, forcing their patients to pay directly for their services.

Efforts to reform American health care fundamentally through national legislative action failed in the early 1990s, as had happened 20 years earlier. Third party payers, mirroring private responses to legislative failures in health-care reform in the 1950s and 1970s, once again created innovations of their own, this time aimed at cost containment. The dominant character of the American health-care system continued to evolve, but it was not clear that these changes had improved the quality of health care or solved the underlying dynamic of its cost.

The issues of the 1970s—cost, access to services, quality control, and humaneness—were far more pressing by 1995. Moreover, there were more than a dozen additional problems, some new, others continuing, that the American health-care system seemed unable to address satisfactorily. These might be grouped roughly into five categories.

First, there is an increase in problems for which the curative strategies of medical science are of only limited help. Since the 1980s the AIDS pandemic has been sweeping the world, including the United States. While some drug therapies are finally available, their cost and the treatment protocols required make them out of reach for most infected persons. In addition, poor nutrition, the use of tobacco, and excessive use of alcohol affect more of the population, leaving many people susceptible to heart disease, strokes, and cancer, the major causes of death in the United States, as well as to serious traffic accidents.[21] Moreover, use of cocaine and heroin in the U.S. increased sharply beginning the 1980s.[22]

Second, the worsening environment is creating serious health problems and the health-care delivery system, focused on offering curative medicine after health has deteriorated, seldom addresses these sources of disease. Air pollution, thinning of the ozone layer because of the release of pollutants from cars and manufacturing processes,[23] radiation hazards, health risks attending the production and disposal of toxic wastes,[24] affect cancer rates. Health hazards resulting from use of new technologies,[25] and those facing immigrants and other poor Americans who work in the growing service sector of the economy and in some of the non-unionized small manufacturing and food-processing plants[26] also receive inadequate attention.

Third, quality of life for the newborn has become a new kind of concern. Teenage pregnancies are an increasing proportion of total births, with higher infant mortality rates and a higher percentage of the surviving babies having serious health problems.[27] Neonatal intensive care units increase the survival chances of low birth-weight infants, at great cost, when efforts to improve prenatal care and nutrition could meet the problem at its source.

Fourth, the distribution of physicians creates major problems in its own right. There is a serious oversupply of medical specialists, whose services too often are used for "defensive medicine" rather than for needed health-care services.[28] There is a shortage of primary health-care personnel in many areas of the country.[29] Moreover physicians, as a group, show little commitment to provide services to low-income and ethnic minority populations in the metropolitan areas where most physicians are living and working.[30]

Fifth, most new financing arrangements for health care simply increase the problems of cost containment. Government regulation of reimbursement rates for hospital, physician, and outpatient services provided to Medicare patients seem to have shifted costs more than controlled them.[31] Efforts at cost containment rarely have been effective for more than two or three years. A major move into capitated payment plans and managed care in the mid-1990s, with hard bargaining for prices by third-party payers of health-care costs, produced an initial slowing of health-care cost inflation, which by 1997, however, seemed to be less effective. Analysts warned that similar slowdowns had occurred before, only to be wiped out by inflationary "cost adjustments" later.[32] There has been strong resistance in the U.S. to using cost containment strategies found in other industrialized countries, because these involve government regulation of health care and caps on total expenditures that will be paid.[33] The reorienting of health-care services toward profit maximization make it difficult to address unsolved health problems. Increasingly, financial resources and personnel are drawn into already developed and profitable areas of health service delivery, leaving fewer resources available to tackle other problems.

Health Care's Contribution to Long-Term Economic Tensions

During the past quarter century American health care has become one of the most important sectors of the economy, a pace setter for economic growth. But because of the way health-care services are organized, that growth has come at a major cost to other interests. It has adversely affected state and federal budget deficits, the ability of American-based manufacturing to compete on the international market, working conditions, and even the number of jobs available in other sectors of the economy. While the development of high-technology health care did not create these problems, it has intensified them. One result has been a growing tension between health-care interests and other major institutional interests in the U.S. Thus an equally serious problem now lies in the changing relation of health care to the rest of the economy.

Why Have Previous Reform Efforts Failed?

Earlier efforts at reforming health-care policy have been ineffective for at least three reasons. First, problems were often tackled piecemeal, as though a single intervention in one area (even a major one) would correct the larger dynamic at work. The few efforts that were made to look at the system as a whole got bogged down in the accommodation of special interests. Second, the more comprehensive reform plans (as seen in Truman's effort to create a national health-care system, in Nixon's and Clinton's efforts to provide universal access to care through health insurance reform, and in minority efforts within Congress to create a Canadian-style health-care system for the United States) assumed that federal regulation, state regulation, or both was the missing ingredient that could guarantee universal access and cost control as the system otherwise continued on with its present emphasis. This roused the opposition of interest groups and the larger public who distrusted government regulation; but even if they had succeeded politically, those proposals probably would not have succeeded practically, because they did not address more fundamental dynamics which were creating the problems in health care. Regulation has a poor track record for success under these circumstances. Third, even though problems in health care were approached using the same problem-solving formulas that were being applied elsewhere in the political economy, health-care dynamics were treated as if they existed independently of everything else that was happening in the political and economic system—a serious miscalculation. The term, *political economy*, as used here, refers to an evolving mix of political and economic developments that shape American social experience. Just as politics does not exist in isolation from economic developments, American health care does not exist in isolation from the larger social dynamics surrounding it.

Many changes in U.S. health care over the past 60 years were in fact responses to a larger set of national and international developments, but the continuing impact of these developments for health-care dynamics was all but ignored by innovators and policy makers. Health-care innovations, in turn, have had a very real impact on national and international life. Had problems not been approached in isolation, but instead viewed in terms of their relation to a larger series of changes occurring in the national and international political economies, a different series of policy options might have been explored. They were not explored, perhaps because most of the analytic strategies popular among academics, politicians, and policy makers fail to observe the system as a whole in ways that let policy makers shape individual choices. Even fewer analytic strategies have made it possible to discuss processes of mutual change that are occurring, or to analyze how innovations fit into larger nonequilibrium dynamics that are developing.

How Might We Proceed Differently?

This book offers a different way to approach health-care policy decisions. It tries to enlarge the frame of reference used to view health-care choices and to extend the range of choices that might be considered.

First, it identifies major national and international influences that have affected American health-care developments.

Second, it examines the process by which major health-care innovations have emerged in response to these developments.

Third, it notes how previous innovations in health care have affected the larger dynamic of change that was occurring—in health care, in the national political economy, and internationally.

Then, after describing factors that have shaped the mainstream of health-care development in this country over a sixty-year period, it examines a series of health-care innovations that developed outside the mainstream, and which are currently being explored by various interest groups in the U.S. This analysis looks for lessons that can be learned from earlier ventures both in the mainstream and at the periphery.

Reexamining current health-care policy proposals in terms of their most likely impact on the broader dynamics already underway, the book concludes by suggesting types of innovations currently feasible that could help move the American health-care system toward a different problem-focus and toward more cost-effective solutions to current health-care problems.

The reader may wish a brief introduction to the broader strategy which underlies the analysis presented in this book. It involves looking chronologically, and then simultaneously, at three levels of social happenings—those occurring internationally, those occurring within the national political economy, and those occurring within health care itself. A few international developments, which emerge as part of the dynamic of evolving international political and economic relations over time, create central problems for Americans. New coalitions arise in response to those developments, introducing different problem-solving strategies. These developments within the U.S., in turn, affect the practice of American health care. Special interests that are particularly affected by these changes then innovate, trying either to solve problems that have arisen or to take advantage of new opportunities that appear. This book identifies health-care innovations that had a major impact on the changing character of health care in the U.S. in different time periods, explaining their emergence in terms of their relation to these national and international developments.

People innovate constantly, but only a few health-care innovations "catch on." Those most likely to succeed are the ones that apply a problem-solving strategy that is already being used more widely by a currently dominant political or economic coalition. When the larger political-economic system is in a state of increasing imbalance, an innovation that seems to offer a way to solve a growing problem which affects many individuals or organizations catches on rapidly. These innovations, in turn, have their own impact on the nonequilibrium dynamic that is emerging. Under such circumstances "the law of large numbers" ceases to apply; that is, the many innovations occurring on the edge of a system do not cancel out one another's impact. Some begin to reinforce others, introducing a new kind of organizing principle that begins to affect the system as a whole, both nationally and internationally.

This, put succinctly, is the analytic strategy that will guide the argument of this book. It will be used to explain the appearance of the dilemmas of health-care reform that we now face, and to suggest some new directions for health-care policy.

(Readers interested in a fuller theoretical description of the analytic strategy which guides the analysis presented in this book will find such a discussion in the end notes for this Introduction.[34])

Political realism proceeds from a recognition that interest groups have the power to veto various kinds of proposals for reform, and that powerful interests within the current health-care system will protect their own agendas as reform efforts proceed. Many approaches that advertise their "political realism," however, are myopic: they focus on what is immediately in view and often ignore the larger picture, thus becoming ineffective in the long run.

Because the health policy agenda and debate of the 1990s is repeating this mistake, and thus is bound to produce disappointing results, this book encourages readers to expand the horizons they take into account. A clearer sense of why the American health-care system is producing the results now seen could free us to proceed more creatively, gaining a clear sense of emerging, alternative ways to approach the same problems, and of interest groups that could help move the system in new directions.

To do this, we must first take a fresh look at the way in which American medical science evolved into the contemporary U.S. health-care industry. We should note, as well, dynamics that motivated reform efforts over the past 25 years, and current regroupings of interests and new explorations that might offer other ways out of the current dilemmas. Locating American health care within a larger context of national and international developments at work may allow more genuinely realistic possibilities for reform to appear.

1

Understanding How We Got Here: Creating a Health-Care Industry

About a century ago each of the industrialized nations of the world reorganized its health-care system to follow the canons of a newly developing, "modern" medical science. As early as 1917, however, the path of health-care reorganization and development in the United States took a somewhat different direction from that seen in other countries. Decisions about national health insurance—and the interest group coalitions that formed around this controversy—created a set of veto groups that would influence health-care decisions thereafter. The contrast in how health care has developed has been especially striking during the 50 years since World War II. Most of the other advanced industrial nations developed some form of a national health-care system (i.e., a government-directed or coordinated program to guarantee health services for all citizens). In contrast, the United States at first created a private, professionally-oriented system focused around the concerns of physicians, who wished to set their own standards of care independent of government control, and to give the highest possible care to patients of their own choosing. About 30 years ago that private, professionally-oriented system evolved into something that, with considerable accuracy, now describes itself as a *health-care industry*. As that name implies, health care in the United States has a unique relationship to the larger economy, and indeed, a unique relation to the social fabric of the nation. Physicians, while still important, no longer are at its center. This chapter seeks to understand how that happened and to identify the kinds of organizational relationships that give the health-care industry its current dynamic.

The central story of what happened does not revolve around the rise and fall of the profession of medicine—that is only one sub-theme of the broader dynamic that has occurred. Nor will an analysis of social inequality, race and class dynamics, or the consolidation of capital satisfactorily explain the changes that have taken place. Many earlier accounts of American health-care developments attempted to fit their analysis into one or the other of these contending frames of reference. Each captures part of the dynamic which has occurred, but misses the larger pattern at work. Professional elites, race and class interests, take on quite different importance and qualities at different points in time, as national and international developments create changing problems, changing coalitions of interest, and new opportunity structures.

In telling the story of what happened, this chapter sketches broadly, a necessary choice in order to cover developments during the 100-year period after modern medical science first appeared in Europe, around 1870, until American health care reorganized itself as a health-care industry, around 1970. Most of the facts that make up this account are well known and often have been brilliantly documented by scholars working from many intellectual perspectives. What distinguishes this account from its predecessors is not its sources of information, but a set of questions that puts together the information others have gathered in ways that let an underlying set of dynamics be seen more clearly.

International Developments Influence the Emergence of "Modern" Medical Science

The half century from 1870 to 1920 saw the rise of modern nation states with international ambitions. These included the new Germany, a reorganized France, and a post-Civil War United States taking its place among the industrial giants. The British Empire's naval preeminence had established a period of relative stability internationally (the Pax Britannica). British bankers were expanding overseas investments, speeding the larger industrialization that was already underway. British bank loans underwrote the economic endeavors of U.S. entrepreneur J. Pierpont Morgan, whose business ventures helped consolidate American business activity and gave rise to a set of giant American corporations that reorganized the American business landscape. Meanwhile the expansion of railway transportation networks all over the world, including a railway system linking the entire United States (a high priority for post-Civil War Congresses) increased the importance of trade. It also created a high demand for steel and became the route by which other American fortunes were made. (Andrew Carnegie's steel mills, for example, provided the raw material for expansion of transportation and industry, and John D. Rockefeller's oil business became a monopoly because of agreements Rockefeller worked out with the emerging private railway system, granting him price advantages over his competitors in exchange for centrally regulated oil production and orderly demand for railway shipping.) In short, it was a time period involving major business expansion and the consolidation of wealth. This broader international pattern, which lasted until disrupted by the First World War, set the context in which "modern" medical science emerged.[1]

The international trade network, which had become much more active as the industrial revolution accelerated international trading during the nineteenth century, had brought in its wake a series of epidemics around the world. This focused attention on infectious disease, and after 1870 led to a reorganization of "modern medical science" around the Germ Theory of Disease. Government encouragement of medical research in France and Germany, and private financing in Great Britain and by some of the new millionaires in the U.S. quickly established the promise of a new, international approach to disease. Research into the causes of infectious disease was conducted on silkworms and sheep, species whose infections were affecting the cost and availability of raw materials for the textile industry.[2] Louis Pasteur in France, Robert Koch in Germany, and other biological scientists in Europe demonstrated the role of microbes, or germs, in the transmission of infectious diseases. They were building on earlier epidemiological research undertaken by civil engineers, who had formed a powerful international Sanitation Movement in the 1850s after they had traced the spread of a cholera epidemic in London to the use of a water source that had become contaminated with human feces from nearby privies.[3]

The germ theory of disease showed *how* filth and contamination produced infection, enlarging the range of strategies available for protecting the public. It enlarged understanding of what was involved in disease transmission and introduced the idea of a specific cause for each form of disease. Medical scientists not only built on the earlier work of the engineer's Sanitation Movement, but gradually absorbed it into their own venture (as the public health movement).[4] Then, a few years later, the British surgeon Joseph Lister used chemistry to discover both antiseptics and anesthesia, which made surgical interventions safer and less painful.[5] The use of antiseptics greatly reduced the rate of infections acquired in hospitals, making the public willing to use surgical corrections for health problems, and to use hospitals for a variety of other services as well.

In short, the international movement into modern medical science as the preferred strategy for dealing with health and disease occurred as part of a much larger set of social transformations that was occurring at the same time. Modern medical science was enthusiastically championed not only by physicians but also by broader coalitions of interest committed to the idea that *applied science* problem solving was the route to progress.

American Particularism

As support for modern medical science grew in most industrialized countries, momentum built to make it the center of a national health-care system, with the state guaranteeing access to its services. That did not happen in the U.S., however. A long-standing tradition of nongovernmental control of medicine had solidified almost a century earlier. Citizens on the frontier had resisted state licensing of professionals, arguing that this amounted to restraint on free trade and that they should be free to find local solutions to a shortage of professionals (including especially doctors and clergymen). Their cause became persuasive when licensed "regular doctors," who did not yet have the germ theory of disease, had problems dealing with an international epidemic like cholera. In contrast, homeopathic physicians who were emigrating from Germany in the wake of the failed revolution of 1848 were having much greater success. For most of the nineteenth century American medicine was treated as a "business" and deregulated. By the turn of the century there was an oversupply of doctors, great rivalry between various medical traditions and the beginning of state regulation. Several states had reintroduced the licensing of physicians, with each medical tradition conducting examinations for the graduates of its medical schools. Meanwhile the free market was creating problems for doctors. Supply and demand in a situation of over-supply had kept fees low, so that physicians' income was similar to that of the rest of the population. Moreover, the expansion of American industry brought with it pressures from corporations to accept fixed-per-capita payment for services provided to a corporations' employees, rather than fees for individual services. With an oversupply of physicians, corporations bargained hard for the lowest rates.[6]

The international movement toward "modern medical science" provided an opportunity for one group of physicians, organized as the American Medical Association (the AMA) to bring a "managed" approach to the development of medicine. The alliances they created and the policy stances they took in the decade before World War I set the direction in which future health-care policy and debate would focus in the U.S. Their way of solving immediate problems confronting doctors as a profession in oversupply set trends in motion that now threaten the health-care system as a whole. Understanding the politics of what occurred will clarify why American health care later became so susceptible to national and international developments outside of health care.

Early in the twentieth century the AMA forged strong links to three groups in a position to influence public policy—to a small set of leading capitalist entrepreneurs and their staffs (especially Rockefeller, Carnegie, and J. Pierpont Morgan), to the presidents of a few elite universities who were advisers to the philanthropic foundations Rockefeller and Carnegie had established, and to leaders in the "non-partisan" Progressive political movement. The Progressives had sponsored antitrust legislation in an effort to control the super-Capitalists' consolidation of holdings but they endorsed applied science and progress as the route to non-partisan planning for the "public good." By forging a coalition around health care that involved most of the contending economic and political forces of the time, the AMA's agenda triumphed swiftly. Because of its county by county organization of physicians and its focus on political lobbying, the AMA succeeded not only in getting each state to prohibit the practice of medicine by unlicensed physicians, but also gained control of the state and national boards conducting the medical exams, thus guaranteeing that no new physicians could gain the right to practice medicine who were not trained in the canons of modern medical science. Philanthropic foundations established by two of the most successful capitalist entrepreneurs of the time—John D. Rockefeller, Sr., and Andrew Carnegie—played important roles in that political process, providing funds that demonstrated the potential of modern medical science and helping manipulate public opinion to build support for AMA proposals.[7]

Surgery was at the forefront of new developments in "modern" medical science, thanks to the impetus set in motion by Lister's work in England, and surgery was most safely performed in hospitals. At the end of World War I the prosperity of the 1920s and the newly created American custom of expanding health services through philanthropic donations provided fertile ground for the expansion of America's hospital system. In 1873 there had been only 178 hospitals in America. By 1909, there were over 4,300. During the next 14 years the number of hospitals in the United States increased by almost 60 percent, the number of hospital beds by almost 80 percent, and the number of nursing schools rose by 50 percent. By 1927, there were 200,000 registered nurses in the nation.[8]

The account of the "medical revolution" in America which occurred in the early part of the twentieth century has been well told from a variety of perspectives[9] and need not concern us in detail here. What is important for us to note is that the establishment of modern medical science as the preferred strategy for health care in America occurred as part of a much larger social transformation, and in a context of political struggle. A new coalition of interests took a political strategy being used to pursue "public interest" in a variety of areas—including anti-trust legislation, tax reform, efforts to end the control of cities by political bosses, and the establishment of public utilities—and adapted it to the task of reforming health care.[10]

"Public Interest" Planning Generates Problems for American Health Care. As medical science triumphed over its rivals, "public interest" problem solving produced a major consolidation of medical training. Graduates of medical schools that did not conform to the AMA's approved curriculum were unable to pass the new medical licensing exams, and the AMA made sure that test scores were publicly reported, by school. Enrollment in schools the AMA disapproved of dropped quickly, and philanthropic contributions to them stopped. As a result, the number of medical schools in the U.S. dropped sharply. In 1906, there had been 162 of them.

By 1915, there were only 95, and the number of students being accepted for training had dropped by 35 percent. By 1929, only 76 medical schools remained.[11]

From the standpoint of planners who wished to see the triumph of "high quality" training in modern medical science, these results were desirable. Moreover, for doctors affiliated with the AMA, this guaranteed the elimination of competition among doctors in the decades to come. Their lessened numbers, and AMA policies of encouraging doctors of a given specialty to set fees in common, county by county, quickly led to a major increase in income for American doctors. For the general public, however, this consolidation of medical training was a mixed blessing. By the 1920s doctors charged higher fees. The number of physicians available to serve minority populations and people living in small towns and rural areas began to decline. Graduates of elite medical schools increasingly chose urban, specialty practices. With lessened competition, fewer young doctors chose to practice medicine in geographically isolated areas or among ethnic minorities or the poor in urban areas. All but two of the medical schools that trained African-American doctors closed, and African Americans were excluded from internships and hospital privileges in most of the rest. The elite medical schools that survived were less likely than their predecessors to admit students who had not gone to the top colleges, thus making entrance into medicine increasingly the prerogative of children from wealthier families. And for many years the surviving medical schools set a quota limiting the admission of women students to 5 percent of their total enrollment. These changes affected the availability of medical care to various population groups in the years to come.[12]

For a while it looked as though the U.S. would follow the path chosen in most other industrialized countries and would create a national health-care system providing universal access to health care. Other nations were guaranteeing access to health-care services for all citizens and were producing a variety of universal health insurance plans to implement these policies. Similar movements were afoot in the U.S. but they were stalled in 1917, largely through the efforts of the Metropolitan and Prudential Life Insurance companies which were controlled by J. Pierpont Morgan, the third preeminent capitalist entrepreneur of the period. Because the wording of Progressive movement proposals for universal health insurance made Prudential and Metropolitan Life fear the loss of one of their major sources of revenue, the sale of burial insurance, these two companies mounted a successful campaign to stop national health insurance. When they persuaded the leaders of the New York Medical Association that universal health insurance would lead to governmental control over standards for the practice of medicine on a day-to-day basis, the AMA mobilized its political clout to block the inclusion of publicly financed health insurance as part of health-care reforms currently underway.[13] With that coalition of opposition (the insurance companies and the AMA) firmly in place, universal health insurance became an insoluble issue in American politics until 1965, when a unique combination of circumstances made it possible to provide government health insurance for the elderly and for people receiving public welfare assistance.

For half a century, solutions to problems of access to medical care could only come through private initiative. The federal government had only a small investment in the funding of health care, primarily through its public health programs. Private philanthropy played a much bigger role. In health care, as in other parts of the political economy, interest groups expanded their turf and most of them spent little time focusing on the unsolved problems in health care that remained. However in 1926 a group of fifteen economists, physicians and public health specialists attending a conference on medical economics in Washington, D.C., formed the Committee on the Costs of Medical Care (CCMC). Soon they had expanded to 50 members, recruiting prominent members of the professions and key interest groups and enlisted the cooperation of the AMA, the Metropolitan Life Insurance Company, and other private organizations.[14] CCMC sponsored a series of studies documenting the rapid increase in the cost of medical care and in problems of access to competent care that were emerging in various sectors of the population. In 1932, at the depth of the international economic depression, CCMC issued a controversial report, one endorsed by 35 of its 50 members, that recommended the promotion of group medical practice and voluntary insurance plans to cover medical costs. It also suggested that local governments "contribute a per-capita share of the cost of group medical plans for low-income citizens of their communities, assisted by the state or Federal government." A minority report, signed by eight doctors and by the representative of the Catholic hospitals, denounced group practice as the "technique of big business [and] mass production" and rejected both compulsory and voluntary insurance as well. It recommended, instead, that "government care of the indigent be expanded with the ultimate object of relieving the medical profession of this burden." When the report was released in November 1932, an editorial in the *Journal of the American Medical Association* (*JAMA*) denounced the majority report and endorsed the minority position. The New York *Times* put its story about the CCMC report under the headline: "Socialized Medicine is Urged in Survey." As Paul Starr has noted, "Coming just as Franklin D. Roosevelt took office, the controversy over the CCMC helped persuade the new administration that health insurance was an issue to be avoided."[15]

"Private Interest" Innovation Sets a Chain of Developments in Motion. Within the next 10 years the basis for health-care development and financing began to change drastically, in directions similar to those recom-

mended by the CCMC. The thrust for change did not come from elite planning groups, or the government, however, but from American hospitals, who were searching for ways to cut their operating losses during the height of the Great Depression. By the 1930s, as Americans' discretionary income shrank, dependence upon individual household funding for medical expenses incurred in private hospitals threatened the continued existence of America's hospital system. As hospitals innovated in order to survive, acting unilaterally at first and then banding together in classic Progressive-style "public interest" legislative reform efforts, they set in motion a dynamic that would change the entire character of American health care.

Innovations in Funding Health Care

Five organizational innovations introduced between 1930 and 1965 had major impact on the changing character of American health care, with 1940 to 1950 a particularly critical period. Most of the innovations concerned new ways to fund health-care costs; however they also had profound implications for the character of actual health-care interventions. By 1965, American health care had moved from an emphasis on doctor-patient encounters to something that increasingly began to call itself a "health-care industry"—a profound reorientation of medical procedures.

The innovations most responsible for these changes arrived in the following order. In the mid-1930s came prepaid insurance for hospital costs. In the 1940s, federal subsidies—for medical research, for medical training, and for hospital construction—were introduced. In the 1940s and 1950s came third-party payments for health costs. Financed by business and industry, these gave American business a growing stake in the funding of health care. In 1965, when the federal government joined business as a third-party payer of health costs (for the elderly and for persons receiving public welfare), the conditions needed to transform health-care services into a "health-care industry" came together. About this time a series of court decisions made malpractice suits easier and thus inadvertently encouraged the growing practice of "defensive medicine." Together, these new ways of organizing and funding health services threw medical costs into a growth-oriented dynamic that has continued unabated to the present. This chapter views those developments as responses to larger trends on the national and international scene. Those trends created special problems—and sometimes special moments of opportunity—for particular interest groups in health care and in the larger political economy.

New International Developments Change the
Context for American Problem-Solving

Major shifts occurring in international political and economic relations helped create the issues that special interest groups within the U.S. tackled during the New Deal and postwar decades. The First World War had ended the era of the Pax Britannica, in which British naval power and control of strategic bases at key transportation routes around the globe reduced the threat of international war. British military and diplomatic strategy, combined with the role of British bankers in controlling capital flow to most parts of the world, had produced a relatively stable international political economy. Britain had been too weakened by World War I, however, to continue that international role, and the U.S. had declined to take it on. Ten years later the international stock market collapsed. Totalitarian regimes, Fascists, Nazis, and Communists, began to dominate much of Europe. After a chaotic period involving opportunistic military and economic plundering by various countries as the League of Nations proved unable to play the role of peace enforcer, a Second World War had emerged. It was followed by the collapse or transformation of most European empires and a new international political and economic order. This new order involved a bipolar reorganization of spheres of influence and trading areas and an attempt by the U.S. (with international backing) to create a replacement for the earlier Pax Britannica, both economically and militarily. This time, however, the new world order also included the United Nations, various regional economic and military pacts, and a multitude of new political states. These larger waves of development had a direct impact on the fortunes of the U.S. political economy, on the economic and health issues it had to address in different decades, and on innovations in U.S. federal policies that became critical for the evolution of American health care.

The worldwide major economic depression of the late 1920s and 1930s, the Second World War of the 1940s, and the U.S. government's decision to create a Pax Americana at the end of World War II created a variety of problems that changed relationships among various interest groups within the U.S. Health care became a focus for many of their negotiations with one another. Coalitions and alliances dating from around the time of World War I created veto groups and avenues of opportunity for advocates of various health-care policies.

Private Response: The Creation of Blue Cross

When private incomes dropped sharply during the Great Depression, the nation's hospitals were threatened. From late 1929 through 1930, immediately following the economic crash, hospital receipts fell from an annual average of $236.12 per patient to $59.26. Since hospitals had relatively fixed operating costs, their operating deficits increased—from about 15 percent to about 20 percent of disbursements. Although the vast majority of hospitals were non-profit and operated as a public service, during an economic depression it was difficult to raise additional charitable funds to meet a deficit.[16]

An ingenious solution emerged in Dallas, Texas. In late 1929, shortly after the stock market crash, the business manager for the Baylor University Medical School's Hospital in Dallas noted a sharp decline in visits to his hospital and began to look for local groups in Dallas who might be encouraged to continue their earlier uses of it. As a former business manager of the Dallas school system, he knew that teachers had guaranteed yearly salaries. Thinking creatively, he approached the school system, suggesting that they offer teachers a low-cost pre-payment plan for hospital usage. If the entire teaching staff were insured, only a small proportion of them would need hospital services at any one time. Thus the monthly rate per person could be low, but the hospital's income level could be guaranteed. He offered to provide each teacher up to twenty-one days of hospital coverage per year for an annual cost of $6 per person. The school system liked the idea and the 1,500 teachers bought it. Soon Baylor extended the arrangement to additional employee groups, and other Dallas hospitals began to follow suit.[17]

As the Depression deepened, the funding problems of hospitals across the country increased. In 1931 only 62 percent of the beds in general hospitals were occupied on an average day. By 1932, the president of the American Hospital Association warned of a possible breakdown in the nation's voluntary hospital system.[18] Then, in 1933, noting the success of the Dallas hospitals, the American Hospital Association recommended that all hospitals in an area cooperate in a joint insurance plan. Thus hospitals entered the insurance business and created a managed market—a strategy that already had been in use by businesses across the nation for the past 50 years.

The CCMC majority report, published in 1932, proposed broader-scale "public interest" solutions to problems of the cost of medical care and dismissed hospital insurance as an inadequate approach to the larger problem. That report raised a storm of controversy, with the politically organized AMA leading the attack. Meanwhile, however, the *private interest* problem of generating operating revenue for American hospitals was reaching a point of crisis, and the Dallas plan offered a simple solution.

During the next two years prepaid hospitalization plans spread from Texas to California, Minnesota, New Jersey, Ohio, and Washington, D.C. Calling themselves Blue Cross, these hospital insurance plans were simple to set up and required little capitalization. However, when hospitals in New York tried to set up a Blue Cross plan, the state superintendent of insurance ruled they would have to comply with all state regulations for insurance companies, including maintaining financial reserves in proportion to the net worth of policies. Hospital and medical leaders then successfully pressed for a special enabling act, which became law in May of 1934. It exempted such plans from the reserve requirement, and required a majority of the directors of the plan to be administrators or trustees of the hospitals that contracted to provide services. This provision guaranteed long-term control of Blue Cross by the voluntary hospitals.[19]

This legislation became the model for enabling acts in other states. In 1937, the AHA received a grant from the Julius Rosenwald Fund to set up a Committee on Hospital Service (later renamed the Hospital Service Plan Commission) to aid community efforts to set up Blue Cross plans. They recommended that plans be supervised by states through their insurance departments, as in New York, and that they provide reserves of service rather than cash. Within two years, 25 states had passed special enabling legislation. By 1940, 39 Blue Cross plans had a total enrollment of six million subscribers.[20]

Blue Cross hospitalization insurance, though it offered major benefits to American hospitals, was far from a perfect solution to the problem of guaranteeing access to medical services. It covered only hospital costs, and was available only to employees of companies or public agencies that offered it. The retired, the unemployed, and most employees across the country at the time, did not benefit from it.

Public Response: New Deal Problem-Solving

Meanwhile, the Great Depression had motivated a new political alignment that introduced some radically different strategies for problem-solving. The election of 1932 broke up an earlier political coalition between the middle class and a wealthy elite who had led the Progressive wing of the Republican Party two decades earlier. The Democratic Party under Franklin D. Roosevelt created a new political coalition linking the interests of the middle class with those of organized labor, farmers, and urban ethnic minorities, who had been disadvantaged by the vast consolidation of wealth that had occurred 50 years earlier.[21] Thanks to the expansion of federal taxation during the Progressive era, major resources now flowed to the federal government. Roosevelt's New Deal introduced the federal government as a deliberate, active problem-solver, using legislation, occasional executive intervention, and the redirection of federally controlled financial resources to introduce new dynamics into the social conflicts of the time.

New Deal innovations included the use of federal deficit spending to bolster the economy and the introduction of massive federal bureaucracies, which established a national welfare system, created public housing complexes across the nation, subsidized private home construction, and operated a set of national research bureaus. Class conflict in America was restructured, first by federal legislation that allowed major industrial trade unions to organize, and then by wartime administrative policies that created a tripartite governing coalition between big business, big labor, and the federal government.[22]

During the next two decades, massive federal spending—for the military, for education (first through the GI Bill and then through continued federal subsidies for higher education), for research, for the mechanization of agriculture in the South through farm subsidy programs, for welfare, and for health (especially after Medicare and Medicaid were created in the mid-1960s)—provided a basis for national prosperity that gradually reoriented the nature of class struggle and social relations in America.[23]

Public Controversy Affects Approaches to Health Problems: The Public Health "Solution". During the 1930s, President Roosevelt was unwilling to test his political popularity in the politically loaded controversy over health-care costs. However, public health projects received attention from his New Deal planners. The 1935 Social Security Act established a federal grant-in-aid program to operate public health services in each state and to train public health personnel. Roosevelt also increased funding for maternal and child health programs. In 1930 the National Hygienic Laboratory had been relocated to Washington and renamed the National Institute of Health (NIH). In 1937 it expanded its research program and set up a National Cancer Institute (NCI). In 1938, Congress provided federal funds to states to investigate and control the spread of venereal disease. And in 1939 the Federal Security Agency was established to coordinate programs being carried out by the Public Health Service and national programs in education and welfare. Thus federal agencies (which later became major channels for the funding of medical research) started as noncontroversial vehicles for extending health services to the public, despite political blockage of health insurance proposals.[24]

Private Innovation: Prepaid, Fixed Per Capita, Total Health-Care Plans. Meanwhile, federal sponsorship of hydroelectric development, and later federal support of the shipbuilding industry during World War II, provided opportunities for private business to tackle problems of access to health-care services in a different way. Some industrial capitalists gained enormously as a result of New Deal policies. One of the most innovative of these leaders, Henry J. Kaiser, built the Grand Coulee hydroelectric dam for the federal government in the state of Washington during the late 1930s. When the Kaiser Corporation moved into small towns and rural areas in Washington to build the dam, it became necessary to develop its own medical services because the size of its construction crews overwhelmed the ability of local doctors and hospitals to serve them effectively. In 1938, working with Dr. Sidney Garfield, Kaiser hired his own doctors and used a variation of the Blue Cross insurance formula to set up his own prepaid health plan. This plan provided all needed medical services for a small additional fee at the time of use. When Kaiser expanded into shipbuilding in cities along the Pacific coast during World War II, he applied the same approach but built his own hospitals as well. His entry into an arena previously controlled by county medical societies was bitterly resisted on a local level, but his influence nationally brought federal rulings that invalidated local injunctions intended to block his hospital projects. When the war ended, the Kaiser-Permanente Health Plan, which hired physicians as employees, began to compete directly with Blue Cross on the West Coast, making its plan available to other employers and offering a full range of health-care services instead of hospitalization alone.[25] Soon the Henry J. Kaiser Family Foundation was educating policy makers and the public about the advantages of total health insurance over hospitalization insurance alone, and about the funding advantages of charging a fixed per-capita fee annually for all services needed, rather than charging a separate fee for each service provided—the traditional practice retained by Blue Cross plans.[26] Kaiser-Permanente could offer a fixed annual fee and prosper because participating doctors were paid salaries rather than a fee for each service performed. It thus was possible to budget a fixed sum for the health costs of subscribers. Doctors had little personal incentive to recommend expensive surgeries or other medical services that might not be necessary, since they gained no additional income from providing such services.

Others also recognized the potential of prepaid insurance plans that cover all health needs for a fixed per-capita fee. During the Great Depression, in fact, several cooperatives in the West had introduced various kinds of prepaid health plans, but few of them had survived the Depression and World War II. Then after the war, in Seattle, Washington, 400 families recruited from members of the Grange, the Aero-mechanics union (in Seattle's major aerospace industry), and local food and general supply cooperatives formed the Group Health Cooperative of Puget Sound. Pledging $100 per family, they joined a group of local physicians in buying a privately owned, prepaid medical clinic's practice and a 60 bed hospital that were for sale because of a slump in the city's economy. As Group Health of Puget Sound evolved through time, it not only expanded its services throughout the state but also developed some new, cost-effective organizational strategies. Their consumer-oriented managed care found high satisfaction both from physicians and their public. With time, Group Health began to integrate primary care disease services with prevention programs and introduced a triaging of care that included self-care advising. They also developed pilot programs to absorb uninsured, lower-income citizens into their consumer service pool.[27]

If the health-care service models introduced by Kaiser and by Group Health of Puget Sound had become widely imitated immediately after World War II, the character of the American health-care system would be quite different than what we see today. Kaiser's programs were clustered on the West Coast, however, and Group Health's geographic reach was even more limited. The model for insurance-based health care that predominated, consequently, was Blue Cross' insurance to cover hospital costs. Its introduction across the nation during the 1930s made it available for use as part of war mobilization planning in World War II. This, then, set the pattern for what followed.

Impact of World War II: Health Insurance as a "Fringe Benefit" of War Mobilization

Once the U.S. entered the Second World War, the federal government mobilized the full resources of the nation for the war effort. This included a major expansion of the armed services (and a concomitant drafting of doctors for military service) and also the conversion of 86 percent of all industrial manufacturing to war production. Making the government into the consumer of most of the industrial production and much of the agricultural production of the nation was a major innovation in the principle on which the American market operated. Soon wartime "czars" were given unprecedented power and discretion to redirect how various aspects of the political economy operated in order to guarantee military victory. Patriotic fervor, and renewed prosperity based on federal subsidization of industry and the military, led to widespread support for sweeping new governmental policies.

The government needed industry to operate at full capacity within a stable economy, one not subject to devastating inflation. To achieve this goal, government officals would have to gain the cooperation of labor and management, who had been at loggerheads for several years because of union organizing activity in the major industrial corporations, which New Deal labor legislation had encouraged.[28] Federal strategies for dealing with the problems of war mobilization unintentionally restructured the funding of health-care services in the U.S.

War planning efforts would be much simpler if wages were frozen and if the government could be guaranteed a strike-free labor force in war industries, with unions themselves acting as enforcers of the no-strike agreements. The federal government achieved this aim by guaranteeing a fixed profit level to firms converted to war-production, in return for their acceptance of labor unions, who, in return, pledged not to strike during the war period and to accept government wage controls. This also helped guarantee union disciplining of the labor force, lessening work disruptions because of racial disputes. (Because of the shortage of available workers, war industries were hiring across the color lines; during their organizing campaigns, in return for pledges by minority communities not to accept temporary employment as strike-breakers, the industrial unions had committed themselves to fight for equal treatment of all workers, without regard to race.)[29]

During World War II, "fringe benefits," including health insurance, became part of a strategy to lure workers into wage-frozen jobs in the war industries, which were shorthanded because of the military draft. In 1942, the War Labor Board decided tax-free "fringe benefits" of up to 5 percent of wages could be offered as an incentive to attract and keep employees in wage-frozen war industry jobs. Since health insurance qualified as a fringe benefit, membership in group hospitalization plans (the only kind of health insurance easily available for a whole workforce) increased from less than seven million to about 26 million subscribers. Blue Cross cornered more than three-quarters of that market and became a giant operation.[30] Equally important, the "fringe benefit" rulings of the War Labor Board paved the way for introduction of health insurance paid by third parties—namely, employers. With the growth of such plans, business and industry would become major investors in the health programs of the nation.

Impact of the War: Federally Subsidized Medical Research

In 1939, as it became clear that Europe was heading towards a major war, a quartet of university and foundation leaders visited President Roosevelt. Karl Compton, James Conant, Vannevar Bush, and Frank Jewett urged him to set up a war planning commission to coordinate industrial production and scientific inquiry—including relevant medical research—for military victory. Roosevelt liked the idea.[31] When Congress refused to authorize funds for it, determined to stay out of the emerging European conflict, Roosevelt turned to the Rockefeller Foundation, which quietly provided a grant. Roosevelt asked Bush to head the planning group.

When the U.S. actually entered World War II, in December of 1941, a mobilization plan was in place, ready to be augmented quickly. One of its key elements was mobilization of the academic community: universities trained specialized military groups and university research facilities were redirected to work on problems strategic to winning the war. Government planners and "war czars" redirected resources and supervised activities in many of these areas. A doctors draft guaranteed that the armed forces had sufficient medical services.

As war mobilization went into high gear Vannevar Bush left the presidency of the Carnegie Institute to become the wartime "science czar" for the U.S., entrusted with directing millions of dollars of federal money into research to aid the war effort—a major new role for the federal government. Through the Office of Scientific Development (OSD), Bush became the major funder of science activity in the country. The OSD's Committee on Medical Research organized 12 major working committees: in aviation medicine, chemotherapeutic and other agents, convalescence and rehabilitation, industrial medicine, information, general medicine, neuropsychiatry, pathology, sanitary engineering, shock and transfusions, surgery, and treatment of gas casualties. Nearly $25 million was spent on these projects over a period of four years. The government also set up the Center for Disease Control, in Atlanta, Georgia, during the war and shortly after the war established the National Center for Health Statistics.[32]

With central coordination of funds, an emotionally united and patriotic scientific community, and a keen administrator, scientific research in the U.S. made quantum advances in both "basic" and "applied" research. Among the most spectacular breakthroughs that resulted from OSD projects were those in atomic research, including the development of the atomic bomb, and the development of inexpensive ways to produce antibiotic drugs—the "miracle drugs" that stopped infectious fevers and could therefore save countless lives on the battlefield. The widespread research on antibiotics led to an explosion of growth for American pharmaceutical companies. After the war their research departments created countless variations on antibiotic formulas, patenting these and marketing them under various trade names. During the 1950s and 1960s the pharmaceutical industry became a major growth leader in the American economy, and the use of antibiotics transformed the practice of primary care medicine.[33]

Vannevar Bush had demonstrated the effectiveness of federal subsidy for scientific research, and there was considerable sentiment in Congress to continue federal funding for research after the war was over. However, Bush had engendered much ill will from rival university presidents and from congressmen whose state universities did not get a proportionate share of the research funds distributed around the country. To quiet his opposition, Bush promised to step down as science czar as soon as the war ended, and to propose a plan for the federal funding of medicine and the sciences that would preclude anyone else from assuming the degree of power over the direction of scientific inquiry that he was exercising at the time.

Bush kept both promises. His parting legacy was the creation of a series of federal agencies to sponsor research, along with rules for how they would decide which projects to sponsor. The plan was adopted by Congress and funded generously. Federal support for the sciences, including medical research, has remained at a high level ever since, funneled through the National Science Foundation (NSF), the National Institutes of Health (NIH), a newly created National Institute of Mental Health (NIMH), and the Department of Health, Education and Welfare (HEW)—which later split into the Department of Health and Human Services (HHS) and the Department of Education.[34]

Under the plan set up by Bush—which is still in operation—no federal bureaucrat could control the administration of research monies beyond his or her special-interest agency. Except in the case of the Pentagon, agency regulations specify the mechanisms by which decisions will be made, in order to preclude undue influence from the administrator of the agency. Most regulations required "peer review" by a panel of research scientists to judge the feasibility and importance of grant proposals. As a result, medical researchers affiliated with major universities or other research centers across the country became key participants in federal funding decisions. They participated in peer review committees to decide which projects should get the funds designated by Congress. They also cooperated with a powerful political lobby of federal agency heads and disease-focused public relations agencies to increase federal funding for research. The American Cancer Society regularly publicized promising research directions as it lobbied successfully for increased appropriations.

As federal expenditures for health were increasingly influenced by these national agencies, informal working relationships were established between federal and state health department bureaucrats, medical school administrators and staff, disease-focused public relations groups, and the American Hospital Association. Significantly, these communication networks bypassed the AMA and its county-by-county organization of doctors, thereby rearranging the balance of power in health care.

Changes in Health-Care Costs. How had these innovations affected health-care costs by the end of World War II? In constant dollars adjusted for inflation, there was a 32 percent increase in per capita expenditures for medical care between 1940 and 1948, as compared with a 12 percent increase between 1929 and 1940. It is hard to judge how much of this change came about because wartime prosperity affected individual decisions about what health services to buy, and how much occurred simply because more people were now covered by prepaid hospitalization insurance. In both 1935 and 1940 total health-care expenditures for the nation accounted for 4 percent of the gross national product. By 1948, health care's share of the GNP had increased very slightly, to 4.1 percent. At the end of World War II, the health-care system's costs were holding stable relative to the rest of the economy.[35]

A New Postwar International Role for the United States
Has Implications for the Economy and for Health Care

As America entered the postwar era, the New Deal problem-solving stance was transformed by a new role which the U.S. assumed in the international arena. In the postwar era the United States assumed a role Great Britain had played before World War I, when the Pax Britannica had provided both military and economic stability internationally. The postwar Pax Americana strategy, combining a New Deal planning approach with international military commitments, included a role as enforcer and stabilizer of international trade and monetary agreements, enforcer and stabilizer of the international military balance of power, and leader of the "free world," with American planning and financing being used to solve problems in the international political economy. The U.S. quickly adopted a strident "anti-communist" stance as a cornerstone for policy making and coalitions of interest, in response to challenges from the Soviet Union, the world's second ranked industrial power, which tried to create its own spheres of interest and captive trading areas. By international agreement in 1944, the U.S. dollar had become the international medium of exchange. American products flooded the international market as other nations struggled to rebuild war-damaged industries. In addition, American trading prosperity was helped by the collapse of old colonial systems, which destroyed some protected trading areas of other countries.[36]

Implications for the American Economy

A high level of postwar prosperity in the U.S. led business and the federal government to think expansively about health-care innovation. Innovations of that period depended for their financial viability, however, on economic relationships that would undergo basic changes as the international political economy evolved. Moreover, some of the arrangements used to guide the growth of the postwar economy generated *new* health-care problems that were largely ignored at the time. For example, health-care innovators took advantage of opportunities being created by the expansion of America's metropolitan areas to build new hospitals and medical office buildings in the suburbs, but they paid little attention to problems of access to health-care services in the center city and rural areas that were being intensified by the suburban expansion.

The reasons for American economic prosperity during this period are complex, involving both national and international developments. Edward F. Denison of the Brookings Institution identified a number of domestic factors that affected economic growth during this period, including changes in the labor force and utilization of labor, in uses of capital, in land acquisition and development, in resource allocation, in knowledge, economies of scale, labor disputes, and in intensity of demand.[37] William Brainard and George Perry pointed to a growing availability of capital stock and energy, higher levels of expenditure for research and development, the growing "quality" of the American labor force which made higher technological production methods practical, and an increased rate of utilization of available resources.[38] Samuel Bowles, David Gordon and Tom Weisskopf argued that an emerging social structure for American capital accumulation made all this possible. It included the Pax Americana, a limited partnership that had developed during World War II between large unions and the management of large corporations, a series of cooperative understandings among America's larger corporations that limited "inter-Capitalist rivalry", and the development of nuclear power sources as a result of cooperative efforts between General Electric, Westinghouse, the Atomic Energy Commission and the Joint Committee on Atomic Energy in the U.S. Congress.[39] The debate among economists about causes of America's postwar prosperity need not concern us here, but three elements which affected the increased flow of economic resources in postwar America deserve more comment.

First, America had a headstart in the competition for trade. U.S. factories, unlike those in other parts of the world, had not been bombed. Moreover, the diversion to war production of 86 percent of the U.S. industrial economy for three and a half years, plus wartime policies that had encouraged a savings backlog among the citizenry, created an initially high domestic demand for both industrial and consumer goods. The return of military forces further reinforced this demand. Thus the postwar U.S. economy got off to a strong start, and it maintained this momentum for a number of years. This high level of demand motivated some managers of major corporations to develop innovative approaches to labor-management controversies that could affect the level of productivity within their industries. Their proposals also had implications for health-care funding.

Second, continued military spending helped stabilize the economy by guaranteeing a continuing federal consumption of industrial products. After an initial military demobilization, federal defense spending rose sharply after 1950, because of the Korean war. Between 1945 and 1960 the government's spending for weapons averaged out at about 10 percent of the GNP. In addition, American military superiority made its armaments attractive to less industrialized "friendly nations," further expanding the market for defense-related manufacturing. An international arms race began. Determined to stay ahead, the American government continued a high level of military expenditures. The combination of high demand for civilian consumer goods and continuing government subsidy for military industries encouraged American industry to undertake a major expansion of industrial capacity.[40]

Third, America's advantageous position for marketing both civilian and military industrial products abroad led to expanded export markets. During the first two decades following the war, 10 to 12 percent of all American manufacturing income came from export trade, and "defense production" accounted for another 10 to 20 percent. Thus, while the exact amount varied from year to year, the combination of defense and export manufacturing provided a fifth to a third of all U.S. manufacturing income.[41]

Creating a New Organizing Principle for American Business

U.S. policy recognized the importance of the export market to American businesses, and balanced this interest against strategic concerns to halt Communist influence in western Europe and Asia. In 1945, 10 to 12 percent of the popular vote in Belgium, the Netherlands, Denmark, Norway and Sweden had gone to Communist candidates, and Communist labor unions in France and Italy were a major force in the early postwar period.[42] Civil war in Greece between Communist guerrillas and other fighters made it clear that Europe was an area of contention between the two major powers, and Communist guerrilla movements in China and other parts of Asia threatened American international interests.

The American government began using New Deal principles of planning and funding to encourage problem-solving internationally. In 1948, the U.S. announced the Marshall Plan, direct aid to European countries to help them rebuild their economies and provide an economic bulwark against Communism. The movement toward politically motivated foreign aid grew even stronger after China fell to Communist forces in 1949, taking the world's most populous nation out of the western sphere of influence.[43] But within four years after the Marshall Plan began to stimulate their recovery, European nations were planning to create a Common Market in which there would be duty-free trade between members but import taxes imposed on products made elsewhere. Since the bulk of American exports were to Europe, this plan could result in American companies' products being priced out of the market—unless they were manufactured in Europe. Congress modified American tax laws, making it practical for U.S. companies to reorganize as transnational corporations whose manufacturing outside the U.S. would be exempt from U.S. taxation.[44]

Efforts of the U.S. government to protect the international trading advantage that U.S. businesses enjoyed, while at the same time encouraging Japan and European nations to develop industrial growth and trade policies that could serve as a bulwark against communist expansion, had two unanticipated consequences. First, the transformation of American corporations into transnational businesses would have profound effects on American society and on the emerging "health-care industry" in the decades to come. Second, by the 1970s the developing economies of Germany and Japan would begin to give American-based economic interests a run for their money, directly challenging the feasibility of patterns for accommodating health-care needs that had been worked out in the 1950s and 1960s.

Broader Changes in America that Affected Demand for Health Services

In the period of early post-war prosperity, expansive planning at all levels became feasible. Industrial corporations expanded their factories and built new ones, and people seeking new job opportunities flocked to the booming metropolitan areas and the new suburbs that were spreading out around them. Elaborate freeway systems were built to link these suburbs to metropolitan centers. Soon new schools, roads, houses, and hospitals were needed, and with the surplus tax revenues that could be anticipated from the new levels of prosperity, Congress was ready to help build them.

In the meantime, federal subsidies that helped mechanize Southern agriculture combined with universal conscription of males for military service and with expanding job opportunities to create a massive relocation of rural Southerners. Governmental subsidies for agriculture were generous during this period, allotted on the basis of the amount of acreage held by a farmer. Owners of Southern plantations invested heavily in agricultural machinery, which displaced a large proportion of southern sharecroppers and agricultural laborers who had previously worked the land. The expanding industrial scene beckoned to those who were being pushed off the land.[45] As the nation's homes and industries began to convert from coal to oil and natural gas, and as coal mines automated to stay competitive, many southern Appalachian residents also joined the trek north and west.

Changing Race Relations and Access to Health Services. As many Americans of color streamed into major metropolitan areas, the non-discrimination clauses in union contracts gave them access to manufacturing jobs that had previously been closed to racial minorities. Access to housing—and therefore to health care, as we shall see—posed a more difficult problem. Excluded from the new suburban housing developments, they settled in older neighborhoods of central city areas. This segregation was encouraged by government housing loan regulations.

Decision guidelines written into Federal Housing Administration (FHA) manuals during the 1930s gave preference for loans to newer neighborhoods that were "socially homogeneous"; older neighborhoods were "red-lined" as poor loan risks. These loan policies allowed real estate agents and banks to discourage minority families from moving into the new suburbs. Because there had been a hiatus in housing construction during the

Depression and the war, many of the neighborhoods open for minority settlement were eliminated from consideration for federally guaranteed loans because of the age of the housing stock. Racial minorities were thus more likely to live in deteriorating inner-city neighborhoods, which were being artificially aged by "red-lining" policies that prevented residents from buying or improving the properties with government-backed loans at low interest. The lower incomes of many inner-city residents had made it hard to get loans in the first place, and red-lining policies made the few loans that were available more expensive, because the federal government did not guarantee their repayment. The dramatic increase in the scale of housing development in the suburbs, which prosperity and G.I. and FHA government loan guarantees made possible, further accelerated the deterioration of these inner-city neighborhoods: most of the available loan money was diverted to newer development areas where the loans would be federally guaranteed.[46] Thus, the growth dynamic in American industry triggered the growth of metropolitan areas in ways that sowed the seeds of racial segregation, the rapid deterioration of inner-city housing, political organization on the basis of race, and unequal educational opportunity between well-financed suburbs and tax-strapped central cities.

Federal Subsidies and New "Class Interest" Splits

Some social critics began to describe postwar America as a "warfare/welfare state" with suburban populations prospering because of continuing military subsidies that guaranteed economic prosperity and the elderly and inner city populations dependent on government-financed welfare programs.[47] While a few studies attempted to document just how important a role military spending played in the postwar American economy, few economists discussed the larger contribution that the Pax Americana was making to American prosperity. Military spending and international trade accounted for at least 20 to 35 percent of the Gross National Product each year. By the time he left office in 1960, President Dwight D. Eisenhower, a former five-star General, was warning the nation to "beware of the military-industrial complex," which he believed had acquired too much power.[48] The prosperity of both the defense industry and what would later emerge as an information-services complex of interests was made possible by federal funding policies toward both wings of the "warfare/welfare" state. Later, when federal funding for medical research, training, and hospital construction was joined by private industry decisions to underwrite healthcare costs for their employees, a momentum was created that later would lead to splits in interest between emerging economic elites.

The profound implications of all this for the health needs of different population groups soon became evident in the morbidity and mortality rates for urban Americans of different racial stock, a disparity that persists today. As the entire scale of activity in metropolitan areas increased, inner-city residents were more exposed to dangers of lead poisoning and to lung damage from smog or other environmental pollutants. As older houses were carved up into small apartments, the health problems that classically follow urban congestion spread to new neighborhoods. So did the effects of stress that come from sound bombardment in crowded neighborhoods, from higher crime rates, uncertain income, and low-cost but high fat and high salt diets. Moreover, doctors increasingly moved their offices to the suburbs, making primary health-care services less available to inner-city residents. By this time, the generation of doctors licensed before the AMA had gained control of entry to medicine was largely gone. The closing of medical schools that had been set up for descendants of slaves, along with racial quotas in the remaining schools, meant that fewer minority physicians were being trained. A serious racial disparity in access to basic goods and services, including health-care services, was beginning to emerge in America's major metropolitan areas, both North and South.

Innovative Failure: A National Health-Care System

By the end of World War II, President Harry S. Truman was ready to follow the lead of other allied nations in setting up a government-funded, national health-care system. It was easy enough to get united support for pieces of a health-care system that did not threaten the autonomy and control of the AMA. Other critical ingredients, however, remained out of reach, as the government planners and the AMA each put together a coalition of special interest groups that might help them win in a legislative fight.

Truman's legislative proposals, which went beyond the publicly espoused social goals of FDR's New Deal, were introduced as part of a Fair Deal for all Americans. In the war of symbols that soon emerged, the AMA mounted a massive public relations campaign that used Cold War imagery to attack "socialized medicine." Given this framing of the issues, opponents included not only powerful special interests within health care, notably the AMA, the American Hospital Association, and National Association of Blue Shield Plans, but also business interests, including the Chamber of Commerce, the Life Insurance Association of America, and the National Association of Manufacturers, the American Farm Bureau Federation, and the American Legion.[49]

Given this line-up of opponents the legislative outcome was not hard to anticipate. Every year since 1939 Senator Robert Wagner of New York (whose 1937 Wagner Act had sanctioned the organization of national industrial unions into the CIO) had introduced a bill to set up a comprehensive insurance system to protect against the cost of ill health. Each year after World War II, Senator Wagner and Representative John Dingell (a Democrat from Michigan, where the CIO's United Auto Workers now exercised a strong political presence) re-introduced some version of that bill to provide federal financing for health insurance. Each year the AMA and its allies opposed the imposition of "socialized medicine". Although Truman wholeheartedly backed national health insurance, arguing for it in his State of the Union messages,[50] the Democratic majority in Congress included a number of conservative Democrats from the South who often voted with their Republican colleagues. Once a proposal got dubbed "socialist", and opposed by the AMA with its effective county by county organization of physicians, one could count on most southern Democrats in Congress to vote with their Republican colleagues in opposition to such a bill. Federally subsidized health insurance remained a dead issue for another twenty years after World War II had ended, thanks in part to the AMA's ability to link such proposals to Cold War ideology.

Federal Spending Begins to Reshape Health Care

Revamping the Hospital System. Despite the warnings of some healthcare experts that hospital construction alone was an inadequate basis for broader planning, Congress passed the Hill-Burton Hospital Construction Act in 1946. Enthusiastically supported by the American Hospital Association and most doctors, the act quickly became part of "pork barrel politics," with politicians scrambling to help local communities get Hill-Burton funds.[51]

As originally conceived, Hill-Burton was to help low-income and middle-income communities acquire new hospitals. In practice, most new hospital construction went to middle-income communities, which were better equipped to raise the matching funds required. The bill authorized spending $75 million annually for a period of five years. With Congressional enthusiasm for local projects and ample tax revenues available, Hill-Burton was kept in place until 1972. During this time it provided $3.7 billion dollars in direct government subsidies for hospital construction and generated an additional $9.1 billion in locally raised matching funds. Between 1947 and 1965 it added 300,000 hospital beds to the American healthcare system, increasing the number of beds available for short-term care in community hospitals by 40 percent.[52]

Subsidizing Medical Training: The Growth of Specialization and "High-Tech" Medicine. Meanwhile, federal funding for medical research and highly technical medical training changed the focus of medical schools and the profile of American doctors. It also provided the impetus for the development of medical treatment using high technology.

Medical schools expanded in size and complexity during the 1940s and 1950s. During the 1940s the number of full-time faculty increased more than 50 percent and the average income of medical schools tripled; during the 1950s the number of full-time medical faculty doubled. As the size of the faculty grew, the number of subspecialties represented increased. NIH research grants were used to develop new research centers and to pay the salaries for an enlarged group of investigators. As demand for research space and clinical facilities grew, medical schools created networks of affiliated hospitals, acquired land in their immediate neighborhoods, and tore down residential buildings in order to build institutes, clinics, and hospitals.[53]

At the heart of this expansion and the trend toward greater specialization lay federal funding. During the four years of World War II, the federal government had spent $25 million for medical research. Thereafter the yearly allocations skyrocketed to $73 million in 1950, $471 million in 1960, and $1.229 billion in 1965. In 1980 the allocation was $7.825 billion—a twenty-twofold increase over 1950, in constant dollars, after controlling for inflation.[54]

Nonequilibrium Trends in Medical Specialization. With research funding also came training grants to train medical specialists. In response, the medical schools began to create networks of affiliated hospitals in which they could place their students for clinical rotations through the "specialties." Thus the expanding hospital system developed teaching roles for the specialists it was sending out into the community; besides bringing additional business into their hospitals, they became part of the training ground, recruiting additional specialists from current medical school populations.[55]

In 1940, one-fourth of American doctors listed themselves as medical specialists. After the war the proportion of new doctors heading into specialties constantly climbed, to 40 percent in 1955, 55 percent in 1960, and 69 percent in 1966. By that time, in other words, more than two-thirds of American physicians were limiting their practice to medical specialties, which offered them substantially higher income and more freedom to set their own hours and conditions of work. The tendency of faculty research specialists to recruit the brightest medical students into their sub-area further heightened the attractiveness of specialized medicine. Ironically, as this was happening America began to develop a severe shortage of doctors available for general, primary health care.[56] But an even more dramatic impact on the character of medical treatment was being made by federal programs for funding medical research, which were stimulating the growth of subsidiary industrial sectors to provide new kinds of medical supplies.

Post-War Public Health Development. In contrast, federal support for the expansion of public health delivery was much more modest. Before

World War II there had been eight graduate schools of public health (at Johns Hopkins, Yale, Harvard, Columbia, the University of Michigan, the University of Minnesota, the University of North Carolina, and the University of California at Berkeley). In 1946, the American Public Health Association developed an accreditation program for schools of public health. Four more schools were established in the next decade (at U.C.L.A., the University of Puerto Rico, Tulane, and Pittsburgh).[57]

Nonequilibrium Trends in Public Funding for Medical Research. Research activities were well funded by the federal government during this time period and the federal public health agencies became the conduit for support of research carried on primarily in the nation's universities and medical schools. The National Mental Health Act of 1946 authorized the Public Health Service to construct a hospital and laboratories as part of the development of the NIH. And the budget for the PHS constantly expanded, from $120 million in 1950 to $300 million in 1960 to $5.7 billion in 1977, with most of the increase going to the National Institutes of Health. The focus was primarily on disease-oriented research, and 80 percent of the funds went as grants to university researchers. There were exceptions to this pattern: in 1954 the Taft Sanitary Engineering Center was established in Cincinnati, the home base of Senator Robert Taft, and funds were granted to state public health agencies and to the Centers for Disease Control in Atlanta. But for the most part, public health grants followed the pattern of medical research seen more generally.[58]

Two factors were responsible for this remarkable increase in funding. The first, of course, was the availability of an enlarged tax revenue created by the general economic prosperity. The second was a highly effective political lobby developed by a private citizen, Mary Lasker. Through the Lasker Foundation (which she had founded with her late husband, a wealthy public relations executive) she worked in cooperation with the American Cancer Society and the American Heart Association to make heart disease and cancer the most popular unsolved health problems in America. Quickly gaining the cooperation of federal officials in the NIH and of medical school research entrepreneurs, the "cancer lobby"—or Mary's little lambs, as Washingtonians began to refer to the venture—became one of the most effective lobbies on Capitol Hill. Always well-informed, Mary Lasker knew how to mobilize national publicity as well as how to tap business friendship networks to influence U.S. presidents and members of Congress.[59] Getting her support became part of medical school strategies for expanding promising areas of medical research, along with securing endorsement of project goals from the new federal health agency heads. Thanks to Lasker's efforts, medical appropriations bills were regularly increased to include additional funding for research on cancer and heart disease. Researchers quickly discovered that the safest way to get funding for more general, basic medical research was to link it with potential implications for these two problems.

Growth Rates for Health-Related Industries

Public funding was not the only source for medically-related research during this time period. After the war, the pharmaceutical industry grew at a record pace. The wartime discovery of an inexpensive way to grow antibiotic medicines in the laboratory encouraged heavy investment in research and new product development. Some medical researchers began to move back and forth between medical school appointments and jobs with the drug companies, or held joint appointments. Soon, a staggering number of patents were being taken out for antibiotics and then for psychotropics, drugs that transformed the practice of primary care medicine and the treatment of emotional disturbance. So many new products were being introduced that *JAMA*, the *Journal of the American Medical Association* no longer tried to evaluate them all. Sales representatives for the drug companies regularly visited doctors, offering free samples of the latest products and educating doctors about the advantages of each new product. By the 1950s the pharmaceutical industry had become a growth leader in the national economy.[60]

Federal money for research also stimulated the growth of companies producing high-technology equipment—new diagnostic machinery and replacements for ailing body parts. The medical school metaphor of the body as a machine became a reality: in addition to the iron lung, which breathed for patients who were paralyzed, dialysis machines substituted for ailing kidneys, pacemakers were installed in ailing hearts to regulate their beat, and external heart pumps were used during operations to circulate blood if the heart was not functioning. Eventually the development of intensive care units in hospitals offered mechanical substitutes for most malfunctioning systems within the human body.

These developments coincided with the availability of federal funds for new hospital construction. Many of the newer hospitals added high-technology equipment, which might be housed in new laboratories, in special wings of the hospital (such as intensive-care units), or throughout the hospital. The new equipment was very expensive, but any hospital that had it available could attract prestigious medical specialists and their retinue of patients.

Institutionalizing "Fringe Benefits":
Third Party Payers for Health Insurance

High-technology, hospital-oriented care became possible because of a parallel development in how day-to-day health-care costs would be funded, the unintended result of private responses to the earlier defeat of Truman's proposal to create a national health-care system. Cold War symbolism had helped mobilize an effective coalition opposing such "public interest" measures as national health insurance or a federally controlled national health-care system. The end of the war left members of labor unions without guaranteed coverage for rising health-care costs, because only 600,000 of the 26 million Blue Cross-Blue Shield subscribers to workplace-based health insurance were covered by plans that had been directly negotiated by unions. In 1946, unions belonging to the CIO, which now represented most workers employed by the major manufacturing corporations, announced that welfare programs, including health insurance, would be a high priority for peacetime contract negotiations.[61] By 1948, Congress had made it clear that it was not about to extend existing Social Security benefits to include health insurance, or to extend present social security benefits to include able-bodied workers. Unions therefore turned to contract negotiations with the major industries as the most effective way of pursuing this agenda.

The first two years after the end of World War II saw a flood of strikes, as American unions began to demonstrate that they were now a force to be reckoned with. Government response to the postwar labor unrest was legislative. The Taft-Hartley Act, passed in 1948, amended earlier New Deal labor legislation and required American labor unions to purge themselves of any Communist leaders. Congress wanted to ensure that American labor unions could never serve as a base for launching Communist political campaigns, as they had in Europe. While accepting the Taft-Hartley amendment to labor legislation strengthened the hand of more moderate factions within the union leadership, it also motivated them to win substantial benefits for their members, in order to retain their credibility as the real voice of labor despite their acquiescence in government sponsored purges of union leaders. By 1948, 10 unions representing 2.7 million workers had negotiated health and welfare plans as part of their postwar contracts. By 1950, the number of workers covered by such plans had increased to over seven million. As union demands strengthened the position of non-unionized clerks and management personnel, some larger organizations began to provide health benefits for all employees.[62]

"Fair Wages". In 1948, Charles E. Wilson, the chairman of General Motors, the nation's largest corporation, entered contract negotiations with the United Auto Workers proposing a formula for deciding what was a fair wage. He suggested that the 1940 wage level, which had been the basis for

wartime wage setting, be adjusted to account for increases in the cost of living, as measured in the Consumer Price Index. In addition to a cost of living adjustment (COLA), to be figured quarterly, workers would receive a "wage improvement factor" that would represent an improvement in their income beyond adjustment for inflation.[63]

About a week after the union ratified the contract, Wilson gave a speech explaining his new proposal: to lessen labor-management strife, the nation needed a fair-wage formula that would help avoid additional inflation, recognize the importance of improving the efficiency of production, and respond to a "distortion in relative prosperity . . . between various elements of the population" which had developed in the aftermath of the war.[64] This was a dramatic recasting of the problem. Wilson was arguing that corporations should begin sharing a portion of their profits with their workers, adjusting wages to inflation levels and tying real improvement in worker income to productivity. The wage scale would thus be adjusted as the efficiency of workers increased.

Fringe Benefits. Two years later, the 1950 GM-UAW contract made this formula more explicit. The union described five economic gains that were institutionalized in the new contract: (1) a jointly administered pension plan; (2) a guaranteed annual wage increase, described by the union as a reward for increased productivity and to be added to the basic wage rate; (3) a continuation of the COLA clause; (4) a hospital-medical plan, with the company paying half the cost of Blue Cross and Blue Shield protection for workers and their families; and (5) an improved sickness and accident benefit program.[65] Contract provisions for increased fringe benefits were preferable to a simple wage increase, since the increase in wages would be taxable and "fringe benefits" were not.

The new GM-UAW contract was in effect for five years. During that time management was free to change the organization of work and introduce more efficient manufacturing machinery. Organized labor, in turn, got for workers a package of "fringe benefits" as the equivalent of social security. They also wanted to be sure that "increasing productivity" would not become a euphemism for displacing workers, and that layoffs could not be used to get rid of union leaders and "troublemakers".

Given the record level of prosperity and management's proposal to share a portion of the profits with workers, union demands were easy to accommodate. Fringe benefits, including health-care coverage, could be part of the proposed profit-sharing. Wage rates could be adjusted to include fringe benefits as well as up-front wages. A "fair" system to deal with possible layoffs could be developed, as well. If layoffs were made, they would be on the basis of seniority: the last hired becoming the first to be laid off. Loyalty to the company thus would be rewarded, with no singling out of individuals for adverse attention during layoffs.

After the UAW accepted the principles being proposed, and the federal government endorsed them as appropriate for industry more generally, the new formula became widely copied. Employer-based hospital insurance was readily available across the country, thanks to the Blue Cross initiatives of the prewar period. There was no other comparable package of services available. Not surprisingly therefore, business-financed private hospitalization insurance became the basic mode of health security in America. After World War II private insurance companies entered the market as well, offering competing and supplementary plans to what Blue Cross was making available. By 1954, 60 percent of the American public had private health insurance.

The offer by management to share profits through wage-setting formulas did more than create a new era of labor-management cooperation; it further stimulated economic prosperity. By granting wage increases rather than keeping wages low, management put money in the hands of people likely to spend it. The marginal propensity to spend out of wages is higher than the marginal propensity to spend out of profits. Economists argued that the expenditure multiplier for wages often results in a five-fold increase as the original wages recirculate through purchase of goods and services. Lower profits from higher wage increases, thus, lead to higher total consumption spending.[66] American prosperity, it seemed, had become self-generating and no longer dependent on international markets and the arms race.

Impact on Health-Care Costs. Because health insurance, as developed under the Blue Cross model, primarily covered hospital costs, patients paid less themselves (and doctors were more assured of receiving payment) if services were provided inside a hospital. While lowering out-of-pocket costs to the patient, this practice increased the total costs for taking care of many health problems. Medical procedures were becoming increasingly high-tech, thanks to federal funding for medical research, training, and hospital expansion. As high-tech equipment (and the high-salaried personnel needed to run it) became available in the newer hospitals, and as these hospitals adjusted their rates to cover construction costs as well as new operating expenses, the cost of hospitalization doubled between 1950 and 1960.[67] Because Blue Cross was managed by boards having a majority of representatives from member hospitals, the hospital insurance companies rarely questioned these increases, simply passing them on to consumers in the form of higher monthly premiums. Businesses were assuming an increasing proportion of the cost of the insurance policies, as part of fringe benefits made possible by the general prosperity; thus individuals covered by the policies had little reason to complain or to question the upward spiral of cost. Neither did the companies, since fringe benefits were tax deductible as a cost of doing business.

Older hospitals which had not "modernized" found themselves at a disadvantage in attracting doctors to refer patients to them. It was the need to modernize in order to keep full occupancy, as well as to maintain prestige within the medical community, that helped create the pressure to extend the Hill-Burton Act far beyond the time span originally envisioned for it. By 1960, pharmaceuticals were not the only pace-setting sector of the economy related to health care; the Standard and Poor's ratings began to single out companies that produced hospital equipment and supplies and managed hospital construction as businesses with high investment potential.[68]

Continuing Problems of Access to Care. After the war, problems of access to health care for inner-city residents, racial minorities, and the poor became increasingly acute. Federal subsidies for hospital construction and medical training were resulting in the location of new hospitals and physicians' offices in the suburbs and in southern communities that until 1963 were not required to admit patients of minority backgrounds. Requirements that a local community raise matching funds to be eligible for Hill-Burton grants meant that fewer poorer communities managed to qualify for these grants. Hospital care was a growing problem for residents of the inner-city neighborhoods, even if they had health insurance. Even more so was access to physicians, for the reasons already described.[69]

This situation began to change for the poorest members of these neighborhoods, however, with the enactment of Medicare and Medicaid legislation that provided government-funded health insurance for the poor and the elderly. Growing racial turmoil, the effective mobilization of the urban poor, and new voter registration patterns among minorities all played a role in getting this legislation passed, overturning a fifty-year stalemate. Changes in the composition of the U.S. Supreme Court beginning in 1953, in turn, became critical for letting this kind of social pressure emerge.

A New Federal Player: The Supreme Court

Political recriminations about the loss of China to the Communist bloc in 1949 led to a major anti-communist reaction in the U.S. In 1952 the Republicans recaptured control of the White House by nominating World War II hero Dwight Eisenhower and Richard Nixon, a young Californian who had gained prominence in 1948 through his "anticommunist" campaign for Congress.[70] During the Republican nominating convention Eisenhower solidified Republican solidarity by offering to nominate the runner-up, California Governor Earl Warren, to be Chief Justice of the Supreme Court. Eisenhower knew little about Warren's judicial philosophy. Warren, it turned out, took quite seriously the Reconstruction Era amendments granting freedom, equality, and full civil rights to ex-slaves. He also believed that the proper role of the Supreme Court was to interpret the *intent* of the U.S. Constitution, rather than to limit itself to a strict interpretation of its language. With Warren as Chief Justice and the appointment of Associate Justice William Joseph Brennan, Jr., the Supreme Court had a majority sharing this outlook, and it began to act as a force in its own right.[71] The Court made a series of rulings that changed the character of social struggle in America. Some of its rulings turned out to be as important for future developments in health care as others were for civil rights. The momentum set in motion by its rulings eventually led to Medicare and Medicaid legislation, which permanently changed the character of health care in America.

Court Decisions Affecting Health Care

In 1953, the Supreme Court ruled that requiring doctors to belong to their county medical association in order to have the right to practice in local hospitals was a violation of their civil rights. Younger doctors became less inclined to join county chapters, and within a few years AMA membership dropped from over two-thirds of all practicing physicians to less than half. Given the new directions in health care, the AMA's credibility as the voice of medicine, and its ability to influence elections through powerful county-by-county organization, was weakened—as was its financial kitty for lobbying, since a portion of county membership dues went to the national organization. Although the Court's ruling attracted little attention at the time, its impact on health-care politics was profound.[72]

The better known Court rulings that became relevant for health-care changes, however, did not deal directly with health issues at all. Rather, they outlawed racial segregation, overturning an earlier Court's ruling that "separate but equal" facilities were allowable under the Constitutional requirement of equal access for all citizens. The Warren Court ruled that racially separate facilities were inherently unequal, and therefore illegal. The rulings began with a decision opening access to schools and quickly spread to rulings prohibiting discrimination in a wide range of social arenas. In 1963, the Courts ruled that it was unconstitutional to give Hill-Burton hospital construction money to hospitals that did not admit members of racial minorities—a ruling that directly affected minority access to medical services.[73] The effect of other rulings was even more profound, because the new Court stance encouraged those who faced discrimination to challenge it directly, knowing that the Supreme Court would ultimately back their right to do so. The escalating racial struggles opened up new opportunities to overcome earlier legislative roadblocks to government funding of health-care services.

Court Decisions, Politics, and the Civil Rights Movement

The new political climate for racial struggles was indeed an ironic outcome of Cold War politics. The Cold War had provided an opportunity to purge the American labor movement of Communist leaders, and the GM-sponsored formulas for setting wages and fringe benefits had solidified a labor-management partnership. Labor union members became increasingly prosperous, though their numbers were shrinking due to automation (and later due to corporate decisions to move manufacturing investments outside the country). U.S. labor split into two segments, the unionized with high wages and benefits, and the rest. As this happened, the poor, the unemployed, and Americans of color who had moved to urban areas became increasingly restive. In place of union spokesmen, Black clergy in the South began to challenge the exclusion of the poor and people of color from access to the privileges and services enjoyed by other Americans.

Earlier, World War II had been presented to the American people as a "struggle for freedom," and the Cold War was justified as an effort to defend the "free world" against communism. Now, in the 1950s, civil rights leaders turned the rhetoric of freedom to their own use domestically. With the Negro churches and the U.S. Supreme Court jointly proclaiming the right to freedom and equality, the movement for racial justice constantly gained momentum. Efforts by southern politicians to label the civil rights leaders as Communists backfired, as ministers held public prayer meetings and led nonviolent "civil disobedience" demonstrations where protesters suffered arrest after massive violation of a law they considered morally and constitutionally wrong. When a southern governor openly resisted the new rulings from the Supreme Court, and President Eisenhower reluctantly backed Supreme Court rulings with a show of force in Arkansas, it became clear that racial struggle had replaced union struggle as the locus of American social controversy.[74]

Political responses to the civil rights campaigns may have been decisive for determining the outcome of the 1960 presidential election. During the fall campaign between John F. Kennedy and Richard Nixon, Kennedy gave open support to Martin Luther King, Jr., when he was jailed in Georgia for civil rights activity. The heavy turnout in northern heavily-Black precincts gave Kennedy his margin of victory in a close election.[75]

Escalation of Demands. By 1960, southern students were staging "sit-ins" in 80 southern communities. Soon, joined by college students from across the country who sympathized with their cause, they were organizing a voter registration campaign across the Deep South, aimed at getting voting rights for Black Americans and at unseating southern segregationist legislators who bottled up civil rights bills in Congress. Civil Rights strategies escalated, focused on bringing legal challenges to southern segregation laws that could be heard by a sympathetic U.S. Supreme Court. Soon southern campaigns of "civil disobedience" against segregation laws were being joined by northern and west coast mass actions of "civil disruption" protesting northern racial discrimination in hiring practices.[76]

The Rev. Martin Luther King, Jr., who had become the most eloquent spokesperson for the movement, then led a Poor People's March on Washington, attended by several hundred thousand demonstrators. Other protest marches, and the 1963 assassination of President Kennedy, coupled with growing evidence that the poor and disadvantaged were becoming increasingly restive, led President Lyndon B. Johnson to put his full weight behind the passage of a sweeping Civil Rights Act in 1964 and an amendment to the U.S. Constitution, which also passed in 1964, outlawing the poll tax. The 1964 election produced a landslide of votes for the Democrats, particularly in northern and western urban areas; liberal Democrats for the first time had a voting majority in Congress. Thus, Johnson's agenda could pass with ease. It included both civil rights and health-care legislation. Coupled together as part of the vision of a Great Society and the War on Poverty, it was difficult for older coalitions of interest to muster enough support in Congress to stop the new momentum.[77]

Legislative Response: Medicare and Medicaid

The solution chosen for dealing with problems of access to health services was shaped by earlier strategies that had been developed in the wake of the defeat of Truman's national health-care system proposal. After federal planners discovered the strength of the coalition that the AMA had organized in the late 1940s to block Truman's proposals for national health insurance, Wilbur Cohen, a New Deal strategist who helped draft the original Social Security legislation and now was working on national health insurance policy, decided national health insurance needed to be recast in a way that would be more difficult to oppose. Cohen and others who worked closely with him argued that since Social Security had become an unquestioned public policy, it would be politically awkward for the AMA to oppose health needs of the elderly, who were also an effective political lobby. Once the principle of federal funding for health insurance was established, they reasoned, it would be possible to extend it to others, including people on welfare and perhaps eventually to the entire public.[78]

For seven years, since 1958, Congress had been deadlocked over various proposals to provide medical services to the elderly poor. There was strong support from well-organized, political constituencies of the elderly for some kind of health-care assistance, but an administration proposal for mandatory hospitalization coverage for the elderly poor, and a competing AMA-sponsored Eldercare proposal limiting coverage to voluntary insurance to pay only for physicians visits, had produced a deadlock on how to proceed. Previously, two conservative congressional leaders, Representative Wilbur Mills of Arkansas and Senator Robert Kerr of Oklahoma, had brought together a coalition of conservative Democrats and Republicans that had effectively stymied executive-branch proposals. At issue was the question of whether health care was a "right" or a "privilege"—that is, whether the government should be responsible for everyone's health needs or only for those of the "deserving poor." The Kerr-Mills proposals, reflecting the view that health services to the elderly were a privilege rather than a universal right, and giving individual states discretion over what health-care services should be given to the poor, had dominated consideration of health insurance legislation for several years. Now, with the liberal Democratic sweep of both houses of Congress in 1964, the Conservatives were no longer in a position to veto legislation or determine its exact content. Representative Mills, who took pride in being the shaper of winning legislation, recognized the new political realities in Congress and abruptly shifted position. Working quickly in the spring of 1965, he combined the two opposing plans for providing health services for the elderly into a single package, called Medicare. Then, in the same legislative package, he added Medicaid, a simple proposal that expanded assistance to the states for the medical care of persons on welfare; it was based on his own earlier proposals and left unspecified much of the detail of how this was to be administered. Thus under this legislation health insurance for the elderly became a "right," while health care for the "deserving poor" became a privilege—a difference largely ignored in the flurry of events. With the contending packages combined, the legislation passed quickly, despite AMA opposition, and President Johnson signed it into law on July 30, 1965.[79]

By addressing the needs of the politically mobilized elderly population and those of the potentially disruptive urban poor, in an atmosphere of national crisis that had led to a liberal sweep in Congress, resistance to federally funded health insurance was finally overcome. Once the AMA discovered what a financial plum Medicare payments for physicians' visits represented, the "socialized medicine" issue disappeared from political debate.

Medicare-Medicaid and Cost Escalation

The U.S. Government had now agreed to fund hospital costs of the aged and welfare recipients, the two population groups most likely to be dealing regularly with severe health problems, and also most likely to use the dramatic interventions available through high-tech medicine. Federal funding for their health care was to be directed toward the American hospital system, which recently had become capable of providing a variety of new medical services using high technology. For hospital administrators, the passing of Medicare/Medicaid legislation provided a new level of challenge for services and an invitation to modernize their facilities.

If the proportion of elderly patients in the caseload increased, laboratory facilities would need to be expanded so that the variety of degenerative malfunctions could be quickly diagnosed. Moreover, if doctors were to adhere to the Hippocratic Oath to preserve life whenever possible, there would have to be an increase in the availability of dialysis machines, cardiovascular operations, heart pacemaker installations, and intensive care machine substitutions for bodily processes in stroke victims. If the urban poor were also to be served, there would have to be intensive care units for newborn babies, an expansion of treatment facilities for children with severe health problems, and the like. Given the extensive mechanization of services that could be anticipated, many hospitals decided to replace their facilities entirely, in order to respond more completely to the new opportunities and demands.

How was all this to be financed? Before 1965, Blue Cross formulas for reimbursing hospital costs allowed hospitals to fold capital improvement costs into the cost of services. Since Blue Cross boards were dominated by members of hospital staffs, they rarely questioned increases in service costs, simply passing them on to the consumer in the form of increased premium charges for the coming year. If Medicare and Medicaid proceeded similarly, there would be no problem for the hospital administrators.

When Medicare and Medicaid were established, government officials sought to avoid conflicts between Social Security bureaucrats and hospital personnel by giving hospitals a choice: work directly with Social Security officials or use an intermediary agency to handle their bookkeeping. Not surprisingly, most hospitals designated Blue Cross as the agency to supervise their Medicare/Medicaid accounts and to deal directly with the government. Also not surprisingly, Blue Cross used its standard procedures for dealing with these new insurance accounts.[80]

The Emergence of a Health-Care Industry

Once Medicare-Medicaid insurance reimbursement became available, a boom in hospital construction began. Hospitals were no longer dependent on Hill-Burton allocations. With government funding through Medicare and Medicaid reimbursements guaranteed to cover their costs, they could issue bonds for hospital expansion or construction and include the cost of both the principal and the interest in the daily operating costs of the hospital, which in turn would be added to the charges for various patient services. In 1965, when Medicare/Medicaid first went into effect, 16 percent of hospital capital funds came from operating surpluses (the income they took in beyond expenses), 46 percent came from gifts and donations from charity or government), and 38 percent came from bond indebtedness. Twenty years later, after the new government-guaranteed bond strategy had developed fully, the proportion of capital obtained from operating surplus had increased to 24 percent, capital income from gifts had declined to 8 percent, and the proportion coming from bonded indebtedness or stock equities had climbed to 68 percent.[81]

Briefly put, hospitals found that the most practical way to expand was to go into debt, adding to the charges being passed on to patients not only the cost of new construction but the interest on money borrowed to pay for it. In order to limit their debt liability as much as possible, they also were increasing charges for other services, in order to generate a higher operating surplus so that a larger proportion of their capital funds came from daily operations rather than from cash borrowing.

Given increased access to funds and an enlarged demand for services by the poor and elderly, the temptation to upgrade facilities was enormous. Moving into a constantly upgraded facility became more than a tempting opportunity after 1969, however. Court rulings made it protective for hospitals, and for physicians as well.

Malpractice

Before 1969, malpractice suits against doctors were relatively uncommon. The AMA had "solved" this problem in the early 1900s by including in its membership pledges an agreement that doctors would not testify against one another in court. So long as most doctors belonged to the AMA, it was difficult to prove that medical care had been incompetent, since physicians would not testify against each other. Since their fees in malpractice cases were usually contingent upon winning the case, lawyers often discouraged potential clients from suing a doctor unless the evidence of malpractice was overwhelming.

This situation changed dramatically in the late 1960s after a series of state court decisions established the right of a patient to sue a hospital for malpractice, striking down arguments that hospitals had "charitable immunity" from prosecution. Courts ruled that hospitals no longer functioned as passive sites where physicians practiced independently; hospitals as well as physicians could be sued if it could be shown that standards of care had been violated in a hospital and that other personnel should have been aware of the problem and intervened.[82] With hospitals eligible for suit, awards also could be larger, and the number of malpractice suits began to escalate. Hospitals pressured academic MDs to testify on their behalf. (Academics rarely belonged to the AMA now that the Supreme Court had ruled this was not necessary.)

As the number of malpractice suits escalated during the 1970s and 1980s, the entire practice of medicine changed. Individual physicians ordered many more diagnostic tests and referrals to specialists, to protect themselves against later suits for having overlooked a rare but possible condition. After surveying private physicians in 1982, the AMA estimated that "defensive medicine" was adding about 10 percent to the costs of services performed by individual doctors.[83] Hospitals, moreover, were finding it both self-serving and self-protective to constantly upgrade their diagnostic and treatment facilities so that they remained "state of the art"; this added to their income and protected them against being found legally negligent. Needless to say, this pushed up the cost of services even more than did the defensive medical practices of individual physicians. Hospitals also expanded their staffs to include a wide range of new technical specialists. In 1960, hospitals averaged 226 staff members per 100 patients; by 1978, the number had reached 370 per 100 patients.[84] With the increasing size and complexity of hospital operations—including the need to make extensive judgments about plant expansion and operation, and to keep elaborate records for the variety of third-party payment groups now involved—the administration of hospitals began to pass out of the hands of doctors and into the hands of professional business administrators. Soon these administrators were introducing cost-accounting methods, business approaches to "growth" and "market shares," and innovative funding strategies into hospital management. The concerns of business became the new standards by which the delivery of health care was judged. This subtle but important shift in emphasis began to change the character of many interactions within the health-care industry.

The result was a major escalation in hospital costs. After Hill-Burton funds stimulated the expansion or construction of new hospitals, hospital costs doubled between 1950 and 1960. After the passing of Medicare and Medicaid, they rose much more rapidly. Between 1967 and 1985, they more than quadrupled. In that period, the general Consumer Price Index increased 322 percent, medical costs as a whole increased 402 percent, and hospital costs increased 710 percent. (See Table 2 of the Appendix.)

In summary, by 1970, the American health-care system had evolved into a health-care industry as various organized interests responded to crises or new opportunities created by changes in international political and economic relations. Innovations introduced by entrepreneurs, at critical moments in the evolving political economy, had become widely copied, changing the circumstances affecting the organization of health care thereafter. "The law of large numbers" prediction, that innovations tend to be too numerous and so disparate that they collectively negate one another's impact, did not apply at such moments: Interest groups quickly copied innovations which showed promise for solving a problem that affected them all. The introduction of prepaid hospitalization insurance, the use of risk pools spread across a firms' employee pool, and employers as third-party payers were not simply innovations in health care; they were strategies created to solve organizational crises created by the international Great Depression, World War II and its after-effects for labor-management relations in America. Had earlier political stalemates not prevented the creation of a nationally funded health-care system, these kinds of health-care innovations would not have been needed. Meanwhile, World War II had created public support for new federal health subsidies for research, for the training of medical specialists, and later for hospital construction. Then Medicare and Medicaid legislation made the government responsible for the health needs of the elderly and those on public welfare, two population groups likely to need high-technology interventions. The transformation of American hospitals, already begun, accelerated quickly. Court decisions allowing hospitals to be sued made earlier AMA strategies for avoiding malpractice suits irrelevant and encouraged the practice of "defensive medicine" using "state of the art" diagnostic and treatment procedures.

American health care was changing, both in form and in emphasis. The health-care industry that was emerging in the 1960s began to play a new role in the economy, thanks to larger changes already underway. As it developed it began to generate serious problems for export-oriented sectors of the industrial economy and for the government, the two groups that subsidized much of its expansion. And the soaring costs of the care it delivered created severe problems for the population groups left unprotected by the new insurance formulas. Health care reform became an important priority in government and business planning. Because health care's relation to a broader set of issues was only partially understood, however, many reforms of the next two decades had little impact. Others actually made the situation worse.

2

First Efforts at Cost Control

By the 1970s American health care had changed profoundly, and its impact on the economy could now be seen. Where for decades its costs had consumed between 3.5 percent and 4.5 percent of the GNP, by 1960 its share of the GNP had increased to 5.3 percent.[1] Since much of the increase was for hospitalization costs which were a "fringe benefit" that would otherwise go into higher wages in the larger, unionized corporations, there was little reason as yet for premium payers to be alarmed.

After 1965, however, the upgrading of the American hospital system to take advantage of high-tech equipment and procedures went into full gear. The cost of hospitalization doubled during the 1960s, and health care's share of the GNP increased to 7.3 percent in 1970, to 8.3 percent in 1975, to 9.1 percent in 1980, to 12 percent in 1990, and onward from there. (These cost increases are presented in Table 1 of the Appendix). The American health-care system's nonequilibrium growth in costs now affected the rest of the economy, including the larger cycle of inflation, Cost of Living Adjustments to wages (COLAs), corporation investment decisions between the U.S. and abroad, and competition between various interest groups for federal subsidies.

Between 1935 and 1965, innovations in the organization of health-care had focused primarily on new ways to secure funds and personnel for health-care programs. In contrast, most mainstream innovations introduced between 1965 and 1980 attempted to apply system management techniques to control runaway inflation. These included (1) government price controls, (2) local planning to avoid unnecessary duplication of services, (3) increasing the supply of primary care providers, (4) lessening demand for hospital services (the most rapidly increasing health-care cost), and (5) shifting from fee-for-service payment toward fixed per-capita spending through the creation of Health Maintenance Organizations (HMOs).

Along with mainstream efforts to control the costs of conventional health care came a more radical questioning of the medical science model itself and the introduction of a mixed model, borrowing less costly strategies from many other medical systems in use around the world. At a less radical level, members of the public health wing of American medicine questioned the *curative* focus for American health care and began to create working relationships with government and business executives to introduce a more *prevention-oriented* model for health care to the American public. In the language used by Thomas Kuhn, it was a period of *anomaly* accumulation, when premises underlying the health-care paradigm began to be questioned. With varying degrees of severity, critics were noting problems which the system seemed unable to solve and were suggesting alternative ways to deal with some of them. For 30 years the health-care system had been tinkered with; now it had entered a phase of accelerated nonequilibrium in its consumption of resources from other parts of the economy.

Major International Political and Economic Developments of the 1960s and 1970s

Three major changes internationally affected innovations in American health care during the fifteen-year period extending from 1966 to 1980. They coincided with important social processes that were coming together to create a period of extreme instability for political, economic, and broader social relations in the United States.

First, the Pax Americana strategy of Communist containment began to bog down. When America replaced the French military presence in Indo-China, the U.S. inherited a colonial civil war from which it could not extricate itself. The accelerating costs of the U.S. military campaign in Southeast Asia[2] combined with health-care spending to create rapid inflation, escalating health-care costs far beyond what would have occurred simply because of the expansion of coverage and the upgrading of medical facilities and procedures that had taken place. Then, within a few years, earlier interventions in Iran, Saudi Arabia and Iraq backfired. By the early 1970s, countries that had been part of major industrial nations' empires or "spheres of influence" formed a cartel of oil-producing states.[3] The resulting increase in oil prices added further fuel to the rapidly growing rate of inflation.

Second, American businesses increasingly shifted investments overseas. Responding to tax law changes made in the 1950s to protect American industry's access to international markets, many major American business corporations had restructured themselves as transnational corporations. Incorporated in many countries, they now paid taxes to many nations, shifting assets back and forth to take advantage of changing wage, tax, and currency exchange rates from country to country. By the early 1970s 10 percent of all American investment capital was going abroad; some key industrial sectors directed 20 to 40 percent outside the country.[4] Between 1970 and 1980 U.S. manufacturing corporations increased their direct foreign investments by $56.9 billion. American transnational corporations as a whole increased their direct foreign investments by $137.4 billion.[5]

Third, European and Japanese firms now began to pose a direct challenge to American economic hegemony. American firms responded to this competition by trying to reduce their own manufacturing costs, "outjobbing"—giving contracts to companies in Latin America and Asia whose low wages let them make products more cheaply.[6] In addition to outjobbing, many American manufacturing plants reduced the size of their remaining workforce by automating parts of the procedure and by requiring "overtime" production in some plants, sometimes reinstituting 48 or even 60 hour work weeks when demand for their products was high. Workers were paid "time-and-a-half" for the extra labor, but the company saved both the fringe-benefit and the unemployment insurance costs that would otherwise have been paid to additional employees as production was adjusted to changeable market conditions.[7] This strategy for meeting competitive pressures from abroad reduced the number of Americans covered by "fringe benefit" health insurance. For many workers whose health insurance coverage remained intact, the higher fatigue and stress levels of the longer work week would have its own impact on the development of health problems over the long run.

As the various strategies used by American companies to lower production costs in response to foreign competition continued, manufacturing became a less dominant part of the U.S. economy. Moreover, the growth rate for profits from American manufacturing (in constant dollars adjusted for inflation) declined, further hastening the flow of investment resources abroad. (Tables 4 and 5 in the Appendix chronicle these changes.)

In the 1960s, international monetary policies had worked to the disadvantage of American firms, accelerating these trends. Because the dollar was used to stabilize other currencies, U.S. prices remained "strong" while other nations could devalue their own currencies in relation to the dollar, thus giving products made in their countries a further price advantage over American-made goods. Not only were wage rates often lower in relation to actual productivity abroad, but currency manipulations and tariff laws often made products from other countries more competitively priced than American-made products.[8] Efforts of the American government to extricate itself from this bind in the early 1970s created a more volatile international trade situation, which lessened American businesses' willingness to shoulder the burden of constantly increasing health-care costs.

Trends in America

At the national level additional dynamics began to interact with these larger international trends, in ways that seriously disrupted the stability of

American social life. The maturation of the "baby boom" generation brought with it a major increase in the size of the potential labor force and the political radicalization of a college generation. The complex dynamics these national and international trends set in motion led to a period of deep urban unrest, new splits in "class interests" in the U.S., and a realignment of political power. All had profound implications for developments in health care. So did inflationary pressures that developed concurrently. This chapter will not analyze those developments in depth, but will acknowledge the importance they had in creating the context which shaped health-care decisions.

Growth in the Potential Labor Force

By the 1960s demographic changes set in motion by the return of the armed forces at the end of World War II were beginning to affect both the economy and demands on the health-care system. The rise to adulthood of a "baby boom" generation expanded the number of adults who were seeking work faster than the economy itself was growing. U.S. corporation profits for manufacturing industries were declining, falling behind the growth of the economy as a whole.[9] Foreign competition in the area of manufacturing was shifting the American economy increasingly toward areas where the 1950s formulas for business financing of health-care costs were not relevant. High growth areas of the American economy during this period were disproportionately in "service" sectors that often did not have labor unions or health insurance coverage as part of their wages. While American businesses continued to grow and prosper, their growth did not keep pace with the demand for additional jobs that population growth was creating. Where 3.8 million adults had been unemployed in 1960, by the end of the 1970s the number had grown to 7.6 million. (See Table 6 in the Appendix.) Economists accordingly began to enlarge their estimates of the size of the unemployment rate that was appropriate for the American economic system.[10]

Meanwhile, as these problems were multiplying, the proportion of tax revenue coming from business constantly shrank. In 1966, 32.7 percent of American tax revenue came from business. By 1980, businesses' share of taxes had shrunk to 19.7 percent. (See Table 7 in the Appendix.) The redirection of American business capital outside the country was increasing the need for federally subsidized services, as the size of the American manufacturing workforce began to shrink in relation to the number of Americans seeking work. The proportion of Americans being covered by "fringe benefit" health insurance decreased at the same time that the costs of health care were skyrocketing. If "welfare" picked up the slack, it would come increasingly from personal income taxes. Given tax shortages, many states limited access to welfare services, including Medicaid. Enrollments did not keep pace with the down-sizing of the workforce. Welfare, and consequently Medicaid, often was limited to unmarried women and their children.

After the mid-1960s both U.S. industrial investment and productivity declined, further undercutting the basis for health-care financing. The reasons were complex, reflecting both investment decisions and problems of the workforce itself. Within many areas of economic activity, despite rapid technological innovation, the productivity and quality of work worsened.[11] Signs of problems could be seen in such indicators as growing numbers of supervisors to production workers, wildcat strikes over claimed "speed-ups" in higher-tech manufacturing facilities, reorganization of work assignments that brought quality control audits and production goal audits into conflict, and widespread attention to "blue-collar blues." Many corporations established "Employee Assistance" programs to deal with alcohol and drug abuse at the workplace. At least as important as any objective decline in the quality and productivity of the American workforce was widespread media attention to the "problem," which helped influence American consumer choices between foreign and American products, affecting the balance of trade.[12]

Radicalization of Political Protest

The "baby boom" generation's emergence into adulthood produced a radical political realignment among the young in the mid-1960s. College students across the country joined the civil rights movement leader, the Rev. Martin Luther King, Jr., and other American clergy as they formed an antiwar movement resisting American military involvement first in Vietnam and then in larger areas of Southeast Asia. Through major internal disruptions the college generation tried to stop the war in Vietnam.[13] As political resistance gathered momentum, a radical counterculture emerged, questioning American values and practices more fundamentally, and attracting many of the young and marginal elite. They challenged the entire approach of medical science and the health-care industry to issues of health and disease and redefined some of the questions that policy makers began to address. At first their efforts seemed to be very much on the fringes of American health care, and it was difficult to imagine how they could become incorporated into the health-care industry. With time, as members of this generation matured and took a variety of jobs in the more established sectors of society, variations on the questions and approaches introduced at the edges of the system began to find their way into the mainstream. During the 1960s and early 1970s, however, the radical student subculture helped to discredit political leaders, affecting transfers of political power and creating a political context in which new policy perspectives came to predominate in national decision making.

Urban Unrest

This atmosphere of discontent spilled over from student unrest to other economic segments of American society. In the late 1960s, the growing poverty in central cities, coinciding in time with the challenges being posed by the civil rights and antiwar movements to public policies and civil order, produced a period of profound urban unrest. From 1965 to 1967, young African Americans in the poorest sections of America's inner cities, rebelling against complex frustrations, but usually responding to incidents of police violence, began selectively burning and looting white-owned businesses in ghetto neighborhoods. The national guard was called out to restore order.[14] Afterward, white residents increasingly left the central cities for the suburbs, and the nonequilibrium dynamics that had been affecting metropolitan areas accelerated. The nature of health problems that inner city residents faced became even more difficult, and so did access to care, except for those who were eligible for Medicare and Medicaid. The Medicaid program used the old Kerr-Mills formulas for fund disbursement, however, which left implementation of such services to the discretion of each state, and also required the state to provide matching funds. Consequently, health services for the urban poor did not increase in proportion to the number of unemployed who were needing subsidy from the government.

Illicit drug use increased rapidly in these areas, further exacerbating problems of poverty and violence, as well as the need for medical services.[15] Citing news reports of CIA shipments of narcotics across Southeast Asia, some radicals accused the government of introducing drugs into the inner cities as a way to curb urban revolt.[16] Liberals dismissed these attacks as figments of radical imagination, but saw the increase in drug use as a sign that the War on Poverty had to be stepped up to avoid the spread of drug use to other segments of the population. Conservatives, in contrast, argued for more severe punishment of criminal elements that profited from the increase in drug use.

The burning of business areas in black ghetto neighborhoods during the late 1960s at first sped up funding for War on Poverty programs and led manufacturers to open up jobs for inner city minorities. This gain was temporary, however. As the pressures of automated manufacturing processes in the U.S., outjobbing, and direct foreign investments abroad picked up momentum during the 1970s, the size of the manufacturing labor force continued to shrink.[17] Since much manufacturing was occurring in unionized industries with a seniority rule for layoffs, the last hired—the young and the inner city residents from minority backgrounds—were the first to be fired. Preferential hiring became preferential firing under a seniority system for job shrinkage. Those who had been laid off from jobs with high union wages often found themselves either unemployed or marginally employed in jobs paying minimum wage (or less). In terms of health care, the marginally employed were worse off than the unemployed, many of whom often were eligible for Medicaid coverage. These developments, in turn, affected political balances of power in the country and helped return the White House to Republican control, as radicals withdrew from Democratic politics and conservative reaction to the civil disruption swelled. After Nixon's election in 1968, War on Poverty programs were subjected to a deliberate federal policy of "benign neglect."[18] The change of political administrations led to important innovations in health care, however, as Republican President Richard Nixon reassessed his foreign and domestic options. This complex web of events allowed new kinds of health policy, including important health-care innovations, to be introduced by a Republican White House. The turmoil of the time and the growing fiscal problems encouraged basic questioning of the entire paradigm that had given rise to the health-care industry.

New "Class Interest" Splits

As manufacturing became less central for the growth of the American economy, a new kind of interest-group split occurred within the United States. Competition for federal funding developed between the older military-industrial interests and a newer set of interests that Daniel Bell has called the information-services complex, of which higher education, computers, and health care are important components.[19] The growth in health-care subsidies was now occurring at the expense of other interest groups.

During the 1950s, the American government subsidized the growth of what President Eisenhower called the military industrial complex: an average of 62.5 percent of the federal budget went for national defense.[20] Industry, in turn, carried the burden of health insurance. In the 1960s, as the health-care industry emerged and an information-service complex of interests developed (with health care, computers, and universities at its center), federal spending evened out a bit. In 1960, 52.2 percent of the federal budget went for military uses and 3.1 percent for health. By 1979, military spending's total share of the budget dropped to 22.7 percent, while the health share increased to 11.7. In terms of federal spending, these two interest groups within the economy were beginning to get somewhat more even treatment.[21]

An even more striking shift was occurring in terms of each group's relative share of the GNP (of which federal spending makes up only one part). In 1960, military dollars outranked health-care dollars about two to one: where 9.5 percent of the GNP came from military development, 5.3 percent came from the health sector. (Ten years earlier the ratio had been three to one.) By the end of the 1970s military spending accounted for 5 percent of the GNP, while health spending accounted for 9.2 percent. (See Table 10 in the Appendix.) The struggle between the two interest groups in the economy was fueled both by changes in their relative standing and by health care's disproportionate impact on the rate of general inflation.[22] Moreover, the competitive pressure for federal funds was felt not only between the military-industrial interests and the information-services interests, but also within the "services" sector itself.

A second split in objective "class interests" was developing among rank and file workers. Those who were employed in unionized industries received relatively high wages and fringe benefits, including health insurance. However many growth areas for the American economy were difficult for unions to organize. In some, employees were paid low wages and given few fringe benefits. Consequently the need for health and welfare services increased. In federal and state budgets, welfare services competed directly against health services (through Medicare and Medicaid reimbursement to hospitals and medical professionals). In short, the growth of health-care budgets came at the cost of other services to the poor and the disabled. In addition, growing health insurance costs to the industrial sector of the economy—and even more important, their impact on inflation and thus on the wage-adjustments that were required under COLA formulas in union contracts—affected the ability of American-based industrial operations to compete with foreign-produced goods.[23]

Inflation

It was a complex dynamic indeed, intensified by an increase in deficit spending, and the escalating effect of the final component in this series— inflation. From the mid-1960s through the 1970s rapidly increasing health-care costs, the arms race, and military ventures in southeast Asia added major inflationary pressures, as did energy price increases imposed by the new oil cartel, OPEC, and echoed by American petroleum industries. The ability to control inflationary trends through federal policy was short-circuited by the new international economic situation. Since the days of the New Deal, government planners had used higher interest rates as a way to slow the flow of money that was creating inflationary pressures. This method was tried in the 1970s, but by mid-decade it backfired. While both prices and wages fell in 1974-75, prices dropped faster than wages, in part because of heightened competition from accelerating imports. Several countries were in the same phase of their own economic cycle, which intensified the price competition from abroad. Lower prices stimulated consumption more than lowered wages dampened it, and much of the spending now flowed out of the country. Because of the price of cars relative to other consumption items, the loss of auto sales to foreign competitors was particularly damaging. In the resulting stagflation, stock market investment in capital expansion of American manufacturing capacity slowed, as well. At the same time, however, increased federal spending for now-mandated social programs further mediated the deflationary impact of higher interest rates. Meanwhile, the high interest rates available from loans in the U.S. stimulated a major flow of OPEC-generated wealth back into the economy. Middle-eastern oil interests began to reinvest high oil profits in Swiss and American banks and in American real estate.[24] This flow of money back into the country, encouraged by high interest rates charged in America in an effort to slow the inflation, simply added fuel to the fire. It was no longer possible to treat the U.S. economy as if it were a closed system, unaffected by developments outside it. (See Table 2 in the Appendix.)

The Impact of Health Cost Inflation on the Economy

Because health care was organized as a private industry rather than as a government service with regulated rates, the price of its services responded to larger market conditions. Health-care costs, which were doubling over and beyond what inflation was doing to health-care prices, affected the runaway inflation rate that began to plague the American economy.[25] These cost increases were only one part of the picture, however. Health care's contribution to the GNP grew steadily during this period, and health care's share of the federal budget was increasing even more rapidly. Manufacturing industries where wage rates were tied to the consumer price index, and adjusted every three months independent of increases in productivity were hit twice: first, in terms of larger budget items for health-care benefits, and second, in terms of health care's impact on the general inflation rate. Cost increases to industry for wages and fringe benefits helped accelerate the move of American investment money out of the country. While economists noted the problems that earlier wage formulas were creating for competitive wages in the new international competition because of inflation, relatively little attention was paid at the time to the role that escalating health-care costs played in this dynamic.[26]

Inflation, of course, was not the only factor affecting the flow of investment money abroad. The European and Japanese economies, rebuilt and modernized after World War II, were giving the giant American (now transnational) corporations a run for their money. Innovations Japanese competitors introduced in manufacturing technology, in inventory and quality control, and in the organization of the workforce, joined with lower wage rates to produce foreign products that combined high quality of workmanship with lower cost. Increasingly, American transnational firms began to purchase goods and services from their international competitors, as well as to expand their own international manufacturing facilities.

As new jobs went abroad rather than to the American labor force, the underlying basis for financing America's health-care industry began to unravel. Private insurance's share of total health-care costs had been constantly increasing, from $996 million (8 percent of the total costs) in 1950, to $64.8 billion in 1980 (by now 27.1 percent of those sharply increased costs).[27] This represented more than a seventeenfold increase since 1950 in health-care costs to business, beyond that accounted for by inflation. (Tables 12 and 13 in the Appendix present a more detailed account of these cost changes.) The new growth areas for the American economy often avoided health-care commitments of the kind seen in unionized industries.

During the 1970s alone, while real dollar health costs for the nation were tripling, employer-borne health costs for American workers (through private insurance premiums) had more than quadrupled. Health-care costs for transnational companies' employees in other countries, however, were much lower. The U.S. had opted for a health industry model for health-care development; it was becoming far more expensive than other countries' health-care systems, while producing poorer overall results. In the past, before international competition became a serious problem, industry might simply have assigned to "fringe benefits" what otherwise would go into direct wage increases, passing any increased costs on to consumers of their products; while this could still be done, it now left American industry at a competitive disadvantage.

Impact on Federal Budgets. Health care's impact on the economy as whole was especially problematic for the federal government. Government costs for health care came directly out of tax revenues. As the total dollar amounts going into health care tripled from 1960 to 1970, the American government's share of direct care costs quadrupled, increasing from just under $7 billion in 1960 to almost $28 billion in 1970; this represented a tripling of costs beyond those accounted for by inflation. Medicare and Medicaid expenses now made up 30 percent of the nation's health-care costs. This put stronger pressure on policy implementers to try to make sure that Americans were getting their money's worth.[28]

A Larger Pattern of Instability

From 1960 to 1980, in short, the American political economy was adjusting to a series of larger international developments that challenged earlier formulas for national and international peace and prosperity. During this turbulent period one U.S. president was assassinated, one announced that he would not run again for president in order to prevent further civil division and disorder, a third resigned to avoid impeachment, and the remaining two presidents were not reelected when they ran for a second term of office. Inflation moved rapidly out of control, and conventional processes for bringing it into check were not used heavily enough to be effective. The sense of instability this created was felt with special keenness in regard to health care.

A Shift in Power and Efforts at Price Control

After winning the presidential election in 1968, early in this time period, Richard Nixon assessed his options. Responding to the dramatic increase in costs for Medicare, he proposed that the national Department of Health, Education and Welfare be given authority to appoint "program review teams" of physicians, other health professionals, and consumers, with power to deny payment for unnecessary Medicare services.

The American Medical Association (AMA) responded by proposing that this task be given to its state medical societies. Critics replied that this would be like asking the foxes to guard the henhouse. In 1970, Congress instructed HEW to contract for Medicare review services with Professional Standard Review Organizations (PSROs) which were to be made up only of physicians. Instead of using state medical societies, however, the PSROs were to be independent medical care "foundations."[29] The new PSROs used computer searches of Medicare records to identify cases that differed from the national statistical norms for their kind of treatment, in terms of length of stay or unusually costly service. Once identified, these cases were investigated to see whether Medicare provisions had been abused. In 1972 AMA pressure on Congress succeeded in getting the PSRO's "peer review" provisions modified. National statistical norms were eliminated as criteria for initiating an investigation. In addition, outpatient services and non-hospital services were removed from this surveillance. Thus PSROs' role became limited to the quality of care in individual hospitals.

Wage and Price Freeze Efforts. In August of 1971, alarmed by a sharp increase in inflation—led by the rapid increase in medical and hospital costs after the enactment of Medicare-Medicaid legislation, President Nixon imposed a general wage-price freeze. This was modified in December with a special focus on medical costs: doctor's fees were limited to an annual increase of 2.5 percent and hospital charges to increases of 6 percent annually, about half of the rate of increase before the wage-price freeze. In January 1973 these controls were lifted for most of the economy, but were retained for health care, food, oil, and the construction industry which was heavily involved in hospital building.[30] For the federal government alone, health-care expenditures had increased from 4.4 percent of the federal budget in 1965 to 11.3 percent in 1973. Cost control for medical services was becoming an ever higher priority for the federal government. (Table 8 in the Appendix shows the growth that was occurring in the size of the total federal budget.)

Ending Hill-Burton Subsidies. By 1972, Congress was persuaded to stop Hill-Burton subsidies for new hospital construction. This action, it was thought, would check the rapid escalation of hospital costs that was threatening to bankrupt the Medicare program. Ironically, it accelerated the inflation of hospital costs rather than slowing down new construction. So many hospitals had upgraded their facilities since 1965, taking advantage of Medicare reimbursement programs and Hill-Burton subsidies, that hospitals which had lagged behind were in danger of becoming "obsolete," with participating doctors shifting their practice (and their patients) to competing hospitals with more modern facilities. Thus, rather than abandoning their expansion plans when Hill-Burton funds became unavailable, hospitals looked for new sources of funds. The easiest solution was to borrow the needed capital, and sell interest-bearing bonds to the public. Whereas in 1968 government and private philanthropy had provided 44 percent of hospitals' capital funds, by the 1980s they provided only 5 percent of the total and borrowed money now made up 69 percent of hospital capital funds.[31]

To compete with other possible investments, hospital bonds had to pay attractive interest rates during a period of rapid inflation. Interest rates constantly rose, as did hospital construction costs. Moreover, the constant expansion of sophisticated, high-tech medical equipment and its costs increased apace. Consequently the indebtedness of hospitals continued to increase rapidly during this decade and became folded into daily operating costs, as had been the custom for some time.

In 1972, Congress added an amendment to Social Security legislation, giving HEW power to deny full Medicare reimbursement to hospitals or nursing homes for any capital investment costs included in their bills which were undertaken without approval from appropriate health planning agencies. This amendment tried to minimize the stimulus that Medicare was giving to hospital and nursing home expansion, by making sure that new construction came in response to generally agreed needs, rather than simply to improve an institution's competitive status or prestige. Two years later Congress moved even more strongly to subject health-care services to review by planning groups.[32]

Defining a "Health-Care Crisis": Questioning the Paradigm

As the health-care industry expanded and its costs continued to increase in the early 1970s, Congressional investigations and public policy planners began discussing "the health-care crisis." Analysts did not frame the problem in terms of the larger international picture, however, except to note that while American health care was the most expensive in the world per person, and set the pace for technical advances in treatment, the health status of the American public had not improved commensurably.[33]

Public debate of "the health-care crisis" moved from the halls of Congress to discussion in special television reports, and responses focused on problems of cost, problems of access to care, problems of quality control (which the burgeoning of malpractice suits was bringing to public attention), and problems of *humaneness*, which the increasingly large and bureaucratic organization of health services, oriented toward cost-accounting, brought to the fore. The AMA was frequently cast as the villain of the piece, a reactionary group interested only in protecting the independence of wealthy physicians. Few noted the new constellation of interest groups that now shaped the direction of the expanding health-care industry: the American Hospital Association, the federal health bureaucracy, the pharmaceutical and hospital equipment industries, and a coterie of prestigious medical researchers and medical school administrators who advised national planning groups.[34] For the first time since the early 1900s, voices began to be heard questioning the direction in which medical science had taken the country.

One of the most noticed critiques came from the priest and social critic Ivan Illich, who wrote a bestselling book decrying *iatrogenesis*, or physician-caused suffering. Illich's book, *Medical Nemesis*, presented such a global and devastating critique of modern medicine that it was largely dismissed by members of the medical establishment, but it received a strong response from portions of the public. The book identified three kinds of physician-caused suffering. *Clinical iatrogenesis* follows from unnecessary surgery, from drug side effects or secondary infections, and from medical mistakes. Illich used medical journals to document the extensiveness of this problem, and his argument attracted particular attention because of the growing number of malpractice suits. *Social iatrogenesis* occurs when the medical system makes individuals depend upon experts for judgments about their daily lives—as in the medicalization of emotional problems, the increasing dependence upon "expert opinion" from health professionals for decisions about life and work, and in the transformation of life and death experiences into depersonalized, high-tech interventions in hospitals. *Cultural iatrogenesis* occurs when physicians encourage the public to pretend that pain and death can be avoided, thereby robbing the society of the depth of experience that comes from confronting its ultimate participation in the life-death cycle that gives meaning to human experience.[35]

Although physicians and medical policy planners paid little serious attention to Illich's critique, Rick J. Carlson, a colleague of Illich who shared his perspective but who framed it more programmatically, was soon attracting elite decision makers to off-the-record meetings held in Washington and New York to consider alternative models and strategies for health care. (These meetings will be discussed in Chapter 6.)

Politically radical critics also spoke up, arguing that the mainstream analysis was wrongly placed. As causes of health problems, they pointed to industrial and environmental pollution, crowded and unsanitary housing, poverty and malnutrition, the marketing of junk foods, and industrial safety hazards. A focus on high-tech interventions after an individual's health has broken down, they insisted, was a poor use of the nation's resources.[36]

In the larger national debate on "the health-care crisis," analysts from the academic establishment argued that a national policy was already in place to address the problems that radical critics had identified. A Housing and Urban Development agency (HUD) had been established in 1965 as part of the War on Poverty to improve the quality of housing available to low-income groups, and in 1970 an Occupational Health and Safety Act (OSHA) designed to reduce health risks at the worksite had become law, as well as an Environmental Protection Act. Health policy planners thus turned their attention back to three concerns of mainstream criticism: cost control, problems of access to care, and quality control. No one seemed to have much sense of how to approach problems of bureaucracy and humaneness.[37] Reformers proceeded with efforts in each of the other three areas, however.

The more radical questioning was not entirely ignored, however. Two very different lines of exploration began to gather momentum outside the mainstream of the health-care industry, among quite different constituencies.

Questioning the Emphasis on "Cure" Rather than "Prevention". In 1968, Congress had established the John E. Fogarty International Center for Advanced Study in the Health Sciences as part of the National Institutes of Health (NIH) complex. As an institution for advanced study, the Fogarty Center sponsored conferences and initiated a series of study reports on medical education, environmental health, societal factors influencing health and disease, geographic health problems, international health and research, and preventive medicine.[38]

The Fogarty Center's work on preventive medicine brought together innovative senior scholars from public health schools around the country and some of the most influential policy advisers in the country, including members of the National Academy of Science, and persons from outside academia, including John Knowles, who had become the President of the Rockefeller Foundation, Walt McNerney, who was heading Blue Cross-Blue Shield nationally, and Clarence Pearson, an executive at Metropolitan Life

Insurance Company, an organization that had continued to play a role in health policy circles since the early struggles about whether to set up national health insurance in the second decade of the century.[39]

Between 1965 and 1970, private health insurance expenditures had increased from $6.5 to $15.1 billion annually as the introduction of Medicare and Medicaid health insurance had set off a wave of hospital expansion and modernization. The federal government's spending for personal health services also had increased dramatically, from $4.2 billion to $10.3 billion. Both public and private third-party payers were jolted by the sharp increase in costs. John Knowles and Walt McNerney felt strongly that something had to be done to lower the utilization rate for hospital services and for medical services more generally. Aware that many visits to physicians are for problems that are not life-threatening, they became interested in the possibility of encouraging Americans to undertake more self-care.[40]

As private households and public and private third-party payers reeled in response to the rapid increase in health-care costs and Congressional leaders discussed the "health-care crisis," communication networks invigorated by Fogarty Center activities introduced innovations that began to move beyond disease-focused health care toward new strategies that emphasized prevention rather than cure. Two new federal agencies targeted toward health promotion were set up within a three-year period; the National Center for Health Education began to promote worksite health improvement programs, and the Heart, Lung, and Blood Institute (NHLBI) of the NIH began funding research and demonstration programs at worksites and in the community aimed at blood pressure control.

These beginnings of an alternative approach to problems of health and disease will be discussed in Chapters 6 and 8. For now it is sufficient to note that the 1970s saw new thinking about health and fundamental experimentation arising both inside and outside established institutions. A new climate of opinion was developing in Washington and among the nation's business elite, one that advocated moving health policy outside the narrow control of the health-care industry. This climate made it possible to create an official, organizational base for disease prevention efforts and began to draw the American business community into active involvement in such efforts.

More Radical Questioning of the Paradigm. At the same time these moves toward a more prevention-oriented approach were getting attention, a parallel movement among radical elites began to reintroduce a mixed model for health care. Inspired by the counterculture that had emerged as part of the antiwar movement of the 1960s and early 1970s, and by the women's movement that emerged shortly thereafter, these critics questioned most of the assumptions on which the modern health-care system was based. Calling themselves members of the holistic (or wholistic) health movement, the women's health movement, or both, they understood "health" to be something much more than the absence of disease, and focused on health-building, even when attempting disease-cure. They challenged the hegemony of medical science, reintroducing into popular "folk medicine" health-care practices from many pre-industrial cultures and from America's own nineteenth-century health care. They experimented with non-bureaucratic relationships for healing, challenging many of the role assumptions of medical science and the health-care industry. Thousands became part-time "healers," and some of them introduced new "health professions" to the folk-medicine scene. Soon, to the astonishment of many in the medical establishment, not only were a number of MDs joining the American Holistic Medical Association, but a past president of the AMA had addressed one of its meetings, and many doctors and some medical researchers began a serious exploration of these alternative approaches to health and disease.

Women's health and holistic health advocates were getting the ear of an important segment of the policy elite. Besides redefining what questions to ask about health and disease, they were demonstrating approaches that could be used to break the hold of high-tech medicine. They attracted sponsors and advocates not only in the counterculture but in various parts of academia, government, business, the media, and even in sections of the health-care industry itself.

As was also true for the prevention movement that was beginning to gain ground, these alternative movements offered a different paradigm for health care, and radically different assumptions about the tasks to be done and ways to do them. These innovative directions in American health care depart sufficiently from the mainstream norm to deserve separate treatment (which will be given in Chapters 7 and 8). Here, it is enough to note that they were emerging at the same time that policy makers and the public were beginning to believe the health-care system was in trouble. Some of the more radical innovations introduced by holistic health participants also gained broader interest and credibility because of foreign policy innovations that President Richard Nixon introduced, which brought non-western medical traditions to the attention of the American public.

International Diplomacy, Acupuncture, and Health-care Reform

Nixon's biggest innovation in foreign policy was to substitute a policy of détente for earlier cold war diplomacy. In place of two-power struggles, détente sought to create shifting three-power coalitions in which two major nuclear powers could jointly counter the expansionist efforts of a third. By 1970, China had joined Russia and the U.S. (as well as France and Great Britain) in the nuclear weapons club. Because China was showing strong signs of rivalry with Russia, Nixon hoped to create a three-nation balance of power, expanding the détente formula so that it applied globally.[41]

With nuclear missiles now replacing reliance on control of the seas as the ultimate military strategy, Nixon hoped to lessen America's investment in cold war defense costs in two ways: by sharing the cost of Western defenses with allies, and by creating an international arena in which Russia and China would balance each other off, rather than working in concert to disrupt Western interests. Ultimately, he hoped, an industrially developing China might open its markets to trading with the West. If Russia began to do this as well, the entire dynamics for international relations would change, and the international market problems that American factories were beginning to experience might improve.

On Nixon's first diplomatic visit to China, in February of 1972, he was accompanied by a New York *Times* correspondent, Harrison Salisbury. During an attack of appendicitis, Salisbury was rushed to a Chinese hospital, where he was treated with acupuncture rather than an anesthetic. He felt no pain during the operation and became fascinated with contemporary Chinese medicine. His news accounts, thereafter, were filled with reports of alternative approaches to health care being used successfully by the Chinese.[42]

America was looking for simple ways to make non-governmental ties between the two countries, and acupuncture and Chinese health programs provided an easy way to reach out. Soon, with active encouragement by the U.S. government, the president's physician, Dudley White, visited China to observe the use of acupuncture, and the American College of Physicians and Surgeons sent teams of doctors to China to observe and assess Chinese use of acupuncture and other forms of health care.

The Chinese had made remarkable improvements in public health since the Communist revolution of 1949. Particularly impressive was their policy of matching the level of expertise to the health demands of a situation, and bringing health care directly to the worksite and the neighborhood. "Barefoot doctors"—health workers with a few months training—visited families, farms, and worksites, providing primary care. The barefoot doctors were supervised by nurses, who handled more complicated medical problems. The nurses, in turn, were supervised by doctors, who handled severe medical emergencies. The barefoot doctors were taught useful techniques for primary care that came both from medical science and from traditional Chinese medical practices, including acupuncture. Indigenous healers, using acupuncture and traditional Chinese herbs for the treatment of a wide range of health problems, also were encouraged to provide health services to the public.[43]

Once medical exchanges began, the Chinese were fascinated by CAT-scan X-ray diagnostic machines and other marvels of western technology.

But the American health-care planners were intrigued to discover the high level of basic health care available to the Chinese population, which had been achieved by scaling down the level of expertise and by providing services designed to *maintain health* rather than cure incapacitating disease.[44]

Each of these Chinese approaches began to find its way into American health practices. Acupuncture treatments became fashionable, and a number of American doctors began taking crash courses in acupuncture after the U.S. medical system gave licensed doctors and dentists the right to practice acupuncture and to supervise other practitioners. Interest in acupuncture increased further after American veterinarians began finding it useful for a wide range of animal health problems. While acupuncture did not replace drugs and surgery as the standard medical intervention in the U.S., its new respectability increased interest in health procedures that challenge the canons of western medical science.[45]

On a policy level, American health planners began thinking about an American equivalent of the "barefoot doctors" approach. By 1970 two-thirds of American doctors were specialists, and both urban riots and nonviolent demonstrations had drawn attention to the lack of doctors available for poor urban minorities. Medicare and Medicaid had made emergency hospital care accessible to many of the poor, but it had not given them access to primary health-care services, which often were in short supply in neighborhoods where the poor live. In addition, people who lived outside metropolitan areas were finding fewer doctors available to serve them.

New federal programs were created to increase access to care. New semi-professional "doctor" roles were created to help fill the gap in primary care services. Nurse-clinicians and nurse-practitioner/midwives were given training beyond that required for licensing and were allowed to practice without medical supervision. Physicians' assistants also were licensed to do primary care under the direction of a supervising physician. In addition, budgets for medical schools were increased with the understanding that women and minority students would be given preference for the additional training slots. Women physicians in America had been much more likely to go into primary care medicine, and the under-representation of doctors from ethnic minorities spoke for itself.[46] In 1972, the National Health Service Corps was established, providing scholarships for prospective health-care professionals in exchange for tours of duty in underserved areas. Its funding peaked in 1978 with $100 million allocated to the program.[47]

Capitation: HMOs

The most dramatic governmental innovation in health care came in late 1973, when the plan Nixon proposed, and which Congress accepted, set up an alternative to both hospital care and dependence upon private physicians. It refocused attention on primary care, but eliminated the motivation to offer ever-more-expensive services in order to generate more income. The name chosen for the new form of care, Health Maintenance Organizations, reflected an almost Chinese conception of the purpose for health care, although the model actually came from the Kaiser health services innovations described in Chapter 1. The parallels to Chinese approaches went beyond the name. The utilization in HMOs of new kinds of health professionals like nurse practitioners, nurse clinicians, and physicians assistants (who cost less) also reflected an awareness that the most effective primary health-care services might be offered by health-care workers with less specialized training than doctors. However, at the heart of the proposal were uniquely American and quite contemporary ingredients.

The HMOs were to be modeled on the experience of American business, and particularly the Kaiser-Permanente program on the West Coast, in providing prepaid general health insurance that would provide a full range of coverage for any services needed. Unlike Blue Cross and other forms of health insurance currently in use, however, health services would be reimbursed on an annual per-capita basis rather than in terms of fees for each service performed.[48] Some HMOs paid a salary to doctors, like Kaiser-Permanente does, while others were organized quite differently. For all HMOs, however, the intent was to limit costs by providing a yearly ceiling on the premiums paid for any single individual. The new form for health care tried to take advantage of the health-care industry's current focus on maximizing income. HMOs would be motivated to "maintain health" rather than to perform expensive curative procedures after health breaks down, it was thought, because an HMO's operating surplus, or profit, comes from spending less on subscribers than the fixed insurance income they provide. The simplest way to do this would be for HMO clinics to intervene early and minimally with their subscribers, to maintain current good health or to correct problems before they become serious. Thus, it was hoped, the profit-building motive that permeated the health-care industry could be used to motivate a shift in emphasis for health care.

The new law setting up HMOs, passed in December of 1973, required businesses with more than 25 employees to offer at least one HMO as an alternative service provider in their health benefit plan, if there were an HMO available in the vicinity. It also provided grants and loans for the development of HMOs. To qualify for these funds, an HMO had to provide physicians' services, emergency care, hospitalization, and laboratory and diagnostic services. In addition, they were responsible for mental health care (up to 20 visits), family planning service, home health care as needed, and referrals for alcohol and drug abuse. Additional, optional, services also were recommended.[49] (Table 14 in the Appendix traces the growth of HMOs during this time period.)

Providing these core services, it should be noted, did not require any change in the basic approach medical professionals were using, except that all care would become available through one agency, the HMO clinic. The most serious change was in the basis of funding. An HMO could only prosper by minimizing use of expensive services. Since hospitalization was clearly the most expensive alternative, HMOs would be motivated to negotiate low rates with hospitals and to use hospital treatment as a last resort, minimizing the length of stay whenever possible. Given this conservative conception of the new enterprise, "health maintenance" became a euphemism for cost-conscious standard care rather than a reorientation of how health issues would be approached.

ERISA

Equally significant for the future development of health care was the decision of large corporations to self-insure for health benefits. Rather than pay out monthly premiums to an insurance company, larger employers paid claims themselves, keeping discretionary use of any "health insurance" funds until actual claims were made against them. Federal legislation authorized this, as part of the 1974 Employee Retirement Insurance Security Act (called ERISA).[50]

The major insurance companies lost their large corporation health insurance market. They adapted in two ways: first, they retained their links to large corporations by *managing* health insurance claims for these companies. Then the five largest insurance companies organized their own Health Maintenance Organizations (HMOs) which competed for the service-provision contracts of the large corporations. No longer able to profit from investing health insurance premiums for short-run gain, they hoped to prosper by providing cost-efficient health care that would allow a profit from capitated payments.[51]

Public Planning for Local Health Needs

In 1974, Congress passed the National Health Planning and Resource Development Act, under which Hill-Burton hospital grants and two earlier programs to encourage regional and national health planning were phased out. In their place some 200 Health System Agencies (HSAs) were set up, to be run by local boards with a majority membership of consumers rather than health-care professionals.[52] These boards were not given decision-making power, however. Their tasks were to draw up three-year plans for meeting the health needs of their local area, to review proposed projects, and to send recommendations to newly created state Health Planning and Development Agencies and to Washington regarding certificate of need proposals that health service providers would be making in their region. Each state was required to enact certificate of need legislation, to set up a State Planning and Development Agency and to establish Statewide Health Coordinating Councils. The act also created ten regional Technical Assistance Centers to help evaluate and plan for upgrading facilities as needed; and at the national level it created a new Bureau of Health Planning and Development and a National Health Planning Advisory Council. The federal government financed the budgets of the local HSAs, but did not directly control their activity. However, it decided whether their contracts for planning and coordinating should be renewed, and set guidelines for the health plans that HSAs and the states produced.

Another Pass at National Health Insurance

The country seemed to be moving toward a rationally planned, nationally coordinated health service. In 1974, President Nixon's annual message to Congress proposed national health insurance as "an idea whose time has come in America." Caspar Weinberger, Nixon's HEW secretary, had concluded that a single coordinated plan would be less expensive in the long run than the hospital-focused programs the federal government was funding. Congressman Wilbur Mills, who had drafted the successful Medicare-Medicaid legislation, and Senator Edward Kennedy, who had been a leading spokesman concerning the national "health-care crisis," both Democrats, cooperated to draft legislation that might get past the opposition of the insurance lobby. Their proposal had insurance companies acting as the fiscal intermediaries for national health insurance, thereby giving the industry income from this extension of services. Their plan also called for consumers to pay 25 percent of the costs covered by national insurance, up to a limit of $1000 per family per year. In a reversal of their traditional positions, organized labor objected to these provisions, and the insurance industry lobbied for passage of the bill.[53]

Meanwhile, congressional attention to health-care policy was diverted by the Watergate scandal, which led to President Nixon's resignation in the summer of 1974. Organized labor and other groups interested in the Kennedy-Mills national insurance bill expected the Republicans to lose control of the White House in 1976, because of these scandals, and urged supporters of national health insurance to wait a couple of years, until a more liberal presidential administration would be available.[54] That moment never came.

OPEC Sidetracks National Health Insurance. By the time the Democrats won the 1976 election, international events had created an entirely different context in which to consider further health expenditures. As noted already, the non-industrial nations who were major oil producers had formed the Organization of Petroleum Exporting Countries (OPEC) in the 1960s. Their first major price-raising activity occurred in 1973, not long after the U.S. had ended its military interventions in Southeast Asia and signaled its readiness to abandon Pax Americana military stances. Despite the cessation of high defense expenditures, inflation increased rapidly. More was involved than simple increases in the prices of energy and health services, but they added important momentum to what was occurring.

During the Carter administration anti-inflationary federal money policies produced a moderate recession in 1979-80 but did not manage to stop the larger inflationary spiral for reasons already indicated. Because of the cost inflation, the size of the federal budget increased 69 percent between 1975 and 1980. (Table 8 in the Appendix traces these changes.) The staggering increase in inflation during this period becomes apparent when one realizes that although federal expenditures had almost tripled during the decade, in constant dollars federal spending increased only 29 percent over the ten-year period. By the mid-1980s, however, the increased debt at high interest rates began to create its own threats to the health of the economy. (See Appendix, Table 11.) There was little enthusiasm in Congress for underwriting further expenditures on national health that might escalate costs as Medicare and Medicaid had done.

Looking back at public policy from the vantage point of 1988, George Kowalczyk, Mark Freeland, and Katherine Levit identified four periods of changing public policy toward rising health-care costs during the fifteen-year period between 1965 and 1979. (1) From 1965 until 1973 there was rapid cost inflation: hospitals expanded rapidly until Hill-Burton funds were stopped, and physicians' fees rose sharply in response to Medicare reimbursement policies. (2) In 1972 and 1973 Nixon's Economic Stabilization Program put a freeze on health-care prices. (3) After price controls were lifted in 1973, an inflationary catch-up by hospitals and physicians continued through 1976. (4) Beginning in the fourth quarter of 1977, the federal government asked the health sector to voluntarily control the rise in hospital costs and physicians' fees so that renewed federal price controls would not be necessary. This led to the creation of cost containment committees in hospitals, efforts by area planning groups to limit recommendations for new hospital construction, the establishment of HMOs to lower hospital use, and government requests that county medical associations limit fee increases. But these voluntary efforts at cost control collapsed in 1979, as cost pressures within the health sector built up.[55]

Assessing Health-Care Reforms of the 1970s

The results were mixed. The new policies aimed at increasing the number of health professionals had succeeded. By 1980 there were 8,000 nurse-clinicians and twice that many nurse-practitioners and midwives. The number of physicians' assistants grew more slowly, but reached 20,000 by 1987. Between 1970 and 1980 the total number of *physicians* in primary care increased by almost 22,000 (from 82,859 to 104,745).[56]

Between 1970 and 1980 the number of practicing physicians serving the general population increased 58 percent, three times faster than the population as a whole. But there was no indication that more doctors were practicing in underserved areas. In 1970, 85 percent of practicing physicians worked in metropolitan areas; by 1980, 88 percent. Moreover, the overwhelming majority of new physicians who went to non-metropolitan areas during that decade were specialists. By 1989 the government had designated 1,944 communities as in need of primary care medicine. Despite the rapid increase in total number of physicians, fewer than a third of the new doctors were offering primary care services. In fact, the proportion of physicians in primary care actually dropped.[57]

In 1975, there were 159 doctors per 100,000 population. By 1980 there were 188 per 100,000 people, but only 69 of them were available for primary health care. Sixty years earlier, when the move toward specialization was just beginning, there had been 92 primary care physicians available per 100,000 people.[58] By enlarging enrollments in medical schools, the country had begun to recover from a serious undersupply of family practice physicians. But so many specialists had been trained at the same time that the move toward specialized medicine actually increased.

Problems of access to medical care remained, despite these programs of the 1970s. Medicare and Medicaid were succeeding in providing access to hospital services for the poor. In 1964, the year before Medicare and Medicaid legislation was passed, people with incomes above the poverty line saw physicians 20 percent more frequently than the poor. By 1975 this had reversed: the poor visited physicians 18 percent more frequently than others and there was an even greater increase in use of surgical procedures among the poor. And whereas in 1964 the white population saw physicians 42 percent more frequently than non-whites, by 1975 this gap had narrowed to 13 percent.[59] Medical care for both the poor and the elderly had become much more accessible. On the other hand, the costs for Medicaid and Medicare had increased dramatically. Between 1970 and 1980 annual Medicaid expenditures rose from $6.3 to $28.1 billion. Medicaid's cost, after adjustment for inflation, had more than doubled. Many Medicaid recipients, by now, were formerly middle-class, elderly persons in nursing homes who had exhausted their savings while paying for health services. The cost increases for Medicare during that same period were even higher, from $7.5 billion to $38.8 billion. Medicare's real cost, in constant dollars, had almost tripled.[60]

The increase in medical costs was not limited to federal government expenditures, for private health insurance charges increased along with Medicare and Medicaid billings, since hospitals used the same formulas to figure charges for the insured, regardless of who was paying the bill. In 1965, health-care costs of American businesses amounted to 14.0 percent of their after tax profits. By 1980 that figure had grown to 42.6 percent, despite the major reduction in proportionate share of taxes paid by American businesses. (See Table 3 in the Appendix.)

The Consumer Price Index (CPI) tracked increases in consumer-paid hospital costs. They were increasing at about twice the general rate of inflation. Table 2 of the Appendix compares relative rates for health care and energy costs during this period.

The HMO alternative to hospital-based care was beginning to catch on. By 1976, some 174 HMOs had been established and had enrolled almost six million patients, primarily in HMOs with 100,000 or more members. By 1980, over nine million patients were participating in HMOs. (See Table 14 in the Appendix.)

The problem of malpractice, and its escalating impact on health-care costs, was not being solved. Between 1960 and 1970, the amount of malpractice awards had quadrupled, from about $50 million dollars in 1960 to about $200 million in 1970. Those figures went steadily upward, and by 1980 there were three malpractice claims per year for every hundred physicians. The AMA was estimating that the practice of "defensive medicine" was adding about 10 percent to the costs of physicians' services across the nation. Meanwhile hospitals continued to upgrade their staffing, equipment, facilities, and procedures, in part to protect themselves from suits.[61] Overall health-care costs had increased, between 1970 and 1980, from $74.4 billion to $249.1 billion. Both the federal government and third party payers (whose costs were financed primarily by fringe benefit payments from business) were absorbing an increasing proportion of these constantly inflated health-care costs. By 1980, cost control had become the major unsolved problem defining the agendas for both public and private health-care funders.

The most important innovations in health care during the 1970s had come from the top, as policy makers reacted to the increases in cost that had been set in motion as a health-care industry evolved from the crises and innovations described in Chapter 1. As each interest group had taken advantage of the new circumstances created by entry of government into the funding of health insurance, costs had escalated dramatically. Policy makers at the national level responded, innovating in ways that changed the opportunity structure for gaining income through health-care delivery. However, health-care reforms of the 1970s ignored some key sources of the demand for ever more expensive services. These included (1) a constantly growing investment in research to develop new, high-tech (and therefore costly) medical diagnosis and treatment procedures and equipment, (2) the fact that training programs were producing an over-abundance of high-priced medical specialists who also increase demand for expensive services, and (3) the fact that the health-care system's focus on after-the-fact disease care largely neglects disease prevention at the individual, social, or environmental level. Moreover, health care was approached as if it were a system unto itself when, in fact, what happens in health care has major impact on the rest of the economy, and vice versa. Reformers also paid little attention to how the American economy was being affected by larger international trends, or to the implications that these would have for public and private funding of health care. Consequently the basic dynamic affecting health-care costs did not change.

3

Health-Care Innovation in a Rapidly Changing World Economy

American health-care innovations of the 1980s grew out of a radically altered climate. New developments, both national and international, created problems that encouraged a major rethinking of how health care was being approached. Older formulas for funding health care were no longer working well. Meanwhile, additional kinds of health crises, international in origin, began demanding new resources that the American health-care system, already the most expensive in the world, hesitated to commit.

Many innovations of the 1980s moved the health-care industry into organizational styles emphasized in the larger American economy. Hospitals, nursing homes, and health maintenance organizations (HMOs) were reorganized as mammoth health-care chains, oriented toward cost control and "bottom-line," profit-oriented decision-making. Physicians became less influential in day-to-day policy making; an increasing proportion of them became employees either of these health-care chains or of other corporations not primarily concerned with health care. Many health-care systems were reorganized as explicitly for-profit ventures. A number of health-care facilities were closed, often for financial reasons. Meanwhile, third party payers tried to impose cost controls. Business-health coalitions, organized in more than 90 metropolitan areas, kept computerized records of health-care costs and the performance of doctors, hospitals, and other health-care facilities. Large businesses negotiated for prices with preferred provider organizations (PPOs) and sometimes invited national health-care chains to enter their metropolitan health-care market. This in turn stimulated physicians to form their own HMOs or PPOs and to offer competitive services not previously of interest to many local doctors.

Health insurance companies began to set "caps" on reimbursement for doctors' services and hospital charges. The government also imposed its own cost control policies on hospital reimbursements for Medicare patients: diagnostically related groups of diseases (DRGs)—related in terms of typical treatment cost—became the new formula for hospital admissions, changing relations between hospitals, physicians, and patients. These cost control innovations created a more adversarial relationship between the institutional funders of health care (business, industry, and the federal government) and providers of health-care services. A more adversarial relation also developed between individual patients and physicians, and between patients and hospitals, seen in escalating numbers of malpractice suits.

The net results of these changes in the organization of health care were discouraging. Costs continued to rise at twice the rate of general inflation. Businesses found health-care costs now approaching the size of their after-tax profits and constantly increasing health-care costs created severe budget crises for federal and state governments. Meanwhile, access to health care became increasingly difficult for many Americans.

New International Developments Affecting Directions for Health-Care Change

International developments significantly changed the implications of health innovations in the 1980s. American industry, seriously challenged even within the U.S. by competitors based abroad, found it harder to pay its share of rising medical care costs. Major net outflows of capital from the U.S. occurred as a serious balance of trade problem developed and the 1970s pattern of making direct investment of business capital abroad continued among formerly U.S., now transnational, corporations. In addition, a major escalation in the international arms race in the 1980s produced strains for the American and the Soviet economies, affecting the federal government's willingness to increase the use of public resources for health care. Eventually, the dynamics behind these changes would combine with events in the Soviet bloc to produce a total reordering of international relations.

Two other international developments added serious new health challenges which the contemporary health-care system was only partially prepared to address. First, a new kind of epidemic, Acquired Immune Deficiency Disease (AIDS), swept through Africa, the U.S., and Western Europe, and began to make its way into most other areas of the world as well. Peculiarities of the HIV retrovirus that produced this health problem began to reorient the way in which medical researchers looked at the health-disease process and forced a reexamination of interventions focused on "cure" instead of "prevention." Second, an acceleration in the international drug traffic produced a growing problem of addiction to "crack" cocaine, first within the inner city areas of the U.S. (hit the hardest by the withdrawal of manufacturing jobs and the deterioration of older neighborhoods), then in the population more generally. In short, *public health* problems, which the after-the-fact, disease-response strategies of the American health-care system could not address effectively, began to consume an increasing share of public revenues.

Balance of Trade and Foreign Investment

Until the mid-1970s the United States sold more abroad than it imported, providing a healthy trade surplus. Because American manufacturing industries were prosperous, it was relatively easy for them to provide fringe benefit health insurance coverage for their employees. In 1975 the U.S. had a balance of trade surplus of almost $16 billion. By 1980 that had shrunk to just over $1 billion, and thereafter the U.S. had to contend with a trade *deficit*. The decline of the American export industry and the growth of imports provides one simple indicator that American industry as a whole was not doing as well as it had in the past. By 1987, the trade deficit had risen to more than $154 billion annually.[1] Some of this money returned, as Japanese, British, and Dutch financial interests purchased U.S. treasury securities and major shares of stock in American-based corporations. By 1987, the U.S. had become a net debtor nation. Within five years the size of that debt to foreign creditors rose to over $600 billion, including about five percent of the U.S. federal debt.[2]

The practical implications for health-care financing of the decline of American manufacturing, seen in the unfavorable balance of trade, were twofold. First, business interests were struggling desperately to lower manufacturing costs in order to be competitive internationally; thus they had a strong incentive to control the costs of health-care benefits. Second, because Cost of Living Adjustment formulas (COLAs) for wage rates in American manufacturing industries called for adjusting wages for inflation four times a year, the contribution of health-care cost escalations to the larger inflation hurt American manufacturing industries' competitive position even more than growing costs for health benefits themselves. These difficulties further encouraged American-based transnational corporations to make direct investments abroad, and also to automate American production so that fewer U.S. employees would be needed. (See Table 5 in the Appendix.)

Combined domestic and foreign investment in the U.S. did not produce enough jobs to keep pace with the increase in adults of working age. Not only did the adult population of the U.S. increase more rapidly than domestic job expansion, but the number of manufacturing jobs in the U.S. actually declined by almost two million between 1979 and 1987. Whereas manufacturing jobs had accounted for 35 percent of all nonagricultural employment in the U.S. in 1946, by 1988 they accounted for only 18 percent.[3] These changes had direct implications for U.S. health care, since unionized manufacturing jobs were most likely to include health insurance benefits. By 1990, 37 million Americans lacked health insurance coverage of any kind.[4]

Escalation of the Arms Race

The erosion of U.S. manufacturing jobs was slowed a bit by a U.S.-sparked escalation in arms expenditures. In the early 1980s the federal military budget almost doubled, increasing from $155.2 in 1980 to $308.9 billion in 1987, a 40 percent increase beyond inflation. Military spending became a major factor in the American economy. During the 1980s the military accounted for 42 percent of federal employment; it also absorbed 45 percent of public and private research and development funds and 38 percent of investment funds for plants and manufacturing equipment. In fact, the military consumed 30 percent of the nation's total goods during the 1980s.[5] This shift in federal priorities clearly benefited American military-industrial interests, helping to stem an erosion of jobs in the sector of the economy most critical for private third-party funding of employee health insurance. The "defense industry" sector of the economy, because of its product, was least likely to shift investments overseas. Its workforce was highly unionized, and health benefits were generous. Without this turn toward remilitarization, the unraveling of earlier solutions to health-care funding dilemmas would have been even more rapid.

The U.S. resumed its earlier stance as guardian of the international political order and opponent of socialist and communist governments and political movements; it intervened more directly in Latin America, where the dynamics of the international political economy were helping to produce massive social unrest, and where a series of political alliances helped intensify a health problem that became ever more serious in the United States.

International Health Problems: Drug Traffic and AIDS

During the 1980s, coca crops, from which cocaine is made, were an important source of revenue in South America, and especially in Colombia. International drug lords targeted the U.S. as the best market for cocaine, and particularly for a new and cheaper form of the drug called "crack." By the end of the decade it had become clear that some Latin American governments were implicated in the drug traffic, and some reports even claimed that certain agencies within the U.S. government were involved. All governments denied these accusations, however, and documentation of political involvement in international drug trafficking was hard to come by.[6]

The sale of "crack" cocaine spread rapidly through the high schools of the U.S. and among young adults, reaching epidemic levels after 1984.[7] At the same time the new international plague, AIDS, was spreading rapidly into the U.S. and throughout the world. These escalating international health problems introduced major sources of health deterioration that could not be corrected by a simple extension of older disease-cure strategies. They escalated demand for many kinds of health-care services.

Ending the Cold War

By 1989, another dynamic was changing the entire character of the international political and economic order. The momentum had begun three years earlier, when Mikhail S. Gorbachev, the head of state, introduced dramatic internal reforms within the Soviet Union and made it clear that he would not use military force to dictate policy to client states within the Soviet trading system. Gorbachev also introduced a unilateral de-escalation of the international arms race, which led rather quickly to more general arms reduction. The Soviet Union's economic empire quickly collapsed, however, as nation after nation in eastern Europe withdrew from the Soviet trade system and made overtures to enter the free market of the West. By 1990, the Soviet Union itself announced plans to drastically reform its own economy, to join the trading system of the rest of the world, and to encourage direct investments from Western capitalists. By 1992, the centrally controlled Soviet political state had collapsed, replaced by a mix of independent states and a loose confederation of former Soviet Republics. The ending of the Cold War forced a reexamination of policy, one that had important implications for the military-industrial alliance of interests within the U.S., which provided an important backbone of financing for American health care.[8]

This highly unstable international scene developed at the same time that the American political economy was reorganizing at a level not experienced for about a hundred years. Older operating alliances and the earlier formulas for labor peace and welfare services were being reexamined. National formulas for dealing with health-care issues were directly affected by a shift in political coalitions and in consequent operating policies that occurred in America during the 1980s.

Changes in America: Realigning Working Coalitions in the 1980s

The election of 1980 marked a turning point in American political life. A new working coalition gained control of the presidency and began to set an agenda that was to have a profound impact on the character of the

American health-care industry. A fifty-year partnership between government, industry, and a coalition of "have not" interests within the American population came into question. The older partnership of labor, management and the government, which had enlarged to include Black urban political and civil rights leaders, now was replaced by a new alignment of business interests and the government, supported by a political coalition of America's wealthy, as well as by white ethnic Americans, religious conservatives, and Southern white voters.[9] Both major political parties had developed internal splits, and political scandals had alienated a large share of the electorate who now did not vote in national elections. This gave opportunity for new alignments of interests to take control.

In 1980, Ronald Reagan narrowly won the presidency on the Republican ticket, getting 50.7 percent of the votes cast, or support from about a quarter of the total eligible voters.[10] Reagan's survival of an attempted assassination in 1982 helped solidify public sympathy for him. When the runaway inflation slowed, after a severe recession in 1982, a wellspring of popular support for his policies emerged. In 1984, Reagan received an additional ten million votes and became the first president since Eisenhower to serve two full terms of office. By the time he left the presidency the character of the economy, class relations in America, and the role of the courts in public life, had changed profoundly. So had the nature of the health-care system.

Reaganomics: A New Approach to Problem-Solving

Reagan's policies marked a major departure from strategies used in the previous 20 years of American government. *Reaganomics* attempted to reverse the Great Society programs that had singled out African Americans and the poor for special attention. While taking care not to threaten the New Deal's Social Security programs which had broad public support, Reagan backed away from support for other social welfare programs. Equally important, he tried to return to the Cold War stance of anti-communism, a strong America, including a strengthened military and related defense industry. Under Reagan, American foreign policy emphasized a strong military presence but abandoned the earlier Pax Americana policy's joint emphasis on a warfare/*welfare* state. *Defederalism* and *deregulation*, replaced a seventy-year emphasis on *public planning for the common good* which had included using federal legislation and taxation policies to control large-scale capitalist activity, or to limit the centralization of financial control. Instead, *supply-side economics* argued that federal policy should encourage capital formation by lowering taxes for the wealthy and ending government surveillance of economic activity. Thus the antitrust legislation of the Progressive period went largely unenforced in the Reagan era. Monetarism fought inflation by setting caps on federal expenditures, reducing the amount of money the federal government put into the economy.[11]

As part of Reaganomics, *defederalism* involved reducing federal taxes and transfers of money to state and local governments. The federal government would abandon responsibility for redressing social inequities, leaving states and communities with the task of finding funds for social programs if they chose not to let market conditions determine who has access to the nation's resources. Enforcement of the Civil Rights Act was all but ignored, as was enforcement of antitrust legislation. Similarly, occupational health and safety legislation and environmental protection legislation were neglected, rather than strongly monitored, because they represented federal regulation that might discourage entrepreneurial business activity. Federal housing programs for the poor also were quietly abandoned to the extent that this could be done through administrative policy. New administrative guidelines shifted funds and personnel away from regulatory activities and into those that encouraged business entrepreneurship.[12]

Dealing with Inflation. A central problem facing the entire country in 1980 was a runaway rate of inflation. Monetarist economic policies slowed the growth of the money supply and raised interest rates, precipitating a deep recession in 1981-82 that led to a worldwide recession. This affected the price of oil, as did the expansion of American domestic oil production. The OPEC cartel's internal agreements to limit their own oil production collapsed, producing a relative glut of oil within a short time, breaking the cycle of energy price increases. This helped slow the rate of inflation due to the cost of energy; in addition, it slowed the flow of foreign, oil-based investment money into American banks. By 1982, the overall rate of inflation had slowed. (See Table 2 in the Appendix.)

Once inflation began to be more nearly under control, supply-side economic policies sought to lower taxes and to stimulate capital investment by freeing entrepreneurs to expand their activity. Corporations' share of federal taxes continued to decline. Where corporations had provided 29 percent of federal tax revenue during the Vietnam period and 22.6 percent during the period of détente, during the Reagan era taxes from business averaged 17.2 percent of total tax revenues. (See Table 7 in the Appendix.) In addition, federal income tax reform sharply narrowed the graduated personal income tax policies which the New Deal had introduced 50 years earlier, which had placed a heavier proportion of federal tax costs on persons in higher income brackets. Equally important, other tax reforms wiped out the automatic increase in government revenue generated as a by-product of inflation. Previously inflation-based increases in income put citizens in higher tax-brackets. Tax reforms now adjusted tax-brackets to inflation, permanently eliminating this source of automatic largesse for the government. Henceforth, voters would have to directly approve any increases in government spending. As a result of these combined influences, the tax base needed to pay the government's share of constantly expanding health-care costs became severely eroded.[13]

The Reagan administration stimulated the economy by enlarging the military budget and placing massive orders with federal defense contractors. In practice, supply-side economics meant that much of the new federal spending went for business contracts, with social welfare budgets frozen in absolute size or reduced. Between 1980 and 1985 an additional $400 billion was added to the federal budget, in real dollars an increase of 65 percent, including over $78.6 billion in additions to federal outlays for the military. Because of inflation, however, the total increase in the federal budget, in constant 1982 dollars, was 28 percent. (See Table 8 in the Appendix.)

The Federal Deficit. The federal government faced real limits on revenue sources. Tax revenues from business and the wealthy continued to decline and Reagan was committed not to raise other taxes. The limits on growth of personal income for less wealthy Americans because of *Reaganomic* anti-inflation measures, and tax reforms that eliminated automatic increases in government income because of inflation further limited federal revenue. Meanwhile, sharp increases in military spending and continuing escalations of health-care costs, which made budget slashing in other parts of the federal budget relatively ineffective, led to sharp increases in the federal deficit and resulting federal debt. When Reagan became president in 1981 the federal deficit had been not quite $74 billion annually. By 1985, it was more than $212 billion annually. (See Tables 8 and 11 in the Appendix.)

The Centralization of Control over Capital

Reaganomics added momentum to trends of economic change already visible in the 1970s, and quickly produced a major redistribution of wealth, power and privilege. Within the larger business community, corporate mergers became the center of attention, paralleling the rise of giant, quasi-monopolistic corporations during the 1880s. The rise and fall of economic fortunes was dramatic. "Hostile takeovers," in which corporate raiders acquired controlling interest in a corporation against the wishes of its management, and "forced buyouts," in which management groups who wished to retain their holdings were forced to buy back stock from investors at considerable loss to themselves, became commonplace. Between 1981 and mid-1988, 41 major mergers of corporations occurred in the U.S., at an individual cost ranging from $2.5 billion to $13.3 billion. One fourth of the major acquisitions were purchased by investment speculators. One out of eight of the major acquisitions went to foreign investors. During 1986 and

1987 alone, there were over 7,500 corporate mergers in the U.S., involving $340 billion.[14]

Deregulation of banking and investment laws encouraged a rapid consolidation of wealth in the country. Between 1976 and 1987 the number of independent banks in America decreased by 59 percent as multibank holding companies doubled the number of banks under their control. Bank failures also accelerated rapidly, especially after the recession of 1982 and the federal response of deregulating banking. Where there had been 53 bank failures under the regulated system in effect from 1977 to 1981, there were 611 bank failures between 1982 and 1987. This pattern soon spread to the savings and loan industry. By 1989, when Congress intervened to save those institutions from collapse, it was predicted that half of the 3,000 savings and loan companies would either close or be merged with multibranch banks within ten years.[15]

Splits in Elite Interests

Reagan's commitment to a military buildup, and his determination not to increase taxes created a clear contest between two interest groups that had emerged in the elite sector of the American economy: what Daniel Bell had called the military-industrial complex and the information-service complex.[16] Each had been dependent upon government subsidy for its growth. Reagan's policy clearly favored helping the defense industry recover its earlier standing. The health-care industry not only fell within the newer, information-service sector, but was a pace-setter for it. In the emerging contest, the government was aligning itself with older sectors of the economy.

In the previous decade the health-care industry had grown rapidly, but manufacturing industries had gone into a dangerous decline. Reagan tried to stop this trend. Where 22.7 percent of the federal budget had gone for "defense" in 1980, 26.7 percent was so allocated in 1985, a return to the post-Vietnam expenditure levels of 1975. In contrast, health care's portion of the federal budget increased from 11.7 percent to 12.5 percent. This change in federal budget priorities was reflected in growth of the gross national product for the nation as a whole. The "defense" share of the GNP increased from 5 percent to 6.4 percent. Health care was financed both by the government and privately, however, and its share increased from 9.2 percent to 10.5 percent of the GNP. (See Table 10 in the Appendix.)

The "Service Complex" Split Between Health and Welfare. Committed to a strong military presence and to a prosperous defense industry, as well as to lowered taxes, Reagan had announced that cuts would have to come from social welfare expenditures. Between 1980 and 1985, however, total federal expenditures for social welfare programs *increased*—from $302.6 billion to $451.2 billion—a 15 percent rise above and beyond adjustments for inflation. Social security total payments increased by 54 percent, and Medicare total payments by 193 percent.[17]

Welfare programs were cut wherever possible. (For example, the health budget for the Bureau of Indian Affairs was reduced by 35 percent.) Federal education programs and veterans' services were held to about half the total overall increase in federal welfare budgeting. Housing programs were maintained at their constant 1980 level, and other health and welfare services were cut. Women's and maternal health became a lower priority. Religious conservatives succeeded in withholding any use of public monies for abortions, in the U.S. or abroad. Child welfare and child nutrition program budgets were cut by 14 percent.[18] Given the political realities of the times, however, Reagan made no attempt to cut social security benefits for the elderly or to disengage from funding their medical costs. The Medicare caseload increased 20 percent between 1980 and 1986, and hospitalization costs, which had been doubling every 10 years, doubled once again within a six-year period.

Larger Patterns of Instability in the Political Economy

A rather disturbing larger pattern was developing for the American political economy as a whole. Health care and military cost increases, decreasing funding of government expenses from business or graduated personal income taxes, increases in the federal debt, the growing redirection of American investment capital abroad, and balance of trade losses marked a shift from the growth dynamic that had been the American economy's hallmark in the earlier postwar period. This shift had begun, in fact, in the 1960s. Now the American economy seemed to be losing equilibrium at an ever-increasing rate.

When systems move away from equilibrium the processes within them often speed up, as the system tries to move back into a more balanced state. In fact, there often begin to be pendulum-like swings in the organizing principles that get emphasized within the system as a whole. Alternating subsets of activities temporarily receive more resources, so that any substantial reorganization to send resources in one direction soon produces a move in the other direction. Over a thirty-year period there were swings back and forth between Great Society programs for minorities and the poor, on the one hand, and Reaganomics programs discouraging these and aiding the wealthy, on the other. Similarly, there were swings from problem-solving through federal regulation to problem-solving through deregulation and back again. There also were shifts back and forth between Keynesian economic policies, in which the government was participant and problem-solver, and monetarism, which tried to encourage problem-solving by private initiative. Indeed, this fits a larger pattern of swings in the economy and in public social policy that has been occurring over a much longer span of time.

By the mid-1970s, however, this seesaw dynamic within the American political economy no longer depended primarily upon internal decisions and policies. Once the world economic system had developed a certain momentum of its own and American corporations had reorganized as transnational economic enterprises, American laws and administrative policies had only limited ability to stabilize economic activity.

Implications for Health Care: New Reform Strategies

Not surprisingly, the health-care industry became part of this broader pattern. Supply-side economics, deregulation, monetarism, encouraging market forces to determine outcomes, and the centralization of capital and control of other resources—all these became important themes affecting health care. Within the health-care industry, management personnel trained in business schools assumed more central roles, directing attention toward policies designed to increase "market share," "cost-effectiveness," and capital liquidity. Whereas the main health policy concerns in the 1960s and 1970s had been quality of care, access to health services, and controlled growth of services, the watchword of the 1980s became "cost control."

Health-policy decision-making in the 1980s was committed to both supply-side and monetarist economic theory. Government policy extended practices being introduced by the insurance industry. Blue Cross and Blue Shield, alarmed by the constant spiral of hospital costs, had begun applying "caps"—fixed ceilings for reimbursing various services provided by hospitals and doctors. Whereas Health Maintenance Organizations (HMOs) provided a fixed per-person fee to cover all primary health-care service costs, regardless of what was done, Blue Cross-Blue Shield continued its fee-for-service reimbursement policy but now applied "caps" for each service performed. The federal government decided to develop its own version of hospital reimbursement limits to use with Medicare, providing a modified combination of the two systems.

Cost Control: DRGs. After a two-year trial in New Jersey, the federal government's Health Care Finance Administration, which was handling Medicare reimbursements, announced its own cost control program, based upon diagnostically related groups of illnesses (DRGs). Admissions to hospitals were grouped according to the diagnosis of the medical problem given as reason for admission to the hospital. A diagnostically related group of admission categories shared in common a similar cost profile for treating that problem, based on past hospital records of treatment costs. The federal government announced that it would not reimburse hospitals for billed expenses, as had been the custom for 50 years with Blue Cross payments. Instead it would pay the "average cost" for treating that illness category as seen in hospitals across the country. If a hospital spent less, they could keep the difference between cost and reimbursement, making a profit. However, if it cost the hospital more to care for a patient than the formula allowed, the hospital would have to absorb the loss.[19]

For-Profit Medicine. Besides trying to impose limits on hospital spending, the government decided to foster greater economic competition within the health-care industry as a whole. Government planners argued that competitive units would be more likely to offer efficient, cost-effective services, and to keep one another from taking improper advantage of the demand for services. Thus the federal government phased out its subsidies and grants-in-aid for establishing HMOs, thereby encouraging private finance capital to sponsor health-care expansion, both for hospitals and HMOs.

The larger life insurance companies, including Aetna, Connecticut General, Equitable, Metropolitan, and Prudential had already moved into HMO planning, administration, marketing, financial support, and underwriting. A number of the Fortune 500 companies had explored setting up their own HMOs, but most companies were more inclined simply to invite HMO chains to do business in their area. This made private financing of HMO expansion attractive to a variety of lenders, and HMO proprietary chains expanded rapidly in the 1980s.

For-profit hospitals also expanded. By 1986 there were 834 for-profit community hospitals in the United States. More than a hundred of these hospitals had gone "for-profit" since 1979. An additional 57 non-profit community hospitals had closed during this same time period. (See Table 16 in the Appendix.)

For-profit health-care corporations expanded into new areas of service delivery, buying nursing homes, surgicenters (freestanding surgical businesses), and emergicenters (providing emergency room types of services throughout a geographic area), offering franchises to local affiliates, and even managing academic research hospitals.[20]

The "non-profit" hospitals also took advantage of new federal policies, offering new kinds of services and often reorganizing themselves as a variety of related corporations, much as the transnationals had done internationally two decades earlier. Few statistics were kept concerning the extent of organizational innovation among these hospitals, but observers reported that many hospitals were reorganizing as mixed non-profit and for-profit ventures. Some were even going multinational.

In the mid-1980s, over coffee, a vice-president of a large, independent metropolitan hospital in mid-America chatted with me about his work. He was supervising the reorganization of his hospital into 16 corporations to take advantage of various growth possibilities. They were now competing both in the for-profit and the non-profit markets, taking over smaller hospitals in their metropolitan area, and providing a variety of subsidiary services. He had just returned from a trip to the Middle East, where his hospital was bidding for a contract to manage the developing hospital system in Saudi Arabia. His major competitor was a West German hotel chain. Healthcare organizations were reorganizing on the model of contemporary corporate life and becoming global in their ambitions. Moreover, they now were facing competition from non-health sectors of the emerging international economy.

Hospital Chains. Even non-profit hospitals were being absorbed into commonly managed, multi-hospital chains. By 1985, some 486 non-profit hospitals were managed on contract by these chains, and over 1,500 hospitals were owned outright by the 249 multi-hospital systems that had emerged. Five large, for-profit corporations owned or managed 624 of the nation's hospitals.[21] They had almost doubled their holdings since 1980. By that year, one out of every six hospitals in the nation was a proprietary, for-profit business venture.

Between 1980 and 1988, over 300 government-controlled hospitals (often those run by city governments) closed or were absorbed by other hospital systems. Five years after the government's DRG cost-control policy was implemented, the American hospital system's capacity had shrunk by 71,000 beds. (See Table 16 in the Appendix.) By 1988, nonprofit private hospitals were managing 50,000 fewer beds than they had at their peak in 1984, a year after the DRG reimbursement policy for Medicare patients first went into effect. There were 34,000 fewer beds available in public community hospitals. For-profit chains, however, had added an additional 14,000 beds to their management, though they did not keep all of them in operation.

Thus the profile of American hospital service was changing. As the total capacity of the system became smaller, the private nonprofit hospitals maintained a steady 70 percent of total bed capacity, adjusting to the reduced demand for hospital services. Public community hospitals, however, shrank from 28 percent of total services offered, an amount they had represented when the Hill-Burton Act went into effect in 1946, to 19 percent of the 1988 total. When Hill-Burton funds for hospital construction were cut off in 1972, for-profit hospitals were operating 6 percent of the total short term hospital beds in service. By 1989, that proportion had increased to 11 percent.

The growth of for-profit hospitals put financial strain on public and non-profit hospitals, because the proprietary hospitals often refused to accept Medicaid patients and closed their doors to patients who lacked private insurance. These patients went disproportionately to the public and teaching hospitals, making those hospitals' financial balance sheets all the more precarious. A survey of 23 large urban public hospitals in 1983 found that they were receiving only 13 percent of their income from private insurers (with some public hospitals receiving only 3 percent).[22]

For-profit health chains were also going international. By 1985, some nine hospital companies based in the U.S. were operating 95 hospitals in 17 foreign countries, and two-thirds of the foreign hospitals were owned by U.S. corporations. A West German hospital corporation, in turn, was operating 26 hospitals in the United States.[23]

Both vertical and horizontal integration of services was occurring on a large scale. In fact, one of the larger for-profit hospital chains, American Hospital, was acquired by Baxter-Travenol in 1986 for $3.7 billion. Baxter-Travenol is a health-care conglomerate which develops, manufactures, and distributes medical products, including pharmaceutical preparations, surgical and medical instruments, surgical appliances, medicinal and botanical products, and fabricated rubber products. In 1997, Aetna Life and Casualty Insurance Company bought U.S. Health Care, Inc., one of the fastest-growing HMOs. Columbia-HCA Health Care Corporation, the largest chain of for-profit hospitals, bought Blue Cross-Blue Shield of Ohio. The health-care industry was mimicking the style found in other areas of the economy.[24]

As the organization of medical services became increasingly centralized and corporate, the independence of doctors declined. By 1985, one-fourth of them were working as employees, rather than as independent practitioners or even as part of doctor-run clinics in which they were partners. Half of all women physicians were working as employees, as were half of all the physicians under 36 years of age.[25] In addition, new lower-paid health occupations were taking over an increasing portion of the primary care practice once offered only by doctors.

Health-Care Cost Inflation

The health-care industry's growth was eating into corporate profits for other business sectors. In 1980, health-care costs represented 42.6 percent of after-tax corporate profits (in contrast to 14.0 percent in 1965). In 1989 the cost to American corporations for health care equaled 98.3 percent of their after-tax profits. (See Table 3 in the Appendix.) These figures, of course, reflect not only the rising cost of health care but also the declining profitability of American manufacturing more generally during this period, as Table 4 of the Appendix makes clear. American manufacturing as a whole experienced a 21 percent decline in inflation-adjusted profits during the ten-year period from 1981 to 1990. The ten-year profit picture for corporations that manufactured durable goods was 32 percent below what it had been in the 1970s. Health-care costs, of course, were only part of the dilemma American manufacturing faced. But that part was significant. If corporations had not been paying employees' health costs, their after-tax profits in 1989 would have almost doubled.

Business Health Coalitions

Business leaders in other parts of the economy that pay for health-care services were being encouraged, by government and their own coordinating organizations, to play an active role in health-care cost control. In 1986, the Health Care Finance Administration, which administers Medicare, began publishing annual mortality statistics, by type of illness, for hospitals that serve Medicare patients. Hospital performance records now could be part of business or private consumer decision making about which hospital to use. By 1985, Business Health Coalitions had formed in 93 metropolitan areas. They monitored costs for health care provided at various health facilities and encouraged the development of Preferred Provider Organizations (PPOs)—health-care providers that offer businesses a set of pre-approved services for a pre-established fee. Fees often are set at bargain rates in exchange for a guaranteed market of health-care consumers. Providers sometimes compensate for the lower price they charge large corporations, however, by charging higher prices to "general" health-care consumers. In addition, the business health coalitions often sponsored the introduction of HMOs into their area, encouraging local physicians to form them. Where local doctors resisted, the business groups often invited national HMO chains to establish services in their area. This frequently spurred local doctors to form their own HMOs as well, and introduced a new spirit of competition into primary care service delivery.[26]

As noted earlier, the five largest insurance companies, who had lost their health insurance market when the large corporations self-insured, set up their own Health Maintenance Organizations and competed for contracts to provide direct health-care services for the corporations' employees. No longer able to profit from investing health insurance premiums for short-run gain, they would reap their profit from providing cost-efficient health care within the capitated payments they received. As insurance companies managed HMOs, a new level of business management and bottom-line profit accounting became part of "managed care."[27]

Cost Control in HMOs. HMOs continued to expand, with the non-profit ones joined by explicitly for-profit enterprises. Whereas HMOs had enrolled 9.1 million subscribers in 1980, by mid-1989 they had almost 32 million participants. (See Table 14 of the Appendix.) Seventy percent of all MD specialists now were associated with HMOs—a self-protective response, given the growing trend and the current oversupply of specialists, and a guarantee of fixed fees per person assigned to them.[28] To increase profitability, some large HMO chains set up physician incentive plans, which reimbursed physicians not simply in terms of the number of subscribers they served but also in proportion to the costs of care given to their patients. If patients were referred to hospitals, or for a number of expensive services, the physician received a smaller bonus at the end of the year.[29]

The increasing number of participants in HMOs lessened demand for hospitalization, as planners had intended. So, it turned out, did imposition of DRG rules for reimbursing hospitals for Medicare patients. HMOs made less profit if they had to pay for the hospitalization of their subscribers, since a fixed fee per capita gave them a finite resource base to spend. Consequently, HMO doctors were less likely to hospitalize their patients. With the DRG reimbursement formulas, it was the *hospitals* that discouraged prolonged stays: since the hospital received a fixed amount of money for each patient, based on the diagnosis given at admission, the hospital came out ahead if Medicare patients remained in the hospital only a short time. Hospitals, therefore, encouraged doctors on their staffs to release Medicare patients as quickly as possible. (Table 15 in the Appendix shows what happened to hospital utilization rates as HMO policies and DRG formulas took effect. Note pre- and post-1982 rates.) Since only hospital *admissions*— not treatments given in their outpatient clinics—were subject to the DRG reimbursement formulas, hospitals also encouraged doctors to treat Medicare patients on an outpatient basis, so that diagnostic work, medications, and the like would not be subject to DRG reimbursement formulas.[30]

The organizational form and character of America's disease-oriented medical care system had changed dramatically during the 1980s, as part of an effort to gain control over constantly escalating medical costs. However, the cost of health care, not counting cost increases due to inflation, continued its upward climb, slowing only slightly. From 1977 to 1982, the cost for health care, adjusted for inflation, increased 22 percent. From 1982 through 1987, it increased 19 percent. (See Table 1 of the Appendix.)

How Effective Were These Innovations?

Between 1965 and 1980, there was a sixfold increase in the actual cost of health services. Business' share of total health-service costs increased from 17 percent to 27 percent, and government's share increased from 21 percent to 32 percent. While the actual out-of-pocket costs had increased enormously for private households, their proportionate share of total health-service costs had decreased from 61 percent to 38 percent. (See Table 13 in the Appendix.)

During the 1980s, DRG policies for hospital reimbursement had been introduced by the federal government, business health coalitions had tried to control health-care cost increases, and businesses began to cover the health expenses of a smaller proportion of the population. Despite these efforts, business, government, and private households continued to pay about the same proportion of the rapidly accelerating health-care bill that they had been paying since 1980. Business' proportion of the costs actually increased slightly as the government's proportion declined; this happened in part because hospitals made up for their losses in Medicare and Medicaid revenue and for uncollectable charges to some of the uninsured by increasing basic charges for services paid under other reimbursement systems. The five-year additional burden for health-service costs absorbed by private households amounted to almost $82 billion. For many of the more than 30 million Americans who lacked health insurance of any kind by 1991, health-care services simply had been priced beyond their capacity to pay. (See Table 12 in the Appendix.)

How had the introduction of HMOs affected this cost dynamic? In terms of cost control, HMOs were not doing much better than the rest of the health-care system. The pattern of health insurance premium increases for HMOs pretty well paralleled what was happening with fee-for-service health insurance. Rates usually were a bit lower than for Blue Cross (sometimes by as much as 5 percent), but with the pattern of rate increases almost identical between the two forms of health insurance, it was clear that health policy planners had not found a way to break through the cost increase dynamic.[31]

Malpractice Trends

Meanwhile, the impetus for use of high-tech medical procedures and numerous tests and treatments due to medical malpractice suits escalated. In 1980 there were about three malpractice claims per year for every hundred physicians. By 1985 that ratio had risen to ten claims per hundred physicians.[32] Insurance agencies found that doctors—anticipating possible suits against them—were reporting 50 percent more medical events that could lead to malpractice suits than were actually being filed by patients.[33]

Although the problem of malpractice exists throughout medicine, malpractice claims vary by specialty. In 1985 psychiatrists fared best (at not quite two and a half claims per hundred) and obstetricians worst (with over 26 claims per hundred). The next most frequently sued specialists were surgeons and radiologists (facing 16.5 and 13 claims per hundred, respectively).[34]

Obstetricians' problems may have been compounded by their increasing use of Caesarean operations to replace birth by natural delivery. Between 1971 and 1983 the number and rate of Caesarean deliveries increased fourfold. By 1986, 24 percent of all American babies were born by Caesarean section.[35] During this time period malpractice claims for permanent injury or "grave injury" to babies nearly doubled, from 13 percent to 25 percent of all malpractice cases. Yet the practice of delivery by Caesarean section continued unabated and indeed, may have been encouraged by physicians' fears of malpractice suits from complications of vaginal delivery.

There was no evidence that pre-delivery circumstances were becoming more precarious for American mothers. Fetal monitoring had been introduced, however, and doctors now were aware of every shift in fetal condition—but with no established record of what changes are normal, and what changes signal trouble. How much of the move toward Caesarean delivery reflected efforts to avoid malpractice liability and how much reflected obstetrician's preferences is unclear. A doctor's preferred delivery method predicted use of Caesarean sections much more accurately than did the mother's or baby's condition prior to delivery.[36] Birth by Caesarean section allows doctors and mothers to avoid certain kinds of possible birth complications, as well as to schedule deliveries at their convenience. But it turns a natural event into an invasive surgery for the mother, adding greatly to the expense and increasing the possibility of damage. Ironically, increases in malpractice insurance rates led many family doctors to quit delivering babies, forcing many parents to use specialists for the birth of their child.

Doctors were not the only ones facing the brunt of malpractice claims. The single largest hospital insurance company reported a 76 percent increase in number of hospital malpractice claims filed between 1979 and 1983.[37] Between 1982 and 1985 malpractice insurance premiums almost doubled for most doctors, and almost tripled for obstetricians. Hospital insurance rates also rose sharply. In 1987 doctors and hospitals paid at least $8 billion in malpractice insurance premiums.

Defensive Medicine. In addition to increasing their charges to cover higher insurance fees, many doctors were practicing "defensive medicine," covering themselves against possible suits for misdiagnosis by ordering extensive laboratory tests and X-ray exams and by referring patients more frequently for consultation with medical specialists. In 1982 the American Medical Association's (AMA's) Committee on Professional Liability estimated that defensive medicine and defensive hospital administrative procedures were costing $15.1 billion that year, about 5 percent of all medical costs. By 1988, the cost of purely "defensive medicine" had risen to an estimated $20 billion annually. Among physicians who responded to an AMA Socioeconomic Monitoring System survey, 40 percent said they prescribed additional diagnostic tests to defend against malpractice suits. One in four also provided additional treatment procedures to avoid possible suit.[38] Often discussions of the malpractice problem estimated its impact on health-care spending primarily in terms of direct costs for malpractice insurance or settlements. Occasionally, however, observers discussed the larger picture. Writing in the *New York Times*, for example, former Secretary of Health, Education, and Welfare, Joseph A. Califano, Jr., claimed that Americans would spend about $155 billion in 1989 for tests and treatments that would have little or no impact on the patients involved.

Califano, who now chaired Chrysler Corporation's health-care committee, reported these health-care costs:

> In 1988, Chrysler spent $700 on employee health care for each vehicle manufactured—twice as much as French and West German automakers and three times as much as the Japanese.... *We are not buying better health care.* The $2,500 we'll spend this year for each man, woman and child in the U.S. is 50 percent more than will be spent in the next highest-spending nation, Canada; more than twice that in Japan, and almost triple that in Britain. Yet each of these nations had lower infant mortality rates and similar longevity.[39]

In short, the pressures that continued to drive up the cost of American health care continued to mount, despite government and business efforts at cost control.

Worsening Problems: 1. The Uninsured

All through the 1980s, as in the 1970s, the proportion of Americans having employer-paid health insurance—or health insurance of any kind—dropped. The changing occupational structure, with fewer jobs in unionized manufacturing industries or other businesses providing health benefits, slowly eroded the basis on which American health care had been built since World War II. During the 1980s the number of Americans whose jobs provided no health insurance coverage and whose incomes were nonetheless too high to qualify for Medicaid, government-paid health insurance, increased rapidly. Between 1980 and 1984 alone, the number of Americans with employer or union provided health insurance decreased by 3,200,000 persons.[40]

By 1990, about one out of every six Americans lacked health insurance of any kind, either public or private. Meanwhile in every year of the Reagan administration the cost of health care had increased faster than the cost of almost all other consumer items, increasing at two to four times the overall consumer price index (CPI) increase (after energy prices began to lower during Reagan's second term of office). While wages were in a stationary pattern, the percent of total expenditures for health care continued to rise for all urban consumer units. For those without health insurance, these trends often created deep personal tragedy when ill health appeared. (See Table 2 in the Appendix.)

Worsening Problems: 2. Health Problems of the Homeless

A second health issue resulted from an increase in the number of Americans who were homeless. A growing number of Americans not only lacked health insurance, but housing as well.⁴¹

The Reagan administration had tried to economize on government assistance with the housing needs of lower-income citizens. The Department of Housing and Urban Development (HUD) changed bookkeeping rules for cooperatively owned low-income condominium complexes built as part of the War on Poverty, ending government assistance for their upkeep. HUD's change in policy forced many of these cooperatives to sell out to private real estate investors, who often "upgraded" the complexes for resale to middle-class home seekers in a booming real estate market. The rapid escalation of real estate values, coupled with the federal government's gradual retreat from low-income housing subsidies, produced a vast increase in the number of individuals and families who were homeless.⁴² So did the closing of many public mental hospitals.

The exact size of the problem was difficult to measure, because of the way records were kept. In 1982 one independent study estimated that 1 percent of the U.S. population, or 2.2 million people, lacked adequate shelter. Other independent sources made estimates that were 10 times as high. During the 1980s, shelters for the homeless, often operated by religious groups, had grown in number and size all over the country. Observers agreed that how many people depended upon such shelters could not be counted accurately. Various centers reported, however, that the number of people using their facilities had increased in four years by 60 to 250 percent, depending upon the location.⁴³ A sizable number of the homeless, of course, did not use public shelters.

The homeless and others without adequate shelter were exposed to many more health risks than the population at large. Although some were eligible for Medicaid hospitalization coverage if they grew ill, others who were employed had no health coverage.

Worsening Problems: 3. Use of Illicit Drugs

The social nexus of health and disease became clearly visible as the sale of addicting street drugs spread throughout the country. Discovering trends in the spread of illegal drugs is not simple. As in the case of statistical evidence about homelessness, the exact extent of increasing drug use in the U.S. is hard to document. However, national surveys of drug use among high school students and young adults, conducted regularly between 1974 and 1990, showed a rapid increase in self-reports of the use of cocaine. In 1974, 2.6 percent of youths under 18 reported having used cocaine. By 1990, the rate of cocaine usage among male high school seniors during the previous year varied by race: 12 percent among whites and 6 percent among African-Americans. By 1987, however, "crack" had made its way into 77 percent of the nation's high schools. Surveys showed that use of cocaine among post high-school young people between 18 and 25 years of age was increasing even more rapidly.[44] Even though surveys showed some leveling off or even decreases in self-reported use of cocaine and other hard drugs in the following three years, the problem continued in "epidemic" proportions.

The health implications from this increase in drug use, as well as from increased homelessness, were immense. Given political priorities, however, little planning was done in response. Caseloads for Medicaid health coverage remained unchanged, at 22 million persons. Despite the freeze on expanding health services to the indigent, between 1981 and 1986 the actual cost of Medicaid had increased more than 60 percent, rising to $45.8 billion. Almost half of the budget went to pay costs for 7 percent of the recipients, elderly persons in nursing homes who had exhausted their savings. Given these resource demands, many states limited the access of younger poor people to Medicaid services.[45]

Worsening Problems: 4. AIDS

Meanwhile, a new and usually fatal health threat, AIDS, was sweeping the world, changing the fundamental character of health problems. In 1981, doctors in the U.S. began discovering patients whose immune systems no longer were functioning. Soon public health officials in many countries were documenting the rapid spread of the debilitating and almost universally fatal illness, acquired through mixing blood, sexual secretions or other bodily fluids with those from a person who is infected. AIDS spread quickly throughout the U.S., Europe, the Caribbean, Latin America, Africa, and into Australia, New Zealand, and Asia. In the U.S. and Europe it at first spread most rapidly in self-limiting populations—hemophiliacs dependent upon many blood transfusions, America's and Europe's gay communities whose subculture encouraged sexual activity with multiple partners, and persons who were drug dependent. By the end of the 1980s in the U.S., however, the HIV virus was spreading into the heterosexual community. It was no longer confined to self-limiting sub-populations of the American public.[46]

This was an international epidemic, not simply an American problem. The most devastating impact was felt in Africa, where labor-force patterns separated families for major blocks of time and produced massive migration of male wage-earners around the continent, with the associated mating patterns that have been found all over the world under such conditions. Customs of polygamy also exacerbated its spread. AIDS swept through Burma and Thailand, where women sex-workers became major carriers of the virus.[47] Worldwide it was estimated by 1995 that 21.8 million people were living with HIV/AIDS. In 1995, HIV-associated illnesses caused the deaths of 1.3 million people, almost surely a major underestimate, given haphazard record-keeping practices in some parts of the world where the plague was widespread. Throughout the decade tallies of AIDS cases constantly climbed, and each new count showed that half of the persons with AIDS had died. No count was kept of survivors who remained alive and relatively healthy, though clinical cases documented the fact that some persons living with full-blown AIDS had done so for at least 10 years.

The number of AIDS cases in the U.S. increased from 199 in 1981 to 164,129 by January 31, 1991, and to 573,800 by the end of 1996, with an estimated additional 600,000 to 900,000 persons infected with the virus but not yet showing disease symptoms. Researchers were finding drugs that postpone the emergence of full-blown AIDS among persons who host the HIV virus and treatments that allow persons with AIDS to survive various opportunistic infections for longer periods of time. With the discovery of expensive, multiple drug therapies that inhibit HIV-reproduction within an infected person, the cost of medical care for American AIDS and HIV-infected patients could be expected to increase sharply during the 1990s.[48]

While the spread of AIDS into the non-drug-using American heterosexual population was much slower than among some higher-risk populations, by January 31, 1991, over 9,000 heterosexually-acquired AIDS cases had been reported to the U.S. Public Health Service's Centers for Disease Control. Some 59 percent of these cases were traced to sexual contacts with IV-drug users or bisexual men, but almost 3,800 of these cases came through other routes. Moreover, more than 7,200 of the full-blown AIDS cases were teenagers or persons who had acquired the virus as a teenager, including 786 young people who had acquired it through heterosexual contacts with persons not in the high-risk groups.[49] Heterosexual African Americans' and Hispanics' risk of acquiring AIDS had become three times as high as white, non-Hispanic Americans and six to seven times as high as that facing Asian Americans. The risk was especially high within low-income neighborhoods of minority communities and among the homeless.

Federal Responses to the Epidemic. During the first six years of the American AIDS epidemic, the federal government had been slow to respond to the social dimensions of the disease. In 1987, however, C. Everett Koop, the U.S. Surgeon General, sent a mailing to every American home describing simply and forthrightly the nature of the epidemic. Koop's pamphlet made it clear that the general public, not simply special population groups, was susceptible to AIDS. It offered simple, nonjudgmental advice about how to avoid the disease.[50]

By 1988, public pressure led President Reagan to appoint a national commission to make recommendations for dealing with the AIDS threat. The original commission, politically appointed, could not work effectively. Eventually it was reconstituted and chaired by the recently retired head of the U.S. Navy. Its final report called for a shift in government priorities, concentrating on limiting the spread of the virus, making control of intravenous drug use a top national priority, increasing both federal funding for AIDS research and agency discretion in how to proceed, and including persons with AIDS in government definitions of the physically handicapped, eligible for services and protections already afforded other physically disabled persons.[51]

The federal budget for 1989 included $1.6 billion for AIDS research and education and $925 million for treatment, a 30 percent increase in funding. The non-discrimination provisions, recommended by the Commission majority but opposed by its conservative members, were included a year later in Congressional legislation dealing with the physically disabled.[52]

Government planning rarely deals with time-spans longer than four or five years. There was little sign that the U.S. Public Health Service Centers for Disease Control's projections of the increased AIDS caseload to be expected for 1992 or the year 2000 were becoming part of systematic health strategizing for the future. (By 1992, the American government was spending $4.277 billion dollars as the federal share of medical treatments for persons seriously ill with AIDS.)

As the epidemic spread, it became clear that medical research was not finding a quick fix that would bring the epidemic to a rapid halt. Persons with AIDS also were developing resistance to drugs normally used to halt the effects of other infectious agents within the body.[53]

In the mid-1990s, new hope appeared when it was discovered that a mix of three protease inhibitor drugs reversed the disease's progression for many AIDS patients and held promise of completely stopping HIV reproduction in the body, if given early on. There was a 19 percent decrease in the U.S. death rate from AIDS between 1995 and 1996, despite the fact that the number of people living with AIDS had increased by 10 percent during that period. AIDS might be on its way to becoming a chronic rather than a fatal disease, and if all newly infected people were given the drugs, it might be possible to slow or stop its spread within the population. These possibilities, however, created a new dilemma: the cost of the drugs frequently ran to $15,000 per person per year, plus doctors' fees and laboratory test costs. An estimated 600,000 to 900,000 Americans already were infected.[54] Treating all infected people would cost at least $10 billion per year, and possibly cost twice that figure. Meanwhile, block grant allocations for treatment of AIDS were quickly depleted. Few private households could absorb the new costs, and private health insurance would face severe cost overruns if it financed much of the new treatment. For most of the world where the pandemic raged most strongly, both the cost and the clinical standards necessary in order to use the new drug therapy placed the new treatment strategies out of reach. Would it be out of reach for the U.S. as well? If not, what else would be given up for public budgets to absorb this cost?

Cost Control and Health-Care Rationing. Reaganomic problem-solving approaches did not work when applied to AIDS. A large, for-profit hospital chain opened the first AIDS hospital, in Houston, Texas, but closed it a year later because it was operating at a loss. Too many AIDS patients were dependent on Medicaid, and government reimbursement rates did not provide a sufficient profit margin to keep private enterprise interested.[55]

People with AIDS, susceptible to diseases triggered by a range of bacteria and viruses that other people handle with ease, threaten the financial base of HMOs, which receive a fixed, per-capita fee for each enrollee and must cover any medical costs involved in caring for that client. Moreover, since both Blue Cross-Blue Shield and the HMOs ensure an entire workgroup, there was no simple way for the health insurance programs to avoid responsibility for the health care of persons with AIDS (as life insurance companies began to do, refusing to insure single men unless a blood test showed that they were not carriers of the HIV virus). The typical AIDS patient of the 1980s incurred medical costs of about $50,000 during the time that he (or she) actively fought the disease before succumbing to it, a cost much higher than insurance premiums for the period would cover. Some of the larger HMO chains developed decision rules to guard their financial reserves: once a person was diagnosed as having AIDS, *basic* health-care services would be offered, but no heroic measures would be undertaken to preserve their life.[56]

The AIDS epidemic thus brought the first application of strategies discussed in health planning circles soon after Medicare and Medicaid triggered the rapid escalation of health-care costs. Anticipating a demand for health services that would exceed availability of funds, Victor Fuchs wrote a book in the early 1970s provocatively titled *Who Shall Live?* Ten years later Paul Menzel continued the dialogue in a book titled *Medical Costs, Moral Choices: A Philosophy of Health-Care Economics in America.* Policy planners assumed that the growing population of elderly persons in this country would become the lever forcing rationing of health-care services. However, it was persons with AIDS who brought the first clear evidence of how this would work in actual practice. It was disquieting. Persons who are socially stigmatized and politically unorganized, who have expensive health-care needs that threaten the financial balance sheet of health-care providers or government agencies, are those for whom full services would not be offered.

Health Care's Contribution to Nonequilibrium Dynamics

The American health-care industry's growth spiral took off just as the rest of the economy, both public and private, was beginning to experience major threats to its continued growth. This clearly was a mixed blessing for the country. On the positive side, high-technology medicine and the expansion of the hospital system had produced one of the few areas of major economic development. On the negative side this was precisely the kind of growth that threatened the interests of both the American government and the major corporations, who were paying the bulk of the new health bill. (See Table 13 in the Appendix.) The expansion of the health-care industry stood in striking contrast to the more sluggish growth in the older manufacturing areas of the economy. The situation for American business was ironic: the transnational corporations were thriving, but their American sub-units were not. Mushrooming health-care costs charged to American subunits within the transnational corporations did not help their competitive situation.

Adding to the competitive problems of American-based manufacturing was the inflation in the CPI, which medical costs helped create. Because wages in America's unionized industries were adjusted quarterly to reflect changes in inflation, rising medical costs hit business twice: first, the increased fringe benefit costs for health care had to be added on to the price of manufactured goods or services; then, in addition, the resulting inflation in general prices, to which rising health-care costs contributed, increased wages independent of productivity, because of the 1950 formulas for a fair wage. These higher wage costs also had to be added on to the price of manufactured goods. (Any inflation escalator, not simply health-care costs, had this effect, of course.)

Rising medical costs affected the overall inflation rate at many levels, but government analysts and academic researchers largely ignored indirect effects on inflation that went beyond the medical care CPI. Direct effects of health-care cost increases on inflation were impressive in their own right. Medical costs now made up 6.1 percent of the total expenditures included in the CPI. Health-care costs rose independently of other inflationary pressures. Consequently, government successes in lowering the overall rate of inflation during the 1980s meant that medical costs played an increasingly important role in inflation. During the post-recession period from 1982 to 1989, the overall inflation rate for the CPI averaged 3.7 percent a year. Despite the federal government's attempt to control increases in hospital costs through the imposition of DRG reimbursement formulas, the inflation in medical care costs averaged 7.4 percent a year, double the overall inflation rate. Thus medical costs contributed 12.2 percent to the overall increase in the CPI during this period.[57] Health-care cost increases contributed to inflation at many levels beyond the ones directly measured in this index, however. As a result, American units of the transnational corporations were paying higher production costs than competing corporations headquartered in other countries, and higher costs than other units within their own transnational corporation. These higher production costs, which hurt American producers' ability to sell their products at home and abroad, further encouraged American-based businesses to invest their profits abroad rather than in the U.S. This flight of American investment capital, in turn, hurt the federal government by lessening taxable American profits that otherwise would have been available to help pay for the Medicare-Medicaid health costs the government now was assuming. In short, the growth of the health-care industry came at the expense of other American industrial sectors and the federal government.

The dominant coalition which had set the agenda both for health care and for the national political economy for a period of 40 years was disintegrating. In its place a new political coalition had introduced a conservative vision and a new stance for problem-solving. That had created opportunities for innovation throughout the economy; these led to a fundamental change in the organization of American health-care services, including a new focus on "for-profit" medicine, centralized control of resources and services, subordination of the medical profession to business interests, and direct intervention by government and business in ways that affected the daily operation of the health-care industry. The outcome of these innovations—each of them aimed at cost control—however was a continuing escalation in the real cost of health care, independent of inflationary pressures. Meanwhile, the increase in the number of Americans without health insurance, in the number of homeless Americans, in the use of crack cocaine, and in the number of AIDS cases posed serious health problems, none of which the existing health-care system could deal with effectively. If there was a single watchword for the American health-care system during the 1980s it had been "cost control." Yet its costs had grown faster than ever. The policy debates which began to form by 1990 proceeded within this context, struggling, in addition, to find a way to provide access to basic health services for the more than 30 million Americans who now were left out of the system.

4

The 1990s: Efforts at More Basic Reform in a New World Order

International developments in the early 1990s were creating a new world order, one with implications for the nature of globally-generated health problems affecting Americans, and for the organization and financing of American health care. National trends set so strongly in motion during the 1980s continued as well, producing their own pressures. Calls for health-care reform reverberated throughout the American political economy.

When the U.S. became the pre-eminent military power internationally after the collapse of the Soviet Union, the size of federal subsidies for military-industrial business activities came under challenge. As military bases closed and defense industries faced cutbacks in government orders, many areas of the U.S. faced economic recession. New jobs that emerged often were for independent contractors or in smaller businesses, areas of employment where health insurance rates were prohibitively high.[1]

The continuing internationalization of manufacturing, already visible two decades earlier, further eroded American health-care funding. Unionized manufacturing firms had provided the base for private health insurance. By 1990 the proportion of the workforce in manufacturing was half what it had been in 1950 when these arrangements evolved.[2] As unions faced pressures from employers to accept lower wages because of international competition, some adopted a new survival strategy. Costs for health care were increasing at twice the rate of general inflation; consequently the United Auto Workers and some other unions accepted lower wage increases in exchange for continuing employer subsidy of health-care benefits. The companies, in turn, bargained hard over health benefit packages. They often compensated for increases in costs by imposing cuts in health benefits paid to retirees and their dependents. Many firms restructured some jobs, reducing labor costs by employing more part-time workers and independent contractors who would be ineligible for health benefits. Employment in a firm known to provide attractive health benefits, thus was no longer a guarantee that one would have access to health insurance. Meanwhile, reduction in the total size of the industrial labor force left increasing numbers of Americans without health insurance coverage. These responses to a changed labor market resulted from the internationalization of business activity. It affected many areas of the economy, not only those directly concerned with export trade. (This happened even among hospitals and other health-care providers, who found health benefits too costly a component of labor costs.)[3]

As the Cold War faded away, the East-West split between Soviet and Free Market trading areas collapsed. In its place came regional trading alliances, including the North American Free Trade Alliance (NAFTA) between the United States, Canada, and Mexico. Its effects on jobs and wages were complex, but they intensified already strong tendencies toward the internationalization of manufacturing.[4] NAFTA's disruption of internal markets in Mexico and Canada made migration to the U.S. (legal and illegal) even more attractive, intensifying public debate in the U.S. about the rights of non-citizens to such public services as schools and publicly-funded health-care clinics.[5] Continuing immigration waves from Asia and Latin America also increased pressures on poorer Americans who lacked flexible job skills, as wage rates for unskilled jobs declined. The underground economy, which included the distribution of illegal drugs, attracted a number of Americans with limited education and job skills, as it had been doing for some years. Drug addiction and an increase in teenage death and violence continued as health issues, and other associated crime problems added their burden as well. International drug cartels now operated openly in Mexico as well as South America. Finding limited success at closing U.S. borders to such trade, American politicians responded by "getting tough on crime," lengthening sentences for Americans caught selling drugs.

As more conservative criminal justice and prison policies went into effect, with much longer prison sentences for involvement in crack cocaine than for drugs popular in more affluent suburbs, incarceration rates for African-American males increased sharply. (Only South Africa rivaled the U.S. in the proportion of its population behind bars.)[6] American prisons are noted for high rates of illicit drug use, and for clandestine sharing of needles. In addition, younger men often become sexual targets for older, tougher convicts. It has been estimated that about a third of the male prison population turns to other male prisoners for sex.[7] Drugs and sexual behavior, thus, make prisons a transmission route for spread of the HIV virus. AIDS had already begun to spread among the heterosexual American population, and especially among the young within poorer communities of African Americans and Hispanic Americans. The temporary imprisonment of many young men from these neighborhoods seemed likely to accelerate the spread of this contagious disease. Moreover, with public revenues frozen because of tax reforms of the 1980s, prison expansion further accelerated pressures on state and federal budgets, competing with demands to expand public spending for health care.

As access to health services for poorer Americans grew more problematic, U.S. Representative Harry Waxman (Democrat from California) had introduced resolutions requiring states receiving Medicaid funds from the federal government to expand Medicaid coverage, including prenatal care, for additional poor people. Added an item at a time, in various sessions of Congress, humane additions to health-care services for the poorest Americans provoked little political opposition at first.[8] Given the continuing inflation in health-care costs, however, these requirements impacted state governments, already strained with increased prison expenditures, and facing voter tax revolts. In addition, the states had to pick up roughly half the costs of nursing home care for elderly Americans when their private funds ran out, and Medicaid costs were increasing at twice the general inflation rate. Both the "war on drugs and crime" and the health-care industry's growth in costs produced enormous demands for public resources. Few states facing these pressures expanded their Medicaid population to absorb younger people who had lost their income and their health insurance in the down-sizing of American businesses.[9]

When the growing number of Americans who lacked health insurance faced health crises, many went to hospital emergency rooms for treatment, but were unable to pay the charges. Hospitals absorbed these costs into overall operating expenses, increasing daily charges to other patients. Daily charges increased further because hospitals had a number of fixed operating costs, but faced lower occupancy rates. (Medicare DRG formulas, discussed in chapter three, motivated hospitals to discharge Medicare patients as quickly as possible. Managed care organizations also tried to limit hospital stays.) All these developments worked in the same direction. They increased the costs of hospital care for all users, accentuating trends already visible in the 1980s. Private third party payers found themselves absorbing the cost of care for many of those left out of the system, paying higher insurance rates because of higher per-patient hospital overhead. While business leaders winced at the sharp yearly increases in health-care benefits costs, few executives attempted to shirk their share of "public" costs. A number of companies bargained, however, for discount rates in return for a guaranteed volume of patients who would use a particular health-care facility. When hospitals acquiesced, many increased the charges to others who were not in preferred provider plans.[10] In short, each "solution" to these systemically created problems with American health care and its financing seemed to add momentum to the acceleration in costs and the consequent exclusion of workers from health insurance.

The health-care problems facing unemployed, part-time and self-employed Americans without health insurance and the increased costs facing third party payers were only part of the challenges affecting health care. Global economic developments were increasing health problems for every one, not simply for those who lacked access to health insurance. The shift of manufacturing to countries with less stringent pollution laws, the release of ozone-eating chlorofluorocarbons (CFCs) into the atmosphere as a by-product of manufacturing activities throughout the world, the continuing fallout from atomic power plant accidents and military tests of nuclear weapons were producing a polluted global environment. Accidents on land and sea and military tactics that poured oil into the ocean or released burning clouds into the air further damaged the global environment. These health risks affected everyone, independent of social or financial status. Cancer rates and other environmentally related health problems were increasing, and with them the demand for expensive medical care.[11] (Chapter 9 discusses this in greater depth.)

Focusing Attention on Health Problems

In 1988, the Democratic presidential candidate had made health-care reform a major theme of his campaign. Although he lost, the issue was now part of the public policy agenda, coupled however with demands to reduce the federal debt, which had grown alarmingly during the 1980s.

By 1990, there was a growing consensus in U.S. policy circles that major changes had to be made in the health-care system, and soon. A National Leadership Commission on Health Care—which included former legislators, governors, and U.S. presidents—and the Pepper Commission, a bipartisan group of current senators and representatives, issued reports calling for important changes in the organization and funding of health-care services.[12] Business interests also were involved: Chrysler Motor Company, for example, paid for ads in the New York *Times* pointing out the cost to American business of current health-care arrangements and demanding major reform. Local business health coalitions presented their own analysis of needed changes in health-care organization and funding. The American Medical Association (AMA) and the Heritage Foundation, a conservative "think tank" in Washington, D.C., each came up with proposals for national health insurance. Meanwhile a number of state governments were enacting legislation to give uninsured citizens better access to health care.

A public consensus seemed to be emerging on four problems. First, all agreed that women and children needed to have access to primary care, and particularly to preventive services such as immunizations. Second, some way to stop the growth in the numbers of Americans who had no health insurance or who had inadequate coverage had to be devised. Third, any increase in the number of people covered had to be coupled with effective cost containment, so that health care would not absorb an ever greater share of state and federal budgets and of the Gross National Product (GNP). If guaranteed access to basic health-care services were to be given to the 30 to 37 million Americans who lacked health insurance in 1990, and to the additional twenty-five million Americans whose health insurance excluded coverage for the cost of their ongoing health problems,[13] it must not overwhelm the economic resources of the federal or state governments or of private business. Fourth, planning was needed to deal with the future costs of Medicare and long-term care, which are expected to skyrocket as the baby boom generation moves into old age, and the ratio of wage-earning taxpayers to retirees—of those who pay for health-care costs to those receiving service through Medicare —is cut in half.[14]

Each of these problems had grown noticeably worse during the 1980s. The decrease in preventive health services for mothers and children occurred because federal budget planners tried to balance increased Medicare and Medicaid hospitalization costs (whose coverage was mandated by law) by cutting other federal health budgets.[15] The number of Americans with jobs providing health insurance declined; as the cost of individual private health insurance became prohibitive, women and children often went without immunizations and other basic preventive health care.[16]

Writing in the *Congressional Quarterly* in February of 1991, Julie Rovner noted that inflation for health care had grown faster than that for any other sector of the economy each year since 1981. By the early 1990s health-care costs made up 12 percent of the GNP. Between 1988 and 1990 alone, health insurance costs to business had increased by almost half (46.3 percent). Health programs' share of the *federal* budget had increased from 11.7 percent in 1980 to 14.7 percent by 1989.[17] If Medicare services to the elderly continued to grow at their current rate, Rovner observed, by the turn of the century Medicare alone would have a larger budget than Social Security or defense, currently the two largest items in the federal budget. By the year 2030 the number of Americans over 65 would double, with the number of persons over 85 years of age expanding from 2.5 million to perhaps 12 million, the number of persons requiring long-term care doubling and the number of persons requiring nursing home care quadrupling.[18]

Between 1970 and 1980, Medicaid's share of state budgets had grown from 4 percent to 9 percent of total outlays. By 1990, Medicaid's proportion had increased to 14 percent, with an additional 3 percent expected by 1995, when Congressional mandates to include preventive health services for low-income women and children would be implemented. States tried to balance their budgets by limiting the number of people accepted for Medicaid and by limiting Medicaid reimbursements to hospitals and doctors, thereby creating budget crises for health-care providers and a sharp adversarial struggle between state politicians and the health-care industry. During the economic recession of 1990-1991, a number of state governments reached funding crises that affected welfare recipients and state employees, as well as the Medicaid system itself.[19]

Health insurance companies and service providers also were under stress. Planning budgets were threatened by the growing costs of long term care of the elderly and by the costs of treating AIDS patients—rapidly growing populations far more susceptible to life-threatening emergencies than was true for the public at large. Efforts to control mounting costs by micromanaging all insurance claims did not stem the tide; instead it increased health-care costs. The administration of health-care claims cost $80 billion in 1990, 12.7 percent of the total health-care budget.[20] Meanwhile many health-care insurers, operating within the context of health-care service for profit, were denying coverage to Americans who might have higher-than-average health-care costs. Efforts to guarantee access to services through laws regulating insurance companies had only limited effectiveness, because many of the larger firms who provided health insurance coverage for their employees now were self-insured, and thus exempt from state-mandated health coverage options. (State laws now were adding as much as 20 percent to the cost of insurance premiums.) The situation, of course, was even more difficult for individuals who tried to purchase insurance independently. "Medical underwriting, experience rating, refusal to cover those deemed 'uninsurable,' cancellation of policies on short notice, and high premiums are common if not almost universal barriers for those seeking individual coverage," noted Emily Friedman in *JAMA*.[21]

Health Policy Issues of the 1990s

The policy debate of the early 1990s centered around four issues: (1) how to extend health insurance coverage to more Americans without creating a major cost escalation for the system as a whole (as had happened when Medicare and Medicaid were introduced); (2) whether to limit costs through the rationing of services—establishing "appropriate" standards of treatment for various diseases rather than maximum possible standards for care, or by establishing rationales for withholding various types of expensive services from particular population groups; (3) ways to influence market mechanisms that affect health-care access and cost, through the establishment of new rules for competition; and (4) ways to make current cost control mechanisms universal so that the entire health-care system had to adjust to them, rather than allowing various segments of the health-care industry to manipulate the market in order to avoid cost-limitation rules or to shift cost increases to areas of service not currently regulated.

The context for public policy debate was shaped by the conservative economic agenda introduced in the 1980s and discussed in Chapter Three. In this context, health care was viewed as a business, with profit maximization assumed to be an appropriate goal for health service enterprises. For-profit health care, and funding health services through private investment sources interested in returning a profit, were taken as "givens" in the health-care debates of the early 1990s. Problems that could not be addressed within this frame of reference often were ignored.

Health-care planners no longer assumed, as they had in the past, that American health care was the best in the world. The health status of Americans on various international health measures had been falling farther and farther behind that found in other industrialized nations.[22] The U.S. and the Union of South Africa were now the only two industrialized countries that did not guarantee access to basic health services for all their citizens. The issue of universal health insurance had been debated in health-care circles within the U.S. since 1917.[23] Finally, after 75 years, there seemed to be consensual agreement, for a time, that it was necessary.

The health-care systems of other industrialized nations were examined with new respect. Canada, Germany, and Japan all have universal health coverage for their citizenry but spend a smaller percent of the GNP on health care than does the U.S.[24] In 1980, West Germany and the U.S. each spent 9.4 percent of their GNP on health care. Ten years later, U.S. health-care costs had risen 33 percent faster than the GNP, while in Germany health costs had increased only 3 percent faster.[25] Comparative health-care costs were even lower in Japan[26] and Canada.[27] Nations vary in the formulas they use to calculate the percent of the GNP that goes for health care. Thus we should be cautious when comparing rates between countries. However, there is no question that other countries spend less per capita for health care than does the U.S. Japan, with the lowest cost per citizen for health care, also has the best health statistics, worldwide. Japanese men and women had the highest longevity; Japanese infant mortality was the lowest in the world.[28]

Federal planners found the German and Japanese systems particularly interesting because both provide work-based health insurance, supplemented by federally funded insurance for those who otherwise would not be covered. Unlike the U.S., however, third-party funders of health care and associations representing providers of services jointly negotiate annual costs, including fixed limits on total per-person costs that will be paid annually.[29]

Business leaders expressed considerable interest in the Canadian system, which relieves businesses of responsibility for administering health-care benefits. Canadian citizens pay a 7 percent tax on goods and services and businesses pay a 1 to 2 percent payroll tax (varying by province). These taxes, plus 13 percent of personal income taxes, fund health services and post-secondary education expenses. Health-care funding is administered by the provincial governments, which negotiate acceptable fees with physicians' associations and reimburse physicians directly for their charges. Canadian hospitals, rather than charging by the patient or by individual services provided, operate on an annual budget. It is negotiated with the Provincial Minister of Health and is based on their costs for the preceding year. The provincial government must approve new hospital construction and the purchase of high-tech equipment. The Canadian system appealed to businesses because of its simplicity, lower costs, and fixed, limited liability to businesses for the health-care costs of employees. Canadian business overhead is lower: there is no need for staff to oversee and administer health benefits, nor do budgets have to be readjusted annually because of increasing health insurance payments.

While businesses were calling attention to the virtues of the Canadian system, the AMA, uneasy about the lower incomes and weaker political position of Canadian physicians, was publicizing potential drawbacks of the Canadian health-care plan. They noted that Canadians tend to get put on waiting lists for such non-emergency matters as elective surgery, unless they pay for this privately. Waiting periods range between one and 72 weeks.[30]

The Canadian health-care plan's provisions exposed the increasingly adversarial interests of the business community and health-care providers. Because of this, and because the Canadian system also eliminates any role for the health insurance industry, which had provided the impetus for veto groups in earlier attempts to develop a national health insurance plan, most of the "political realists" who offered U.S. health reform plans largely ignored the Canadian model.

None of the three models for health care used in Germany, Japan, or Canada, however, fit the American scene exactly. All three countries differ from the U.S. in their mix and distribution of physicians within the population, an important factor affecting access to health care. All three have a higher proportion of physicians who provide general health care rather than specialized services, and they are distributed more equally within the population. The cost of medical education for students in these countries makes training accessible to a wider population group and lessens pressure to recoup education costs through high fees for services. Similarly, malpractice insurance costs are of a qualitatively different character in these systems, so that price negotiation with physician groups becomes easier. The three systems also are less complex in their organization of health-care providers; none involves the mix of per-capita and fee-for-service organizations found in the U.S. Where multiple insurance sources exist, their origins come from consumer groups rather than from service providers or for-profit business interests. Thus no country offers a blueprint for health care that would fit the American situation without some major changes.

After Michael Dukakis, the 1988 Democratic presidential candidate, made universal access to health care a central theme of his campaign, a number of federal agencies began to address the issue, including the Department of Health and Human Services, the Steelman Commission of the Social Security Advisory Council, and a joint committee from both houses of Congress. In addition, individual congressmen and various national policy groups began to make proposals, and fifteen state legislatures began to act on their own. The proposals that generated the most public attention and policy level support came from the bicameral Pepper Commission in Congress and from the state of Oregon.

The Pepper Commission

In 1988, Congress established the U.S. Bipartisan Commission on Comprehensive Health Care, popularly known as the Pepper Commission. Made up of six senators, six representatives, and three presidential appointees, it was asked "to develop recommendations for workable and enactable legislation that could resolve...the problems facing the health care system."[31] In September of 1990, after two years of hearings and discussion, the Pepper Commission issued its report. In the words of Senator John Rockefeller IV, one of the commission members:

> "The commission concluded that....health insurance coverage must be universal....We can neither patch nor replace current coverage. Rather, we must secure and extend the combination of job-based and public coverage we now have into a system that truly guarantees adequate coverage for all Americans and that ensures effective and efficient operation in private and public coverage alike."[32]

Although the Pepper Commission did not reach consensus on how to achieve these objectives, a majority report recommended that all businesses with more than 100 employees be required to provide coverage for all their workers and for their employees' non-working dependents. The private insurance market would be reformed by forming community risk pools for small businesses that seek health insurance. This guarantees access for small businesses and their employees to a minimum health benefit package at rates comparable to the insurance costs for larger companies. For a five-year period, small businesses were to be offered tax credits as an incentive to acquire health insurance for their employees. If small businesses had not done so within four to five years, they would be required to pay into a government health insurance program replacing Medicaid and including all persons not covered by private insurance through employers, using the same rules for reimbursement that apply to Medicare.

In the Pepper plan employees pay 20 percent of the costs for their health insurance. Preventive services are provided without co-pay requirements. Fifty percent of outpatient mental health services charges and 80 percent of the cost for other basic services are paid for by employers' insurance policies, once an initial deductible charge of $250 per person or $500 per family has been made. No individual or family, however, pays more than $3,000 per year in cost-sharing for medical services.

The entire federal system uses Medicare reimbursement formulas. A new federal Agency for Health Care Policy and Research collects data, sponsors outcomes research, and develops practice guidelines and quality assurance mechanisms that could help both public and private consumers of health-care services use their money wisely.[33]

The Debate Takes Shape

The Pepper Commission Report set the stage for serious debate of reform proposals, thereafter. The May 15, 1991, issue of *JAMA, the Journal of the American Medical Association* published Rockefeller's arguments in favor of the Pepper Commission majority report, along with a dozen alternative plans for reform sponsored by various interest groups within health care, including a proposal adopted by the AMA. Sponsors of the various proposals included the American Heritage Foundation, the Medical Schools Section of the AMA, the Urban Institute, Physicians Who Care, Physicians for a National Health Program, and U.S. Representative Edward Roybal, who argued for a national health insurance plan consolidating public and private health insurance into a single program, as in Canada, administered nationally by a new federal agency, the U.S. Health Administration.

Most of these proposals for universal coverage anticipated an overall increase in costs. To help the government subsidize costs for the poor, some plans lowered or eliminated current tax exemptions for health insurance benefits.

All plans included some kind of cost-containment strategy. Most included one or more of the following methods:

1. Lowering insurance premium costs for those who now are charged higher rates, either through community-wide rate setting or by setting up state wide pools to insure persons and groups currently lacking access to competitive insurance rates.
2. Requiring co-payment for individual services, to discourage overuse of the health-care system.
3. Making Medicare reimbursement formulas universal, so that different reimbursement systems could not be played off against one another.
4. Introducing negotiated payment levels established annually between payers and service providers, encouraging managed care budgeted at a per-capita rate rather than on the basis of the number and type of services provided.

5. Negotiating annual hospital budgets based on types of services provided in a given year, to replace the present fee-for-service remuneration for hospital services.
6. Saving on administration costs for health insurance by providing a single payer that reimburses on a capitation basis, with federal contributions tied to changes in the GNP.

These various methods differ in how they would contain costs. Some give consumers more responsibility for monitoring their need for services; others spread costs more evenly among all consumers. The rest give payers a larger role in negotiating which services are provided, at what cost, and/or simplify administration so that annual budgets can be calculated realistically.

While some plans involved government insurance programs, others mixed public-private insurance plans, and still others would absorb Medicare and Medicaid in the private market. The autonomy of service providers differed widely, as well. This is not the place to compare these individual proposals in detail, other than to note that each protected the particular interest of the group that sponsored it. Taken together, these proposals reflected the range of special interests that divide the American health-care system.

From Policy Discussion to Political Advocacy

The Health Care Reform bills introduced into Congress by the Democratic leadership in May and September of 1991 closely paralleled recommendations of the majority report of the Pepper Commission. During the 1992 Presidential primaries every Democratic candidate produced his own variation on health reform proposals and the incumbent Republican President, George Bush, announced his own plan for reform. It included a voucher system which poor families could use to pay for health insurance and tax credits to middle class tax payers to offset costs for basic health insurance. The winning presidential candidate, Democrat Bill Clinton, made health-care reform and reduction of the federal deficit twin centers of his campaign. Shortly after his election he announced the formation of a Health Care Reform Task Force, to be headed by his wife, Hillary Rodham Clinton, and co-directed by Ira Magaziner, a specialist in corporate reorganization and "bailout," and by Judith Feder, who had been staff director for the Pepper Commission and was now the principal U.S. Deputy Assistant Secretary of Health and Human Services, with responsibility for planning and evaluation. The Clinton Task Force invited over 500 public health academics, state health system staff members, and a few persons from other backgrounds to produce position papers, which the leadership of the Task Force would then accept or reject as a proposal was crafted.

As a bevy of proposals had surfaced all over the nation earlier, Paul Elwood had quietly convened an informal network of major figures in America's health-care industry. (Elwood, a major health policy adviser to Nixon and Bush, was considered the "father" of the public policy which created Health Maintenance Organizations—per-capita fixed fee, managed health care, which Nixon had sponsored.) The "Jackson Hole" invited-network of health-care elite met together monthly at Elwood's retirement home in Wyoming and began to explore their own preferred solutions to the current health-care crisis. They had become key advisers to President Bush and now assumed that role with the Clinton Health Care Reform Task Force. The "Jackson Hole Group" endorsed Alain Enthoven's argument that "managed competition" should become the new formula for joint government and private solution of national problems. In 1993, the Progressive Policy Institute, which had advised presidential candidate Bill Clinton in 1992, also had endorsed a plan that would rely on "managed competition" to reform health care. Magaziner and Hillary Rodham Clinton, both newcomers to health-care policy, accepted the recommendations to use "managed competition." It became the basis for the Clinton administration's health-care reform proposals.[34]

"Managed competition" represents a synthesis of liberal and conservative management philosophies. The liberal, New Deal, approach to social problems had involved an "activist stance" by government. The federal government identified major social problems that needed attention and intervened directly, using its resources to try to solve the problem. In contrast, the conservative policies followed by the Reagan and Bush administrations took government out of an active role as problem-solver, depending on the workings of the free market to deal with social problems. Both of these approaches had serious limitations: America's changing economic situation and declining tax revenue base now made depending on either state or federal tax revenues to finance social reforms problematic. On the other hand, free market approaches to problem-solving had produced vast inequities of access to health care and other services, as well as a serious federal deficit.

"Managed competition" would combine features of both strategies. The government would take an activist stance, identifying social problems that need addressing. Rather than depend on public funds and government bureaucracies to correct a problem, however, new laws would change the conditions for competition, so that a "managed market" would be motivated to act in ways that addressed social problems more creatively. Government agencies would monitor outcomes, recommending changes in regulations or new laws to provide incentives for private interests to act in ways that correct current social problems.[35]

The Clinton Task Force started with the general framework of the Pepper Commission majority report, adapting and enlarging it to restructure the American insurance market (i.e., creating managed competition) to encourage the following objectives: (1) to give all Americans access to basic health services; (2) to share the costs of doing this equitably; (3) to limit consumption of services so that costs would not become excessive; (4) to negotiate the best possible prices, consistent with high-quality care; and (5) to control the inflation of health costs over time.

The Task Force went to work, guided by these goals, the earlier work of the Pepper Commission, advice from "managed competition" advocates, and examples available from the successful health-care systems now operating in Germany, Canada, and Japan. Many Task Force participants favored federal regulation of health care as the most practical solution to the nation's problems, arguing for a single payer system similar to Canada's. When they discovered that the Clinton administration was committed to "managed competition" with the *market*, rather than federal regulation, as the major vehicle for reform, task force members adapted their proposals. Since the Clintons favored state by state experimentation as a way to discover in practice what works best, advocates of a single payer system focused their energy on making sure this could happen at the state level, designing legislative proposals that would free each state to develop its own approach to health-care reform, within broad federal guidelines. Eventually, a massive national plan for health insurance reform, running to 1,400 pages of detail, was prepared by the Task Force and proposed to Congress by President Bill Clinton in the fall of 1993.

Table 4-1 (next page) identifies which strategies the Clinton Plan intended to use to accomplish each of the goals stated earlier.

At the heart of the Clinton plan to reform health insurance lie three regulatory strategies. First, all employers are required to provide health insurance for their employees. This Employer Mandate provides the funding base for most health insurance. Tax subsidies reimburse businesses whose health insurance obligation become excessive (i.e., beyond 3.5% to 7.9% of their payroll, depending on the employer's average wage). Medicaid and Medicare continues to provide insurance for the elderly and those on public welfare.

Second, a National Health Board has power to oversee health spending budgets and standards for health-care provision. A guaranteed package of Health Benefits would be established. Health-care providers need approval from the National Health Board in order to be eligible for insurance reimbursements. To get this, they must provide a specified set of services and make service delivery available to all citizens in a large geographical region.

TABLE 4.1   Goals and Underlying Strategies in the Clinton Plan for Health
Insurance Reform

Goals	Strategies
1. Services for all	Providers eligible for reimbursement only if they a. provide region-wide delivery of services, and b. enroll all applicants for their service plan
2. Equitable cost-sharing	a. Employer Mandate to provide health insurance b. Employee co-pay (20%) c. Tax subsidies for • excessive employer insurance costs, and • insurance for the unemployed d. Community-rated premiums (the same cost for everyone in a community)
3. Discouraging Over-Consumption of Services and Resources	a. A guaranteed, but limited, benefits package of covered services b. Lower prices for plans that have a fixed annual cost for all services and which use professional "gatekeepers " to control use of benefits
4. Securing Reasonable Prices	a. Quasi-Monopoly Purchasing Alliances create a Buyer's Market b. Incentives for users to enroll in capitated payment plans (fixed annual cost)
5. Controlling Inflation over Time	a. National Health Board sets annual Global Budgets (in consultation with Congress) b. National Health Board vetoes price-bids if they will exceed the Global Budget

Third, the Clinton Task Force planned to create health-care purchasing alliances to negotiate rates and services charged to businesses and government for the employees' health-care benefits. Preferential rates would be offered for "managed care" plans with fixed per-capita charges. Cost incentives, thus, were to be used to move Americans out of fee-for-service relations with doctors in private practice and into "managed care" that could allow caps on third-party spending for health benefits.

Large employers could choose between continuing their existing benefits services or joining the health alliances; participation would be mandatory for smaller employers who, however, would gain the price advantages available to large employers (because the combined employee pool would spread risks of high cost medical care over more persons).

Insurers could only sell through the health alliances and would be prohibited from excluding coverage for pre-existing medical conditions. A single, mandatory, community premium rate was to be charged to all participants.

To guarantee that health-care inflation did not become excessive, the National Health Board would establish a Global Budget for total health spending, in consultation with Congress. The National Health Board could veto rate increase requests from providers, insurers, or purchasing alliances if they would produce national health-care spending that exceeded the established Global Budget.[36]

Responses to the Clinton Task Force Plan

When the Clinton Task Force proposals were announced, political conservatives expressed alarm at the degree of governmental regulation involved. They also were troubled by the extension of entitlements similar to social security to larger portions of the public. (In addition to creating ongoing federal obligations, they believed new entitlements would create additional patronage relations between the federal government and the private citizenry, relations likely to strengthen long-term loyalty to the Democrats who sponsored health-care reform.) Given widespread support for universal health-care coverage even among the more centrist Republicans and the public at large, however, this theme remained muted in the opposition strategies which followed.[37] Meanwhile physicians, managed care plans, insurance companies, and business interests responded in terms of their own potential gains and losses.

After the Clinton Task Force proposals were announced, health-care providers adopted a two-pronged strategy. Professional associations and business groups lobbied Congress for changes that would benefit them. Meanwhile, health-care providers began to regroup, forming new partnerships that could survive and thrive under the proposed new market conditions. Providers of health care were expected to serve *all* citizens of a region, including many who previously had been ignored or avoided. To protect themselves against catastrophic costs in caring for those now left out of their care networks, hospitals and HMOs should operate region-wide and have a very large pool of subscribers for their services. They also would need more primary care providers and less specialists than most hospitals now had on their staffs.

Inspired by the proposed changes, but independent of legislative action, a massive restructuring of health-care services began. Networks of service providers formed, with formerly competing hospitals and HMOs now entering into cooperative agreements that sharply reduced competition. Hospitals prepared for an upsurge of HMO enrollment, trimming their staffs to lessen the number of specialists, and hiring more primary care physicians, nurse-practitioners and allied primary care providers. If the legislation passed, they would be ready. If it did not, they would be in a stronger position to bargain with the business alliances that had formed in over ninety metropolitan areas. Meanwhile physicians found themselves in an increasingly defensive position; the oversupply of specialists left those physicians especially vulnerable. As hospitals tightened their lists of approved physicians, "old boy networks" influenced who remained. Minority physicians often found themselves left out of the smaller pools of approved physicians that were being kept by the new hospital-HMO alliances. HMOs increasingly bought up private physicians' practices, gaining greater control over the day-to-day practice of medicine.[38]

Congress Reworks the Plan

As these changes, inspired by legislative proposals but independent of the legislative process, began, a major struggle emerged in Congress over the Clinton health insurance reform proposals. One of the most trenchant, yet comprehensive analyses of the ultimate legislative failure of the health-care reform efforts set in motion by the Clinton Task Force has come from Sallyanne Payton, who had been legal counsel to the Clinton White House for health care and a member of the Clinton Task Force, as well as a consultant to the National Governors' Association and to various Republicans in Congress.[39] During Task Force deliberations Payton had predicted trouble in Congress, seeing a mismatch between the comprehensiveness of the President's proposal and the fragmented nature of Congressional decision making. When Congress created five committees to deal with health insurance reform rather than forming a single, joint committee to deal with this legislation, she has argued, chances for passage went down. Legislative responsibility was shared because various details of the comprehensive Clinton Plan fell within the jurisdiction of different committees of the House and Senate. This opened up greater opportunity for legislative disagreement while lessening the likelihood that a bill could be crafted and passed before a new congressional election. That is precisely what happened. One congressional committee rejected the Clinton proposal entirely reporting out a modified single payer plan which would fold all of the uninsured into Medicare, Part C. Other congressional committees working on health insurance reform became dominated by coalitions of more conservative Democrats and centrist Republican members who opposed a mandate that employers provide health insurance for their employees. These centrist Republicans were willing to look for methods to expand private health insurance coverage and were willing to find resources to support coverage for persons with low incomes. However, they wanted to keep employer freedom of choice and thus resisted both employer mandates to provide insurance and compulsory employer membership in giant purchasing alliances. They also distrusted global budgets set by the federal government.

The real death knell for the proposal, Payton believes, came when top officials of the largest corporations, whose health and benefits officers earlier had been supportive of Task Force efforts, did their own cost-benefit analysis of what they would gain and lose in terms of health benefits spending and taxes if the comprehensive insurance reform plan went into effect. They concluded it would cost them more than they would gain. Both the Business Roundtable and the Chamber of Commerce withdrew their support for the legislative proposal in February, 1994. With this loss of support it became difficult to push even modified forms of the Clinton legislative proposal for health insurance reform through Congress.

Many special interests began to attack the plan, but two had special impact on Congress. Small business associations predicted the Employer Mandate would raise the cost of doing business, forcing marginally profitable smaller businesses to eliminate a million jobs. Meanwhile, an association representing smaller insurance companies worried that the health insurance proposals would benefit the larger insurance companies but run the smaller ones out of business. The small insurance companies sponsored a series of nationally televised ads to raise doubts about many details of the plan with the American public.[40]

With these signs of growing opposition, congressional Republicans, sensing a moment of opportunity, decided to stall passage until after the 1994 Congressional elections.[41] A conservative coalition of right wing Republicans swept the election, a vote widely interpreted as a public response of "no confidence" in the regulatory focus of Clinton health reforms. The "Contract with America" espoused by the winning coalition of conservatives was endorsed by a voting electorate similar in size to the support incumbent President George Bush had received two years earlier when losing to challenger Bill Clinton; now the number of American voters choosing not to participate in this election gave conservative Republicans their chance to reshape basic government policy. Health-care reform would take a back seat. Incremental reforms, not comprehensive restructuring of health insurance, would be the order of the day. With one party in control of congress and another in control of the White House, each with quite different agendas, federal solutions to the health-care dilemma would be politically difficult.[42]

The Clinton proposals for health-care reform went down to defeat, but the national discussion the proposals generated had its own impact on private responses to the health-care cost challenges. In addition to the consolidation and centralization of control that was occurring among health-care providers, an important group of third party payers repositioned themselves.

Employers responding to the national debate about "managed care" as the route to cost control, increasingly restructured their employee benefits packages to push their employees to get health care from HMOs and other "managed care" preferred providers. By the end of 1995, 71% of all employees with private (third party-paid) health insurance were enrolled in "managed care" plans. Meanwhile both state and federal governments made plans to shift more of the Medicaid and Medicare patient load to "managed care" providers.[43] The health insurance reform debate accelerated trends that already were in motion, consolidating power and control among health-care providers and leaving "managed care" providers in position to structure market demand for services more generally. Thus the impact of the Clinton proposals for health insurance reform was profound, independent of its eventual fate in Congress.

Reforms of the 104th Congress

The 104th Congress was controlled by the right wing of the Republican party, whose policy agenda included ending deficit spending, reducing taxes, eliminating the federal welfare system and reducing the role of the federal government more generally, instead leaving it to the states to deal with their own social problems. Health-care reform had a much lower priority, but was not totally ignored. In fact, federal health-care spending became a target for budget reduction. Continuing the conservative economic policy of containing costs through supply side choices, Congress voted to limit federal spending for Medicare and Medicaid over a seven-year period and to set up economic incentives that would move more elderly Americans into managed care health plans. In the House of Representatives, conservative Republicans championed measures they believed would create market incentives for wiser consumption of health-care services by health-care "consumers". In these proposals current low-deductible health insurance would not be abandoned but would be challenged by the creation of medical savings accounts as an option for consumers who wished to make their own decisions about which services to purchase, and to keep any savings that might accrue if they did not over-consume.[44]

Instead of relying solely upon "gatekeepers" from the health professions to limit consumption of health services (as is done in "managed care") medical savings accounts would offer direct financial benefits to the health-care "consumer" for wise purchasing of services. The proposal raised a storm of controversy, with opponents raising two, quite different levels of objections. One set of opponents feared the medical savings accounts would encourage portions of the population to neglect early treatment of health problems, leading to lowered health for that portion of the population over time and to higher costs for treating the health problems at a later stage of illness. Other opponents feared that medical savings accounts would be chosen by the healthy but avoided by those most likely to have health problems. This would shrink the health insurance risk pool, sharply increasing the cost of health insurance for those who remained in it. The resulting rise in the cost of health insurance premiums, in turn, would lessen the number of businesses offering health insurance to their employees.

As the debate gained momentum, conservatives argued for an incremental approach to health-care reform, rather than for comprehensive restructuring of the total system. If universal access to services is the central problem to address, they argued, then address the problem, itself. There are a variety of reasons why different segments of the public lack access to basic health services, they insisted. Rather than develop a monolithic plan to deal with this problem, it would be preferable to introduce a series of incremental reforms, addressing each specific problem. Introduce small reforms and see how much of the problem has been met before doing more. Limit government subsidies for health care to the small core of uninsured who remain after incremental reforms have encouraged the market to make health insurance more accessible to the public. Table 4-2 (next page) identifies eight groups within the public who have difficulty getting basic health-care services, along with the proposals made in Congress to address their problems.

Between them, the various incremental reform bills introduced into the 104th Congress addressed access problems faced by six of the eight groups who currently have difficulty getting basic health-care services. Not surprisingly, given the political climate, the problems of middle-class Americans now left out of health care were addressed more effectively than the problems of the poor.

No proposals addressed the problems of unemployed Americans who do not have Medicaid nor of the working poor who lack health insurance. (After proposals to have an Employer Mandate to cover them met strong political opposition, their plight remained unaddressed.) It was not clear how well proposals to shift Medicare and Medicaid recipients into capitated payment plans would work, either for the recipients of care or for providers, who would now receive a fixed annual payment and become responsible for populations known to often have higher-than-usual needs for care. Reports from states that have tried this approach uncovered a number of care providers who offered minimal services while collecting the capitated payments.[45]

TABLE 4.2   Incremental Reform Proposals During the 104th Congress:
             Breaking Down Access to Care by Market Segment Affected

Who is Now Left Out?	*Proposals to Deal with This*
1. The Unemployed who are not on Medicaid	(Ignored in Incremental Reform Proposals)
2. The Working Poor who lack Health Insurance	(Ignored after failure of Employer Mandate)
3. People with Pre-existing Medical Conditions	Exclusion would be illegal (Bipartisan Senate Bill)
4. People Who Change Jobs	Portability of Insurance (Bipartisan Senate Bill)
5. Small Businesses and the Self-Employed	Include in Federal Employees Health Benefits Plan (Clinton Proposal) Voluntary Purchasing Pools (Bipartisan Senate Bill)
6. Many Medicaid and Low-Income Medicare Enrollees (because primary care physicians often will not accept government discounted payment rates)	Incentives for Medicare Enrollees to Join Capitated Payment Plans (Republican Proposals) Transfer Medicaid Recipients to Capitated Payment Plans (State Legislation)
7. Inner City Residents Who Lack Access to Primary Care Physicians	(Ignored)
8. Citizens Who Live Outside the Standard Metropolitan Areas	(Ignored)

In addition to addressing problems of access, supporters of incremental approaches to health-care reform also tackled the problem of cost containment. Resisting price controls, conservatives instead targeted sources of excess spending, applying "supply-side" strategies to lessen funds available to be used in these ways. Table 4-3 summarizes the proposals for cost containment under consideration in the 104th Congress.

TABLE 4.3   Incremental Reform Proposals During the 104th Congress:
Lowering Costs By Lessening Consumption of Health-Care Services

Targeted Source of "Excess Spending"	*Proposal to Reduce Expenditures*
1. **Federal Medicare and Medicaid Budgets for each of these programs (Deficit Reduction Bills)**	Set Caps on Federal Expenditures
2. **Providers Use of Benefits Packages**	Consumer Incentives: Voluntary Health Savings Accounts (Archer, McIntosh, Porter Bills, H of R)

Between them, the various incremental reform proposals tackled a wide range of access and cost issues. However, most of these problem-solving efforts had their own dangers. Budget reductions that ignore the content of services invite providers to withhold services rather than to provide needed services more effectively. Eliminating federal requirements that all persons below a poverty minimum have the right to health care, leaving servicing of the needs of the poor to the discretion of each state, almost surely would lead to lower services being provided the poor, and for many states, abandonment of some segments of the poor who did not have strong political clout or support. Encouraging the healthier, wealthier elderly to leave Medicare and/or to go into managed care plans would heighten the per-person costs for federal care to those who remained behind, lessening federal access to funds from the healthier elderly, fundamentally changing the character of the risk pool for whom government subsidy was required. Similarly, as noted earlier, offering optional medical savings accounts (as contrasted with shifting the entire health insurance market in this direction) also changes the risk pools for private insurance. The healthier choose medical savings accounts; those with high health costs stay with low-deductible insurance, as private businesses that have tried this have discovered. As a result, costs for the remaining health insurance risk pool become prohibitive, since only the more expensive users of health services remain in the risk pool. Moreover, one runs the danger that individuals and families strapped for cash will ignore early danger signs of health problems, using the money instead for other purposes.

Most of the proposals showed ignorance of how insurance markets work or of past experiments with similar proposals. Thus they threatened to increase current problems, rather than to resolve them. Similarly requiring insurance companies to cover all medical conditions without creating universal access to insurance seems sure to increase the number of people unable to afford health insurance. Premium costs must rise. As health insurance costs go up, the number of private employers who offer their employees health insurance plans goes down. Purchasing alliances that bargain for rates closer to those offered large employers would help, but how these two reforms would jointly affect the number of Americans having health insurance coverage was less clear. However, increasing the rates for insurance (to cover the costs of previously excluded conditions) and making Medicaid insurance an optional decision for state governments seemed sure to intensify the problems of low-income Americans, rather than to resolve them. Independent of their eventual legislative fate, these bills demonstrated the vulnerability of poorer Americans when incremental reforms are attempted that do not change the basic dynamic affecting health-care funding and delivery decisions.

Few members of Congress wished to face the 1996 elections having done nothing about health-care reform. The Senate passed the Kassebaum-Kennedy health insurance reform bill, a bipartisan "minimalist" package coming out of the Senate Labor Committee addressing concerns of middle-class voters: It guaranteed portability of insurance coverage from job to job, with minimal waiting time before eligibility for health insurance coverage went into effect for new employees. It made it illegal for health insurance companies to refuse coverage of pre-existing conditions. It also provided encouragement for the establishment of voluntary health insurance purchasing pools, so that small employers could join together to create large risk pools and be eligible for lower health insurance premium rates.

The House of Representative's health insurance reform bill introduced medical savings accounts as an option. President Clinton threatened to veto the health reform bill if medical savings accounts were included, arguing they would destroy the health insurance market. Conservatives in the House of Representatives refused to vote for a bill which did not include medical savings accounts. A compromise eventually was reached, allowing medical savings accounts among the self-employed, for a limited time period, to allow assessment of their impact on the health insurance market. In addition, the Health Insurance Portability and Accountability Act of 1996 (PL 104-91) required access to mental health benefits, and mandated development of a standardized, electronic billing and accounting system for the health-care industry.[46]

The reforms of 1996 seemed guaranteed to increase health insurance costs, and consequently to decrease the number of employers offering health insurance to their employees. The 25 million Americans who had no coverage for pre-existing medical conditions were benefited, however. What the balance of gains and losses would be for Americans covered by health insurance was unclear. It was quite clear, however, that the Kassebaum-Kennedy Health Insurance Reform Act of 1996 had not solved the basic problems affecting access or cost for the U.S. health-care system.

The 105th Congress. The 105th Congress added an additional $24 billion to the federal budget to provide health services to children from low income families without health insurance. This was an improvement, but still left millions of low-income Americans without funded access to health care.[47]

State Health-Care Reform

Meanwhile, 16 state legislatures were working on health-care reform legislation of their own. Several tackled directly the problem of providing access to health-care services for uninsured citizens in their state. One state had already done this. In 1971, Hawaii required all employers to provide health insurance for their employees and established community-wide health insurance rates that are uniform for all employers within a community. This legislation closely resembles the Pepper Plan. In addition, however, Hawaii established numerous public health clinics to guarantee access to primary health-care services to all state residents. With access to services guaranteed through these two provisions, Hawaii now has the lowest infant mortality rate and the highest life expectancy rate of any U.S. state. Perhaps because only two insurers have entered this market (Blue Cross-Blue Shield and Kaiser-Permanente), making enforcement of reimbursement rules simpler, costs for health-care services have increased more slowly than on the mainland. Heads of small businesses, however, have complained that the insurance law limits expansion of the Hawaiian economy. Hawaii's reforms preceded ERISA legislation. Other states, because of ERISA, are not free to follow Hawaii's example of a two-pronged policy (of universal employee health insurance plus easily accessible primary care facilities available to all) that makes the Hawaiian system effective.[48]

The most widely discussed state plan for health-care reform was crafted in Oregon. The Oregon plan dared to tackle the question of health-care rationing head-on, rather than approaching it by default. All citizens of Oregon would have access to a basic minimum of health-care services, but not to the maximum possible services. The state took responsibility for funding health services for people who lacked access to employer-based insurance or Medicare, but hoped to remain financially solvent by deciding what kinds of medical procedures would be available to persons whose health insurance was paid by the state. Oregon prioritized both types of treatment and categories of people who would have access to various subsidized services. Maternal and child health care, for example, would take precedence over expensive procedures for the elderly. Other expensive procedures like organ transplants would be available only to those who paid for them privately. Early plans called for public funding of care for AIDS patients to be phased out as the disease progressed, but this had to be revised later because of widespread objections. A basic minimum of care would be available to all citizens, rather than costly care for a few.[49]

National planners avoided the Oregon solution, arguing that needed services should not be withheld unless it becomes absolutely necessary. Because the American health-care system is much more expensive than those of several countries who cover all needed services for citizens, many planners argued that the U.S. also could pay for all needed services, if it eliminated unnecessary waste and duplication in health-care delivery. As the health-care reform debate went forward it seemed possible that the states would provide a natural laboratory for observing the consequences of different health insurance policies in action. A number of states abandoned their own health insurance reform bills, however, after the congressional election of 1994 stopped the national momentum for health insurance reform.

For a year or so after that election, a number of observers suggested that the public and private "managed care revolution" and the voluntary restructuring of the private market to adjust to capitated payment pressures would bring health-care cost increases in line with general inflation. However, that victory proved as short-lived as had previous cost containment efforts. By the end of 1995, two of the major health benefits management companies reported that costs once again were rising and that the annual cost of health benefits now averaged $3,821 per employee.[50]

Can Any of the Proposals Solve the Dilemma?

The last time national health insurance had been debated, in the mid-1970s, policy analyst Rick J. Carlson had urged Congress not to set up a national health insurance system. He argued that it would absorb all available funds and freeze in place an already antiquated approach to health-care problems, a disease-focused, curative medicine model of proven inefficiency. He had argued for a mixed medical model, that would combine conventional health-care services with more radical approaches to the causes of health problems and to the social-psychological-physiological interactions that are part of the health-disease process.[51]

Fifteen years later the broader health-care revolution that Carlson and others had tried to introduce and institutionalize still has not jelled. Now the increasing number of people left out of the health-care system, with no viable alternative for meeting their immediate health needs, creates another kind of health-care crisis for the nation. The health-care system's insatiable appetite for resources, and its ability to circumvent cost-control strategies, give a prescience to his earlier warning. Indeed, insurance is only one part of the problem, and cost estimates for reforming the system, which ignore known escalators of cost that will be arriving shortly—a spreading AIDS epidemic and an aging baby boom generation—give contemporary relevance to Carlson's earlier warning. Yet the growing number of persons with inadequate access to health care would make current advice to avoid national insurance, with no viable alternative in sight, unconscionable.

The challenge for policy analysts is clear. They must find a way to provide real access to health-care services for those most in need of them, while at the same time helping the nation move beyond the health-care industry's current approach to disease, which has created the cost and access problems.

A careful look at the range of proposals for health-care reform being discussed in the 1990s provides little grounds for optimism that effective cost containment will be possible under the kind of reforms now considered politically feasible.

Enlarging the base of the insured seems likely to escalate health-care costs still more, threatening the financial stability of states and federal governments and of business interests. Even more discouraging, the proposals for national health insurance coverage do not address access problems created by the distribution of physicians geographically, or by specialty, and the problem of race and class biases in medical practice. These problems will not be solved by the creation of new health insurance programs.

It is time to step back, looking more analytically at basic strategies for containing costs, maintaining quality, and guaranteeing access to services, noting how these underlie the range of proposals currently under debate. Can any of these approaches solve the problems we face? Or all of them together? Or is a still more basic strategy needed? If so, what might it be like and what must it accomplish? Chapter 5 explores these questions.

5

Contending Strategies for Reform: Underlying Principles, Unanticipated Consequences, and Unmet Problems

Most Americans share a common set of values about health-care reform—i.e., that everyone should have access to health care, that it is important to contain costs, and that reforms should not diminish the quality of care they now receive. They differ, however, in the priorities they set when these values compete with one another. They also differ about what kinds of strategies for problem-solving actually work. In the debates that rage currently, battle lines often get drawn by forcing analysis of health care into pre-existing formulas for broader problem-solving, including especially arguments about the advantages and disadvantages of federal regulation or market competition. As a consequence, the range of potential solutions under discussion gets artificially constrained.

Health-care reform advocates have split into three camps. Some want a national health-care system similar to that in Canada. (The Canadian system leaves provision of services in private hands but funds it through public taxes. All citizens have guaranteed access to health-care services. Provincial governments regulate prices and reimburse health-care providers.) Others want to rely on a free market to supply services for which there is sufficient demand. Most, however, have tried to reform the present mix of *public and private* financing for health-care services, while leaving the provision of services in the private market.

Advocates of a Canadian-style health-care system make access to services for everyone the highest goal, and are willing to levy new taxes to fund this and use government regulation as the route to cost control. Advocates of free-market approaches give access lower priority, stressing the importance of cost-efficient care that encourages economic prosperity. Consequently they oppose new taxes and endorse measures to encourage flexibility and innovation among health-care providers (which they believe government regulation discourages). They point to failures in trying to force health-care professionals to obey regulations that conflict with professionals' own basic values—i.e., providing the highest possible standards of care and preserving their own income. Rather than embark on what they see as a lost cause of trying to regulate the providers of care in the name of cost control, advocates of free market approaches to health-care reform look to supply-side economic policies: Limit the supply of money available from various funders and let individual providers of care adapt to the new circumstances innovatively!

Neither of these ideological perspectives has carried the day. The frozen tax base of the 1980s and 1990s has limited government income, and the public has demonstrated its hostility to new forms of taxation. Moreover, a broader public policy move toward *deregulation* of business, widespread doubts that regulators can ever effectively control the regulated, and the emergence of conservative political coalitions in both the Republican and Democratic parties, have left advocates of a Canadian-style health-care system for the United States in the minority. Meanwhile, evidence has grown that "the market" heads toward opportunities for maximum financial gain rather than public service, if left to its own devices. The constantly increasing recruitment of new physicians into higher paying medical specialties rather than into primary care delivery, the down-sizing of the American hospital system to increase profitability rather than to guarantee access for all the population, and the continuing growth in the number of Americans who lack access either to funding for medical expenses or to care itself, point up the limits of free-market solutions to problems of access to health-care services.

The majority of health planners, consequently, have opted for a middle route, acknowledging the political constraints and practical problems that block development of a Canadian-style health-care system, and the inadequacy of coverage that results when one leaves everything to the free market. They have sought a mix that lies somewhere between these two principles, often finding somewhat awkward compromises between regulation and free market strategies, or between containing costs and guaranteeing access to care.

Chapter 4 focused attention on strategies that advocates of "managed competition" recommended in the early 1990s as solutions for the American health-care crisis. The Clinton Health Insurance Reform Task Force, building on the earlier work of the Pepper Commission, tried to create a comprehensive plan that would leave intact the mosaic of interests in the American health-care industry, but redirect them toward achieving better solutions to the following five goals: (1) giving all Americans access to basic health-care services; (2) sharing the costs of doing this equitably; (3) limiting consumption of services so that costs do not become excessive; (4) negotiating the best possible prices that are consistent with high quality of care; and (5) containing the inflation of health-care costs over time. Their proposals combined strategies used by regulatory, single-payer health-care systems (such as that found in Canada) with other strategies proposed by those who believe health care works best when organized as a competitive, free market. The Clinton Plan's overall strategies borrowed much from the German and Japanese health-care systems, each of which combines features of both regulatory and free-market traditions. Perhaps not surprisingly, advocates of single-payer plans found the Clinton proposals overly cumbersome and accommodating to established interests in health care. Free market advocates, in turn, were appalled by its ultimate reliance on regulation and bureaucratic supervision.

It is time to move beyond the politics of these unfolding events and to look more carefully at the three contending strategies for health-care reform. How are they similar? In what ways are they different, with what implications for health care? For the public? What principles do they use when pursuing the five goals articulated by the Clinton Task Force's plan? What consequences might we expect if national health-care policy was able to pursue any one of these three approaches in a consistent manner? Would unmet problems remain? If so, how would unmet problems differ between the three approaches? What additional questions need to be asked if we are to find a more workable solution to the current dilemmas of American health care? These are the questions this chapter will address.

Single-Payer Plans

Canada, like Sweden and other governmentally-regulated, single-payer health-care systems, makes access to basic health-care services for every citizen a high priority. Adequate care for all takes precedence over the highest possible standard of quality in service delivery, when limited resources bring these two goals into conflict. This seems to work. All these health-care systems outrank the U.S. on a number of measures of the health status of the population as a whole.

It is not clear that these better health outcomes result from funding and organization of health services. There are also important differences in the total population's access to education, employment, nutrition, and housing. Nonetheless, there are important and striking differences in how health services are made available to the public. In Canada, the government pays for medical care, taxing both personal incomes and business operations to get the necessary funds. As the single payer for services, provincial health departments set the terms under which payment will be made. Hospitals must provide services to any citizen who comes to them. Rather than bill the government for each patient (as happens in the U.S. with Medicare and Medicaid) hospitals are given an annual budget, based on their operating costs the preceding year, plus any upgrading of services or equipment that is approved by the provincial health department. Private physicians bill the provincial government for services performed and in turn take responsibility for the care of particular patients. The provincial government sets the fees they will be paid for these services, after negotiations with physicians' organizations.

Table 5.1 provides a brief overview of how government-regulated, single payer systems organize their resources to meet the five goals articulated by the Clinton Task Force planners. An asterisk identifies features of the strategy that are shared in common with the Clinton version of managed competition. Single-payer plans have the virtue of simplicity in organization, in funding sources, and clarity in lines of authority. Principles underlying the strategies that are used to achieve each goal for health-care reform require little explanation, other than to explain that in the Canadian model hospitals receive annual budgets, rather than reimbursement for particular patients, and are required to serve all who come to them. These budget constraints slow the acquisition of high-tech equipment in Canadian hospitals. In order to operate within their budget constraints Canadian hospitals also have explicit triage rules for handling medical emergencies and more optional care. Persons wishing to have elective surgery, for example, often must wait their turn—sometimes for many weeks or months. Other kinds of care seem to be superior to that in the United States: Pregnancies and births, for example, receive high priority for treatment and care is given without additional cost to the family.

TABLE 5.1   Goals and Underlying Strategies Used in Single-Payer Plans

Goals	*Strategies*
1. Services for All	Hospitals Serve All Who Come (Primary Care Maldistribution Not Addressed)
2. Equitable Cost-Sharing	Taxes* (taxes on goods and services, payroll taxes, personal income taxes)
3. Discouraging Over-Consumption of Services and Resources	A. Benefits Package* B. Hospital Annual Budgets C. Triage Rules for Services
4. Securing Reasonable Prices	Enforced by Single Payer
5. Cost-Management Through Time	A. Global Budgets* B. Provincial Health Board Rations Technology

Critique

Some observers have worried that a Canadian-style system would lead to lower standards of care for Americans. It is not at all clear that the overall quality of care suffers under this kind of system; nonetheless the constraints imposed by single-payer budgeting would force some adjustments in the kinds of care given some Americans—as is also happening under the broad imposition of privately run managed care plans. Some rationing of care will occur under both systems. The Canadian approach, however, is vulnerable to another level of criticism. It lacks strategies for dealing with some unsolved problems of the American health-care system that affect access to care.

The Canadian model presents no simple way to deal with the severe maldistribution of service providers found in the United States. Not only does the U.S. have an oversupply of medical specialists, but *all* doctors are in short supply outside the standard metropolitan areas, and few physicians provide primary care services for poorer neighborhoods of the metropolitan areas.[1] Some advocates of a single-payer system argue for a national health-care system in which health-care professionals would be government employees, who could be assigned to locations of need. Others argue for subsidizing all medical education (as is done in a number of other countries) in return for tours of duty in underserved areas as part of debt repayment. Neither of these proposals, however, nor the more general strategy of having a single payer set health-care policy, suggests how such a system in the U.S. would secure cooperation from health-care professionals and service institutions. Not only their income but their professional standards and personal autonomy, as well, would be challenged by these kinds of rules for payment and for service delivery. In the past U.S. health-care professionals have been able to subvert the intent of various control measures imposed on them. A single-payer system, consequently, would need to develop effective strategies for gaining the cooperation of health-care professionals. Control of payment is not sufficient to secure the active cooperation of a professional group.

An equally serious challenge would be that of securing a sufficiently large tax base to fund health-care costs. For the past quarter century national and international political and economic developments have eroded the American tax base. Public opinion polls suggest that Americans would be willing to increase taxes in order to make sure everyone has access to health care. It is not clear, however, that there is widespread public support for major tax increases to fund the entire health-care system.

If the Canadian model were used in the United States, its advocates say, a number of current problems would be solved. Costs would be lower because the health insurance industry no longer would add its margin of profit to health-care expenditures. Setting annual hospital budgets would slow the growth of the sector of the American health-care industry that has set the pace for cost-increase. Business would be freed of responsibility for administering health benefits.[2] (Businesses would still have to figure health-care costs into production costs, however, since they would pay taxes to help support health services.)

Advocates of a single-payer system argue that Americans would be willing to pay higher taxes if their overall household expenses went down. Much of the income for the Canadian health-care system comes from value-added taxes rather than from personal income tax. This affects the price of goods rather than coming as a direct assessment from the government affecting private households. Since overhead costs for health benefits already affect the price of goods, advocates argue that it should not affect prices nor the competitiveness of American-made goods on the international market and thus would not be experienced by American citizens as a burdensome tax that came directly out of their paychecks. A single-payer system could lower health-care expenditures, advocates argue, as well as eliminate insurance profits as part of health care and it would remove layers of administrative bureaucracy in private business and the government now devoted to the complexities of administering the American health-care system. These cost savings should be more than sufficient, they insist, to allow wage increases that would offset any small additions in personal income tax that might come if Canadian tax formulas were used.

Critics of single-payer plans warn, however, that the projected economies would have serious consequences of their own. Since hospitals have been an important growth leader in the U.S. economy, and are a major employer, stopping their economic growth would have repercussions throughout the economy. The problem with hospital costs is not that they keep going up, these critics argue, but rather that they go up as a captive cost to business, government, and private households. As hospitals prosper, consequently, other interests are put in jeopardy. If hospital growth came from free consumer choices that did not require business or governmental subsidy, they argue, there would be no problem so long as the entire public had access to the services they needed. We have to be careful, they continue, not to weaken the economy in the name of health-care cost control.[3] That logic extends, as well, to contraction of the insurance industry.

Other critics note that if a single-payer system on the Canadian model were adopted, business would be largely removed from the health-care playing field—an institutional interest group that has sponsored fundamental innovations in health-care delivery and cost containment. Government has played a very different role, and the health-care industry itself is focused in another direction. Perhaps Americans should think twice before advocating the removal of business as a major institutional player in health-care change, they warn.[4]

In addition to these objections and defenses of a single-payer plan, some observers voice an additional concern. They note that in the U.S. political system those being regulated often end up controlling their supposed regulators. (Regulated industries regularly hire government officials when their terms of service with the government ends, and they also are skillful at crafting agendas for negotiation that produce governmental decisions to their liking.)[5] This perspective produces skepticism that single-payer strategies could produce either the cost savings or more "consumer-oriented" service delivery in the U.S.

Again, noting the past ability of health-care providers to circumvent efforts to regulate their behavior, some doubt that government directives would succeed in getting American physicians to shift locations for practice or their medical specialties in order to provide for the health needs of the currently underserved. Thus they question the ability of a single-payer system to deal effectively with problems arising from the current maldistribution of physicians in the American health-care system.

Both defenders and opponents of single-payer plans for American health-care reform agree that there are limits to what a single-payer system could accomplish. A single-payer plan seems unlikely to make major inroads on the maldistribution of health-care services in the U.S. Nor, given the current strong opposition to single-payer plans among many American health-care providers and their professional associations, is it clear how a single-payer system could secure the cooperation of health-care providers and institutions, who are in a position to undercut reform goals.

Even in Canada, where institutional relations have a different history, opponents point out, the single-payer system has not succeeded in its efforts at cost control. Canada's health-care costs are second only to those of the U.S., and Canadians are cutting back on their benefit packages in an effort to limit cost increases. In short, despite some real advantages, single-payer models also have serious difficulties.

Currently, the political prospects for a single-payer plan do not look promising. Some observers greet this observation with relief. Instead of supporting a single-payer solution to America's health-care dilemma they advocate a more sophisticated use of competition, of market incentives and of market force to motivate physicians, hospitals, and other health-care providers to provide services where they are most needed, at a competitive price. The great advantage of market incentives, they argue, is that people act in terms of their own self-interest and thus do not try to outsmart the system or circumvent its goals.

Market Competition

More conservative policy analysts resist government regulation as a route to reform. Instead they rely on the creation of incentives that will motivate innovators to provide needed services for less cost as a way of furthering their own financial wellbeing. They prefer to let innovation emerge from the normal dynamics of market activity whenever possible, but they are willing to use legislation to make it more likely that this will happen.

The following strategic approaches are favorites among those who advocate market competition as the best route to reform. First, they favor supply-side approaches to cost containment: limit the amount of money available, and let providers innovate to offer more services than their competitors for that amount of money. Second, they prefer to leave innovation to the private market, rather than to regulate it. They do, however, favor using public funds to increase possibilities for profitable innovation. Because of these preferences, they often leave untouched those problems for which market solutions have not yet appeared, such as getting services to the unemployed or to the working poor who now lack access to primary health care; they want to disturb market dynamics as little as possible. Table 5.2 summarizes the strategies for health-care reform currently sponsored by advocates of free market competition. The principles of using incentives and shared risks to motivate behavior lie at the heart of many market competition strategies for health-care reform.

TABLE 5.2   Goals and Underlying Strategies in Free Market Plans

Goals	Strategies
1. Services for All	(Strategies Vary by Market Segment that is currently left out of the market) A. (Voluntary) Purchasing Pools* B. Provider Incentives* (Medicaid to Capitated Payment) C. No strategies for working poor or unemployed not on Medicaid
2. Equitable Cost-Sharing	(Often Ignored)
3. Discouraging Over-Consumption of Services and Resources	A. Managed Care* B. Consumer Incentives (Health Savings Accounts)
4. Securing Reasonable Prices	A. (Voluntary) Purchasing Pools* B. (Capitated) Payment* C. Shared Risk (High Deductible Insurance)
5. Cost-Management Through Time	Market Competition

These ideas may be less familiar to some readers than the more intuitively obvious regulatory strategies of a single-payer system. Put most simply, market incentives involve opportunities for financial gain that make one behavior more attractive than another. Negative incentives involve threats of loss if particular organizational behaviors are chosen or continued.

Shared risk is a more complex market strategy used to divide potential gains and losses equitably and it is used to set insurance premium costs. An accident, illness, or the like can involve high costs. Insurance protects against financial loss at such times. If the risk of loss is shared between the insurer and the insuree by requiring a high deductible before insurance benefits begin, the annual premium costs less. Both parties share the risk of loss, and both gain in years when no claims are filed. (That year, the insurance company keeps the premium and pays out nothing on this contract, but the insuree pays less *every* year than if the policy protects fully against possible loss.) This principle applies to all insurance, including health insurance. High deductible policies cost much less than policies which reimburse for all health costs, because the insured assumes some of the financial risk for illness. How market-oriented policy advisers would use incentives and shared risk to reform health care is discussed below.

Provider Incentives

If providers are neglecting a segment of the public one can create either positive or negative incentives for them to get services to these people. An offer to put all Medicare and Medicaid enrollees into HMOs creates a positive incentive for capitated payment plans to enroll this population—if they think they can serve the total Medicare and Medicaid population for less than the capitated payment that is offered.

Many market advocates dislike health-care agreements which include Benefits Packages that guarantee payment for treating all health problems—or even a designated list of health problems. These create a positive incentive for *providers* to use more expensive treatment options, cynics argue, a "pork barrel" of services that providers are free to prescribe with full assurance they will be repaid. Professional medical ethics call for the highest standard of care for every patient, which encourages a preference among medical professionals for costly "state of the art" diagnostic and treatment interventions. When combined with a guaranteed benefits package, this creates strong incentives to use "the best"—whether or not less expensive alternatives would work just as well. As protection against this tendency, some capitated payment plans have created their own counter-incentives for the physicians who act as "gatekeepers" in primary care plans (i.e., for those who must approve referral to specialists, use of more expensive diagnostic tests, referral to hospitals, or other higher-than-usual expenses). Some capitated payment plans now withhold about 15 percent of a physician's salary or expected fees until the end of the year. This, then, gets treated as a "merit increase". Physicians whose patients cost less than the average receive a larger proportion of these funds. Those whose patient care costs were higher than usual get less than average from the pool.[6] This controversial practice creates an incentive to withhold expensive care unless it is critical for the patient's health.

Consumer Incentives

When the bill is paid by a third party, there is little incentive for a patient to question the need for services, thus leaving decisions entirely in the hands of the medical professional. Two strategies are widely used to give consumers more incentive to use only the services they need. First, research has shown that requiring a co-payment by the patient each time care is received acts as a deterrent to consulting a medical professional about minor matters. The lower the income, the higher the deterrent from a co-pay charge for an office visit.[7] Asking patients to pay 20 percent of their medical costs, with an upper limit of liability, represents a further extension of the principle of using negative incentives to discourage overconsumption.

Health savings accounts represent a positive incentive for individual consumers of health services to make economical choices. Health savings accounts are set up for employees, who then pay for all services they receive up to a fixed maximum (e.g. $2,000 or $3,000 per family). Insurance covers services beyond that amount. When less is spent in a year, the individual or family can keep the balance of the account for personal use. Only one family in eight spent $2,000 in 1992 for medical services in the larger metropolitan areas, and only one family in eleven spent that much in the less-expensive metropolitan areas. Moreover, only one family in eleven spent $3,000 that year for medical services in the more expensive metropolitan areas and only one family in 16 did so in the other metropolitan areas.[8]

With health savings accounts employees receive a larger portion of their wages in cash rather than in payment for insurance premiums. The possibility of converting health benefits into personal savings creates an incentive to use fewer medical services. Health savings accounts also save administrative costs, since most households spend less than the insurance deductible, and thus pay for services directly rather than submitting insurance claims for their health-care expenses. Conservative Republicans, seeking a reform that puts more decision-making directly in the hands of the individual consumer, introduced three bills into the 104th Congress to allow health savings accounts as a supplement to catastrophic insurance coverage.[9]

The proposals faced wide opposition. Labor unions and some public health professionals opposed the idea, arguing that it would encourage poorer health and more expensive health-care expenditures in the long run—they argued that individual health-care consumers, unable to judge what they do and do not really need for good health care, would be tempted to postpone early services that could identify health problems while they are simple to treat. Colleges, businesses, and other organizations that had experimented with the idea warned that its optional use could destroy the insurance market. Some had tried giving employees a choice between using conventional health-care insurance or health savings accounts backed up by catastrophic insurance. The healthy opted for the health savings accounts while persons with ongoing health problems opted for conventional insurance. This destroyed the insurance pool, making insurance premiums prohibitively expensive.[10] (Insurance prices are set by spreading the risk of expensive use of the policy over a large pool of people. The premiums paid by people who make no use of their insurance, or minimal use of it, cover the costs generated by those people whose claims far-exceed the amount of money they have personally paid in premiums. If the low-users of insurance all leave the insurance pool, those who remain are people whose costs typically exceed the amount of premiums they have been paying. Consequently the price of insurance premiums has to increase sufficiently to cover their expenses. The net result is that health-care costs more in total: the healthy get back their portion of insurance costs that previously helped pay for persons who were sick; meanwhile, the cost of care for persons in poor health remains the same, requiring a larger outlay for health benefits.)

It would be possible to modify proposals for health savings accounts to make a combination of health savings accounts plus catastrophic insurance the standard form of health insurance. This would preserve the insurance pool necessary to keep premiums affordable. Conservative advocates of health savings accounts, however, have been ideologically committed to freedom of choice. Thus this alternative has not been strongly considered.

There are, in short, a variety of ways to use incentives to reduce tendencies for both health-care providers and health-care consumers to overconsume services. Each proposal has both advantages and clear risks.

Shared Risk as a Strategy for Lowering Costs

An even more controversial strategy to encourage better use of health-care resources transfers the entire responsibility to pay for most day-to-day health-care costs back to individual households. Insurance only pays for catastrophic health-care costs, rather than for more routine care. Policies that require a high deductible before reimbursement is paid—i.e., those that involve shared risk between insurer and insuree—cost considerably less than policies that cover most expenses. Thus the cost of insurance to third party payers would be considerably less. Health insurance premiums go down rapidly as the deductible goes up because only a few households have high medical expenses in any given year. If one can afford the risk, buying insurance with a high deductible can save considerable money. Conservatives in Congress earlier recommended substituting "catastrophic insurance" for the present low-deductible insurance for Medicare recipients with higher incomes. Popular outcry against losing a Medicare entitlement and increasing the amount of unprotected risk that each family would have to absorb made such legislation impractical.[11]

For the employed population there are ways to combine shared and protected risk so that *employers* bear more risk (and potentially share in the cost savings) rather than individual households. In 1994, for example, a number of small businesses in Michigan bought high deductible health insurance policies for their workforce. The *employer* paid the first $1,000 of health-care costs for an individual employee, or $2,000 for a family, before insurance reimbursement began. (Some shared this deductible cost with the employees, others paid for it themselves.) The annual cost of health insurance premiums was $600 less for each family covered. Employers absorbed a risk that they might spend $1,400 more than they normally would for some families before insurance reimbursement went into effect (i.e., they took responsibility for any expenses up to the $2,000 deductible for each family, minus the $600 premium reduction for that family). Most employers reduced that risk to themselves further, by requiring the family to pay $200 to $300 of the deductible before they could receive reimbursement from either the employer or the insurance company. Employers who bought this high-deductible health insurance gambled that most families would have medical expenses that were lower than the deductible, so the employer's total spending would be less. That gamble paid off: Cambridge Partners, one of the early companies to use this plan, reported a 44 percent reduction in health benefits costs during the first two years of participating in the new plan.[12] As this news spread among employers, high-deductible health insurance became a popular option among small businesses in Michigan. Since both the employer and the employee remain protected against *catastrophic* health-care costs if a major health problem develops, overall savings are likely to continue, despite variations from year to year in how much risk the employer actually absorbs.

In this example of how shared and protected risk can be recombined, employers become the major risk-taker, and potential gainer from shared risk. Under these circumstances they have an incentive to bargain for lower rates for services and to encourage employees to make prudent use of them. Variations on this strategy can also be used to increase *employee* incentives to use services wisely. For example, it would be possible to reduce employee co-deductibles, or to share savings with employees, as health-care costs go down. If this were done, both employer and employee would have motivation to use health care wisely. Shared and protected risk, in short, can be regrouped in a variety of ways to decrease over-utilization of disease-care services. Some put individual households at risk while others do not.

Critique

Market-oriented approaches to reform have one major advantage over regulatory approaches: Those who participate in the reforms do so out of a sense of self-interest, convinced that they have a chance to improve their own situation. Regulatory approaches, in contrast, can feel coercive to those who do not share the social values that lie behind the regulatory intent. Self-interest can motivate the regulated to evade or "outsmart" the system, in order to protect or improve their own situation. This advantage of the market approach, however, also creates a dilemma. Market-oriented strategies do not work well for getting goods and services to the entire population. The market rarely works to the advantage of everyone. There are winners and losers, as the principle of shared risk makes clear. The market-oriented strategies for health-care reform listed above could work well for some segments of the population, while leaving the poor little better off, or perhaps worse. Some proposals, including especially shared risk market proposals that provide positive incentives to avoid use of health-care services, could inadvertently lead to worse health and to more costs for disease care.

These problems with market-oriented health-care reform, most observers agree, are quite serious. Some, however, believe these problems are not insurmountable. There could be ways to combine shared and protected risk, they suggest, and to build safety nets into some of the potential cost-saving strategies. It also might be possible to combine market approaches for segments of the population that are not financially vulnerable with more protected strategies for lower-income populations.

We should not dismiss market strategies out-of-hand, any more than we should dismiss the concerns and advantages found in single-payer systems. We must understand, however, that market-competition approaches to health-care reform often involve substantial risks both for gain and loss. If market strategies are to be used, they must be chosen with great care, and with full awareness of vulnerabilities that must be protected.

Managed Competition

As these approaches are now spelled out, neither regulatory single-payer plans nor market-competition approaches to health-care reform seem likely to solve the problems confronting Americans. What happens when one combines the approaches? As Table 5.3 makes clear, the "managed competition" approach articulated in the Clinton Task Force Health Reform proposals borrowed evenly from both of these traditions. Of its eight key proposals, half were shared in common with single-payer plans. The other half came from market-competition strategies.

How the Clinton Task Force proposed to use these elements to secure access to care for all Americans at a reasonable cost was discussed in Chapter 4. The proposal used both positive and negative market incentives. Consumers got lower prices if they chose capitated payment service plans that offered "managed care." They had a negative incentive to use unnecessary services: they would pay 20 percent of the cost of any services used, except for some preventive care. (There was, however, a maximum annual liability per family.)

TABLE 5.3   Comparing the Three Approaches

	Strategies		
Goals	Single Payer	Managed Competition	Market Competition
1. Services for All	Hospitals Serve All Primary Care??	Region-wide Providers must Serve All	Does not address
2. Equitable Cost-Sharing	Taxes	Employer Mandate Employee Co-Pay Community-Rating Taxes Supplement	Often Ignored
3. Discouraging Over-Con-sumption of Services	Benefits Package Hospital Annual Budgets with Triage Rules	Benefits Package Managed Care	Savings Accts. Managed Care
4. Securing Reasonable Prices	Single Payer Enforces Price	"Monopoly" Purchasing Alliance Capitated Payment	Voluntary Purchasing Pool Capitated Payment
5. Cost-Management	Health Board Global Budget	Health Board Global Budget	Market Competition

Similarly, providers of care were motivated to reach out to now-avoided populations through a negative incentive: If they did not offer services to the entire geographical region of a purchasing alliance, and accept all enrollees who applied, most providers would be ineligible to compete for the rest of the market. The positive incentive for *individuals* to choose capitated payment plans became a negative incentive pressuring *physicians* to offer primary care services: Most specialists would have to affiliate with capitated payment plans to survive. Since there are now more specialists than are needed, some would lose their current source of income and would have to switch to primary care.

The Clinton Plan used a three-pronged market strategy to keep prices at a reasonable level. First, purchasing alliances would hold near-monopoly control over access to the purchasers of services, and they could refuse to consider bids for services from providers who set prices beyond a level acceptable to the National Health Board.[13] Second, employers would have to offer employees three competing service plans, but could choose which three to offer.[14] Third, the 20 percent co-pay required each time individuals used health-care services, except for some preventive services and the annual maximum liability, would help discourage frivolous use of health-care services by individual households.

However, the three elements of the Clinton Task Force plan for "managed competition" which were most critical for its operation all relied ultimately on regulatory power. The Employer Mandate would make employer-funded health insurance a legal requirement, rather than optional, as at present. The purchasing alliances that secure common health insurance prices for firms of different sizes would be quasi-monopolies. Everyone who marketed health-care services or insurance in a given geographic area thus had to do business with a single alliance. The National Health Board established global budgets for health-care spending and would be empowered to veto price bids if services would cumulatively exceed the global budget. Thus despite some elements in common with a market-oriented approach, the Clinton Plan relied ultimately on regulatory strategies. This version of "managed competition" could not secure sufficient political backing to become law. If it had, it is not clear that it could have succeeded in getting services to all without a major cost increase.

Critique

A key element of the Clinton approach to cost containment seemed likely to increase rather than decrease prices over time. In order to get services to everyone in a geographic region, the Clinton Plan would require health-care providers to offer services throughout a purchasing alliance's geographical area. They would have to include high cost users of care in their plan along with everyone else. Health-care providers, thus, would need to enroll large numbers of people, so that the costs of serving now-avoided groups would be balanced out by the costs of serving others who need little care. Only large provider networks could do this. Thus only a few large providers would survive in each metropolitan area. Competition among providers, consequently, would be minimal. Under those circumstances there will be little market incentive for providers to offer services at substantially lower costs than competitors are charging.

With everyone paying the same community rate for services, and only a few competitors setting prices, critics predicted, costs would rise to the top of the level acceptable to the National Health Board. Patients' 20 percent co-pay requirements would be the only real disincentive for costs to rise, and relying on this for cost containment is a risky strategy: many patients defer to their doctor's judgment when a diagnostic test, referral, or treatment is recommended. Low-income families would be the most likely to ignore doctors' recommendations, but often to their detriment; cost rather than judgment about the personal utility of the service would motivate their choices. Managed care provides no solution to this dilemma. In a market with few competitors, managed care gatekeepers can preserve the profit margin of service providers by withholding unneeded services, but this is not likely to lower the overall *price* of care. The combination of community rated premiums and large provider networks, thus, creates an open invitation to cost increase. The National Health Board could veto rate increase requests, but Congress would be free to change the ceilings on the Global Budget for health-care expenditures. One can count on heavy political pressure from health-care providers to increase the spending ceiling. If these pressures are resisted, and providers are given capitated payments, they are likely to respond by decreasing services. That, then would create pressure from the public to lift the spending ceiling so that a better quality of services can be provided.

When costs of health insurance rise, if there is an Employer Mandate to provide health insurance for every employee, fewer marginally profitable businesses will be able to pay for health insurance. Some will go out of business. Others will reduce the size of their workforce. Others no doubt would bring pressure to increase government subsidies to share the costs of health insurance. In all three cases the effect on the public treasury is the same: there will be an increased need for government-funded health insurance as the number of unemployed increases, or as more businesses are subsidized for part of their health insurance costs. Meanwhile, no new source of tax revenue to pay for this has been generated.

In short, the Clinton version of "managed competition" would have created new problems for the American health-care system. These pressures, then, would have seriously undercut its effort to provide health care to all Americans at a price the nation can afford. Access to care, cost, or quality of services (or all three) seems likely to have grown more problematic.

Comparing the Three Approaches

Single-payer plans have the virtue of putting the provision of health-care services first, when values for health-care reform come into conflict, but they do not take sufficient account of how the current American health-care industry affects the vitality of the economy as a whole. The free market has the virtue of flexibility in responding to new conditions, but opportunities for profit take precedence over making sure that everyone gets the health care they need. Thus it has the opposite strengths and problems from those found in single-payer plans. The Clinton reform plan's version of managed competition hoped to use the strengths of each of these approaches, while avoiding their fatal flaws. Unfortunately it did not succeed. The Clinton Task Force produced a rigid plan for reform, in many ways akin to the logic of large corporations or the mainframe computer. What was needed was a way to capture the strengths of each approach that works more nearly on the logic that has led to the proliferation of smaller businesses or the personal computer revolution. Both small businesses and personal computers have the advantage of providing flexible solutions to immediate problems, rather than locking everyone into mammoth structures that centrally control all resources and provide fairly limited, and rather rigid, options for problem-solving. Something similar is needed for health-care reform.[15]

Could Any of these Contending Strategies Work?

Probably not, as now formulated. All three of these approaches to health-care reform use principles of economics that relate to supply, demand, risks, and incentives to influence the *business* of providing *disease care services* to the public. None of them questions the focus of attention on disease management nor on the use of high technology as the preferred strategy for care. None of these strategies provides a way to attack sources of disease. Instead, they take levels of need for disease-care services as a given, not as something that could be varied through public policy. Similarly, all accept without question the current medical preference for using high technology to diagnose and treat disease. Unfortunately we now are headed in directions that reflect a "mainframe computer" or giant corporation mentality. Although the Clinton plan was not adopted legislatively, many of its recommended features have become part of current health-care trends. A massive shift of both public and private health insurance enrollees into capitated payment plans is occurring. The development of massive networks of health-care providers, which buy up private physicians practices and create monopolistic or semi-monopolistic health-care markets, is transforming the nature of competition in health care, but not improving either cost or access to care.

So long as health-care remains disease-focused and is approached primarily in economic terms, we will be fighting a losing battle with increasing costs. This would be true even if levels of technology remained constant; social and demographic changes now on the horizon, and the deteriorating quality of the global environment will sharply increase the need for disease-care services in the next few decades, as Table 5.4 makes clear.

TABLE 5.4   Five "Growth Areas" for Disease-Care Services
During the Next Two Decades

What?	*Why?*
1. Elder Care	The elderly population is growing in size.
2. HIV/AIDS	Four to five million HIV carriers will progress to full-blown AIDS and additional people will become carriers.
3. High-cost chronic illnesses	The baby boom cohort are reaching middle age.
4. Cancer	Environmental deterioration increases risk.
5. Health problems from use of addicting substances: nicotine alcohol narcotics	Legal markets target vulnerable populations (e.g., minorities and the young)
	International trade agreements (e.g., NAFTA) make control of illegal substances more difficult, while the down-sizing of businesses forces more people into illegal economic activity

The social and demographic developments listed in Table 5-4 will sharply increase the need for disease-care services. As the volume of demand for services increases, pressures toward higher costs for care are inevitable. The American economic system no longer can afford to be organized around demand-driven health care, with government, businesses, and private households being captive payers as costs increase. We will have to find ways to have an impact on sources of disease problems, not simply find ways to pay for their consequences. In the past, demand-driven health-care growth was not a problem. As health-care costs have become more expensive, however, we no longer can afford that approach to health-care planning. In the first decades after World War II—when the U.S. economy was robust, when tax revenues were high, and tax laws let inflation produce surplus tax income that then could be used for governmental problem-solving—efforts at health-care reform were clearly *demand-driven*. Businesses' health benefits packages and public Medicare/Medicaid formulas tried to give everyone all the health-care services they might want or need, and let service providers set the level of demand. Federal medical research budgets generated an exponential growth in knowledge and in the use of increasingly high-tech medical interventions. This approach set in motion a treacherous cost dynamic, as the developments chronicled in chapters two through four have documented.

There are at least three problems with demand-focused health-care policy. First, if sources of disease are not addressed, the need for services can grow more rapidly than the resources to pay for them. Second, need and demand are not the same, and can operate independently of one another. Public demand is quite elastic, able to increase out of all proportion to real *need* for services. Third, professional medical values encourage the best possible care, which has come to mean using "state of the art" strategies for diagnosing and managing disease.[9] These increasingly involve high-technology and consequently have become quite expensive. This professionally-oriented emphasis gets reinforced by profit goals, which further increase service providers' demands for costly services that they prescribe and patients accept. The end result: an explosive growth in costs.

Since 1972, beginning with the introduction of federally sponsored capitated-payment plans to finance health-care services, American health-care policy increasingly has moved toward *supply-side* strategies for cost containment. (Limit the supply of money, and providers will adapt.) Providers have done so. Capitation rates of payment and managed care organization of services motivate providers to control patients' access to services. However, when *profit* is an important end value for service provision, supply-side economic policies for cost containment sometimes lower services and eliminate access for the economically vulnerable. This is not acceptable. We need additional strategies that lessen both the need and the demand for expensive services.

Economic concepts like *supply and demand, incentives,* and *shared and protected risk* are helpful for understanding some aspects of American health care, but they cloud our ability to see other dimensions of what is at issue. It is true that the American health-care industry is a vital part of the economy, and that it responds to the same factors that influence other economic competitors. Health care, however, is much more than an economic commodity. Good health is key to effective functioning and a good life. Health care, consequently, cannot become simply an economic commodity whose distribution is left to the vicissitudes of market forces. Instead of simply replacing demand-driven strategies with supply-side controls, we must change the *need* for higher-cost services and then influence *demand* for them by changing motivations toward consumption. Future debate about health-care policy must examine strategies for cost containment that reduce unnecessary expenses rather than diminish the quality of care. Only as costs become manageable can Americans provide a high quality of health services to all. The contending political and economic strategies of single-payer plans, market competition or managed competition, with or without managed care, seem unlikely to succeed in taming costs; as now formulated none of these approaches address the sources of disease that create a need for care. They also do not provide any alternatives to the cost-dynamic which the increasing trend toward high technology medicine keeps in motion. We will have to approach the problem of health-care reform more fundamentally.

TABLE 5.5   Some Guiding Principles for Reform

---

1. Deal with SOURCES of DISEASE, including
   - Individual Behaviors that increase
     susceptibility to disease
   - Social and Organizational Practices
     that affect exposure to health risks
   - Environmental Changes that affect health

2. Deal with SOURCES OF COST INCREASE in
   caring for disease, including
   - Funding arrangements that increase costs unnecessarily
   - Overuse of high-tech medical diagnoses and
     interventions, and of medical specialists

3. Redirect public and private resources to GET BASIC
   SERVICES TO UNDERSERVED POPULATIONS

4. Approach Health and Economic Policy Issues Jointly

It is time to shift our point of intervention in the health-disease process. It is much less expensive to keep people well than to cure them. Our present system finances disease care by taking health insurance premiums from the well and giving them few services to maintain their health. Instead their financial contribution is used to pay for other people's sick-care. We need to develop a system of *health* care that can supplement or replace our current *disease*-care system.

Fortunately there is more to the story of American health care during the past half century than the emergence of the *health-care industry*. The same large social, economic, and political dynamics that produced the responses which jelled as the health-care industry also produced counter movements that directed attention to *health*.

Thomas Kuhn has argued that scientific knowledge develops as a series of revolutionary leaps of thought. As problems arise that should not be there—if things worked the way we have been assuming—Kuhn argues, innovators begin to ask more fundamental questions, daring to challenge the assumptions on which current knowledge is based. Occasionally a shift of attention alerts inquirers to new questions, and new ways to deal with old problems.[16] Something like that seems to have been occurring in health care in the past few decades. As both the promise and the unsolvable dilemmas of the health-care industry's version of medical science have been seen more clearly, other interests have begun to direct attention to health, rather than disease. They have demonstrated some ways that disease care can encourage the body's own health-building. A number of institutional interests nationally and internationally also have focused attention on a broader sense of health and disease than is captured in biochemistry, identifying processes and relationships that strengthen or weaken health—i.e., the optimal functioning of the self (body, mind, and spirit) within an interactive social and physical environment. These developments have been spurred on by changes that were occurring in scientific inquiry, in the international political economy, and in the global environment itself, which was being monitored in new ways. New coalitions of interest, often developing outside the health-care industry but occasionally within it, experimented with different ways to provide health care. None has produced a model that can replace the health-care industry. Indeed, like the health-care industry itself, each experimental path has its own strengths and weaknesses. Some of the experiments, however, have important lessons to teach us. If we incorporate some of their discoveries more fully into our current health-care system, some of the dynamics which now lead to ever-more-expensive health care could begin to change. Moreover, a focus on health could begin to lay a safety net that would make some current proposals for economic reform of health care much less risky for the American population.

It is time to retrace our steps, to see how some of the same political, economic and social developments that led to the establishment of the health-care industry also produced quite different coalitions of interests, ones that asked new kinds of questions about health and disease. Their questions, and the potential answers that they began to explore, open up a different kind of agenda for problem-solving in health care. While we are not likely to adopt their demonstrations as a simple replacement for the health care industry, we have much to learn from them that will be useful for mainstream health care reform. When the focus shifts to *health*, a variety of new possibilities for problem-solving emerge, and it becomes possible to approach the economics of health care in new ways.

6

Origins of New Health-Care Perspectives

The development of the American health-care industry and the failure of efforts to tame or reform it are only part of the story. Over the past 30 years, a series of independent developments in scientific research, in various national and international social movements, and in mainstream institutions internationally (including transnational corporations, European parliaments, NATO, and the United Nations) have opened up new ways to understand the health-disease process. The new conceptions extend far beyond the confines of biochemistry and reorient our sense of the legitimate domain for health-care policy. At first, because explorations went in so many apparently unrelated directions, critics often dismissed them as irrelevant. Only now are we beginning to understand what each has to contribute to a more basic reorientation of approaches to health and disease that seems to be occurring. Scientific research, social protest movements, international political and military alliances, philanthropic foundations, and transnational corporations have all contributed to an important shift in conceptual frameworks that is developing as one response to an emerging global social order.

International Developments That Changed the Context for Problem Solving

Several international developments noted in earlier chapters have helped create the circumstances in which social movements could introduce new principles for social organization, problem identification, and problem-solving. Because the worldwide economic depression of the 1930s, followed by World War II, had made it difficult for young couples in many countries to start their families, the end of war led to a "baby boom" in many parts of the world. These children grew up in special circumstances, created by the size of the new birth cohorts and the economic, political and social changes that were occurring globally. As they grew to adulthood, a much higher percent of them went on to study in colleges and universities. The common experiences of young adults in most countries, and the easy communication and travel that became part of the international scene in the 1960s, gave them an outlook that often differed strikingly from that of their parents, a "generational perspective" more global in focus and more critical of contemporary institutions and practices.

The collapse of European empires during World War II, and the emergence of non-aligned "third world" nations proud of their pre-colonial histories, made young people aware of the strengths of non-European traditions previously viewed as primitive or inferior. Cold War realignments that attended the demise of the colonial system, and especially the American military ventures in Southeast Asia during the 1960s and 1970s, became a focus for questioning and resistance by the new generation.

Meanwhile, escalation of the international arms race—involving the development of nuclear weapons by several major powers, new military strategies that affect the environment, and new information-gathering potential from spy satellites—focused attention on international policies that threatened not only localized populations, but the health of the entire planet.

As this was happening, the industrialization of Eastern Europe and certain areas of Latin America and Asia—when added to earlier industrialization in Western Europe, North America, Australia, and Japan—produced major changes in worldwide demands for energy, and raised the levels of environmental pollution caused by emissions from manufacturing processes and burgeoning automobile traffic. These environmental changes were now easier to monitor because of worldwide surveillance technologies available to the military and because of international scientific cooperation coordinated by the UN.

Finally, the postwar demilitarization of Germany and Japan had left them free to develop their economies without the burden of arms race expenditures. The growing success of German and Japanese competitors motivated American-based transnational corporations to experiment with new approaches to health care (which was consuming an increasing percentage of their profits). In addition, the different political arena in Germany allowed its baby boom generation to raise a series of questions that began to resonate around the world, helping spawn international movements that addressed issues of environmental health.

National Developments

The impact of these broader international developments was reinforced by independent American trends. After World War II the U.S. federal government continued to increase its funding of scientific research (as described in Chapter 1). Greater resources for medical, biological, and atmospheric research, and for the social sciences as well, produced important shifts in how a new generation thought about issues of health and disease. At one level, medical research continued to proceed from the metaphor of the body as machine, producing more high-tech medicine and a proliferation of medical specialties, thus encouraging the directions in which the health-care industry was already developing.

This increased funding for scientific research coincided with introduction of a new paradigm for explaining biochemical events and with break-through discoveries about how viruses operate. Discovery of DNA's simple formula, and its presence in all living creatures, revolutionized our under-standing of health processes (as will be discussed in Chapter 9). Medical science began to understand health dynamics in terms of information trans-fers, a major reformulation of the earlier germ theory of disease.

Meanwhile, atmospheric researchers began to uncover disquieting evidence of health hazards that were being created by manufacturing pro-cesses and by the proliferation of automobile exhaust emissions. As epide-miologists traced the incidence of disease problems among populations who were exposed to various kinds of atmospheric pollution or lived in proximity to toxic waste sites, it became clear that treatment strategies based on the germ theory of disease were missing the mark.[1] Then, as additional researchers demonstrated the role of stress in the etiology of many disease states,[2] it became apparent that purely biochemical descriptions of disease processes and treatment strategies based only on biochemistry or surgery were inadequate and inefficient for disease control. Federal funding kept U.S. researchers in the forefront of knowledge breakthroughs; and their discoveries in the physical and medical sciences constantly enlarged our understanding of the health-disease process and led observers outside the health-care industry to question its prevailing emphases.

Concurrently, groups of scientists and physicians joined a larger de-bate examining the political developments leading to World War II and the ensuing atomic arms race. After World War II European social critics un-dertook an agonizing reappraisal of the strengths and weaknesses of Euro-pean civilization. As they tried to understand how death-dealing totalitar-ian regimes—fascist, nazi or communist—had become so influential in twentieth-century European life, they saw how science and technology had been used to enslave and destroy whole populations. The questions they raised were echoed in organizations of scientists and physicians who tried to counter the destructive impetus of scientific inquiry.[3] Shortly after World War II, nuclear physicists warned of the dangers of the arms race. Later, organizations such as Science for the People and Physicians for Social Re-sponsibility kept similar policy issues alive, noting that the health and wellbeing of the entire world's population was being placed in jeopardy by international military policies.[4]

Funding for the social sciences also had its impact. As several leading American universities systematically strengthened their social science de-partments, a younger generation developed a comparative, international perspective that frequently questioned the assumptions on which Western imperial policies had been based. One assumption strongly challenged was the belief that Euro-American culture and the Western scientific viewpoint that epitomized it were inherently superior to all its historical predecessors. The dominant theoretical position in the social sciences during the 1950s and early 1960s was functionalism, a perspective first introduced into anthropology around the time of World War I in an effort to overcome ethnocentric bias when analyzing practices found in other societies.[5] These practices were to be understood in terms of what they accomplished within a given cultural context, rather than ranked in comparison to the practices of Western European or American traditions, or of scientific, technological society. During the 1960s and 1970s the functionalist perspective was challenged by critics who noted its tendency to accept the status quo and to ignore conflict and interest group struggles;[6] nonetheless, it helped create a deeper respect for non-industrial cultures and for non-scientific frames of reference.

These philosophic and social theory debates influenced students in American universities, who observed the political controversies of the mid-1950s through the early 1970s with intense interest, and often applied the favored intellectual arguments of the time to political analysis and action. Students on elite campuses across the country became involved in the civil rights struggles led by Martin Luther King, Jr., and by the Student Nonviolent Coordinating Committee (SNCC). Many then joined King in linking civil rights struggles with opposition to the undeclared war in southeast Asia, and later participated in a series of "liberation movements" concerned with the rights of various minorities or disadvantaged elements of the population.

As we shall see, by the late 1960s these various themes came together in surprising ways; students and other radical critics were questioning the assumptions of the health-care industry as well as those of the political establishment. Freeing themselves of the assumption that scientific medicine, or Western technological society, was superior to practices of other cultures, they critiqued the assumptions on which "modern health care" is based and actively explored health strategies used in other cultures. "Popular medicine," thus, reintroduced a mixed medical model for American health care, ending the monopoly medical science established in the second decade of the century. It offered radical alternatives to approaches used by the health-care industry.

Emergence of a Generational Perspective in the 1960s

Those who shared the new generational perspective seemed to have five things in common, regardless of where they lived or how they expressed themselves. First, their concerns were not only international, but global: members of this "social generation" thought about the planet as a whole, not simply about political units and their relationships. Second, they abandoned the assumption of earlier generations that the current world order is necessarily superior to what preceded it; while not rejecting science and technology, they looked with new respect at practices and philosophies from pre-scientific, pre-modern social orders. Third, they were less concerned with efficiency and productivity than with the humaneness of institutions and problem-solving strategies. Consequently, they questioned the basis for social coordination on which much of the current social order was built; not content with attacking specific practices, they challenged bureaucracy, patriarchal bases for relationship and social order, and scientific and technological "imperatives" to which people were expected to adapt.

Fourth, in contrast to pragmatic approaches that break problems down into small components, members of this social generation thought systemically about relationships (how each relates to a whole) and looked for integrative dimensions that apply to many levels of analysis. Finally, instead of seeing economic or materialist goals as the only basis for policy choice, they saw humans as part of a larger whole. They came to understand themselves, their relations to one another and to other species, and their relations to the global environment *ecologically*. This ecological-environmental frame of reference, combined with the other four generational vantage-points, provided a code of ethics that mobilized them to confront and challenge many practices of their societies.

With time, many members of this social generation came to question the simplicity of their youthful efforts to reform society. Many now viewed their earlier ventures as naive. Nonetheless, as they took on adult leadership roles in various American organizations and institutions many continued to use the broader orienting frame of reference. Although they no longer saw the world from a "New Left" political perspective, they often approached problems globally, ecologically, and 'holistically'—understanding the "specifics" of a situation in terms of their relation to a larger whole. They continued to show a deep respect for the contribution of other cultures and to consider science and technology only one among many ways to solve problems. As they sought ways to make organizations and institutions more humane they often reworked strategies that had developed during their period of youthful rebellion.

In the 1960s this generational perspective was articulated most clearly by college students and recent college graduates of the world's more elite educational institutions. All over the world, during that decade, university students challenged the privileges and practices of their elders. They held in common a disrespect for "technocracy" or bureaucratically organized professional expertise—particularly when it was used to create special privilege for the experts or to heighten "system productivity" at the expense of human values. These were issues that had not been addressed by the class-focused struggles of an earlier period. The "new generation" was as critical of socialist and communist bureaucracy as of technocratic developments in the West.[7]

Originally, as leaders of these protests noted, they represented a new kind of "class interest," in the sense of having a unique relation to means of economic production.[8] In the early 1960s, many baby-boomers were economically in limbo, attending colleges and universities, postponing their entrance into adult economic roles. Many avoided such roles for a number of years.

Although their most articulate spokesmen and women often identified themselves with the social role that Marx had defined, the members of this generation responded less to economically defined class interests than to what Max Weber had described as status interests. They mobilized around life-style issues, and around their responsibilities as a privileged elite, identifying with racial and ethnic minorities, and assuming special responsibility for their wellbeing. The new social generation first became visible in the U.S. in the 1960s, when efforts of African-American college students in the South to end segregation captured the attention of university students across the country, who often supported their struggles. From an initial American belief in equality and championing the underdog, many students moved to a more fundamental questioning of the coalitions and power interests that supported an "outmoded" system like racial discrimination.[9]

The questioning gained intensity as politicians escalated military aid in Vietnam into an undeclared war in Southeast Asia, drafting young people to serve in one of the most unpopular military ventures of American history. As this happened, young adults now found their life chances directly affected by political decisions with which they disagreed. Many college students began to see the war not as an isolated "mistake" but as an inevitable—and tragic—expression of the dynamics that energized the dominant American culture. They began to see the civil rights struggles and the anti-war movement as different facets of the same underlying problem. For these students problems of "peace" and problems of "freedom" became inextricably linked.[10] They challenged educational institutions to abandon value-neutrality and to champion the oppressed.

In the U.S., where a split was beginning to develop between military-industrial and information-services alliances of interest, the activities of this radicalized college student generation helped to reorient the attention of adults within the information-services complex, creating widespread opposition to the war. Student resistance to the military campaign in Vietnam grew into a more general opposition, to criticism of "imperialism" in

U.S. foreign policy as well as in the policies of other nations, and to a concern for "liberation" issues more widely. Gradually this concern spread to health and the environment as well, themes which began to resonate much more widely with the American public. While the new social generation did not persuade older cohorts to adopt a dialectical political outlook, its activities helped to establish new conditions for larger problem-solving.

This generational perspective emerged in the U.S. among college students and young adults who called themselves the New Left. They were Left because they called into question the dominant ethos of international capitalism. They were New because they went beyond earlier socialist or communist ideological critiques, condemning bureaucratic technocracy in socialist countries as well as in the West, and demanding a humane, person-centered social order. As increasing numbers of American students studied and traveled abroad and international students came to the U.S., a constant exchange of information, values, and tactics for common action took place internationally among young adults of the baby-boom generation.[11]

The New Left political ventures of the 1960s developed a unique style, reflecting their relation to other social developments of that time period. As part of that style, they introduced new strategies for social coordination that have persisted and by now have been modified by other interests, including transnational corporations, and parts of the health-care industry. These strategies represent more than generational differences in style. These ways to coordinate activity overcome some of the limits of more conventional organizational behavior.

These developments are most easily understood by tracing each of the new strategies back to their common origins in the protest movements of the 1960s and then noting how each evolved. This chapter, consequently, moves back and forth in time, identifying each development that emerged in the 1960s, noting its evolution and later relevance for health care, and then doing the same for other elements that originally developed as a common, coherent strategy for social protest.

The style of New Left protest movements was influenced strongly by the southern U.S. civil rights movement of the late 1950s and 1960s, in which other students from across the country participated. "Moral confrontation" became a defining characteristic of the student ventures. To this they added several unique contributions: a mode of decision-making that they called "participatory democracy"; an alternative to bureaucratic coordination which has come to be called "networking"; and an alternative to the particularistic focus of science and technology—a more holistic and ecological framework for understanding how individual activities relate to systemic wholes, an approach captured in the motto, "Think globally, act locally." These four approaches to problem-solving gave a special character to social protests, internationally. Over time, each has been adapted for use by other interest groups in the international political economy and has come into use within health care itself.

Moral Confrontation

The organizing tactic that most fully characterized the major social movements of the 1960s was moral confrontation, which developed within the civil rights movement of the 1950s and influenced the style of many "liberation" campaigns thereafter. Through mass confrontations they hoped to inspire opponents to change their behavior, and if that did not work, to coerce them into doing so. These movements were ethics-oriented; they revolved around demands for justice and freedom for people who were being denied these "rights." During the next two decades many social movements adopted the strategy of moral confrontation. Moral confrontation simplifies complex realities, identifying one ethical issue as the most critical aspect of a situation, demanding that others pay attention to this and change their own behaviors. Critics sometimes objected that moral confrontation campaigns over-simplified issues. They accused the moral crusaders of being self-righteous and smug. However, by redirecting attention to the ethical implications of the activities of daily life, moral confrontation crusades often succeeded in changing practices that offended their participants. Once institutionalized, this strategy found its way into controversies about access to medical services. By the early 1990s, for example, opponents of abortion blocked the entrance to abortion clinics, accusing doctors and the pregnant women who came there of participating in the murder of unborn children.[12] Act Up, an AIDS direct action group, was staging dramatic moral confrontations that influenced budget allocations, peer-review choice of recipients for some federal research grants, and the way clinical trials of new drugs were conducted.[13]

The concept of moral confrontation was adapted for use in other kinds of health interventions, as well. Families and friends of alcoholics or drug abusers were mobilized to confront the substance-abuser en masse, making it clear that the entire relevant subcommunity would not tolerate continued behavior that damaged them.[14] As research evidence on the negative effects of smoking on non-smokers became public, non-smokers began to mobilize to demand respect for their rights as well. Some cities, some airlines, and eventually national legislation banned smoking in many public places. Many workplaces also adopted no-smoking policies after non-smokers mobilized to demand their health rights.[15] Thus this approach to problem-solving, developed by social movements of the 1950s and 1960s, continued to evolve as it spread to new interest groups within the population.

Participatory Democracy

Both the civil rights and anti-war movements encouraged grassroots action (as well as actions planned more centrally). Despite occasional difficulties of implementation, they subscribed to a creed of democratic decision making and called their coordinating strategy "participatory democracy."[16] The crux of the new approach was reliance on localized decision-making, taking advantage of information, "expertise," and judgment possessed by those most directly involved in the moment-to-moment activity of a particular project. "Leaders" were listened to with respect, but the people who would be carrying out the details of a protest demonstration made on-the-spot decisions about how to proceed that took into account rapidly changing situations and their own needs as well as the agenda of the leadership.

The ideal of radical equality that underlay the New Left's participatory democracy soon led to efforts to insure equality and respect for all citizens, including those needing health care. The New Left focused attention on the poor and ethnic minorities, noted their lack of access to health care, and joined with others who were demanding more equal access to health services; these collaborative pressures, which the New Left supported (but did not originate), eventually resulted in Medicaid legislation. Medical students set up free clinics in urban neighborhoods, demanded community control of health services for their neighborhoods, and introduced the concept of "patient advocates"—people familiar with the health-care facility would help patients articulate any dissatisfactions they had with services, confront medical practitioners when needed, and help resolve differences between them to the satisfaction of the recipients of health-care services. This practice gradually became institutionalized in many hospitals across the country.

In time, the principle of participatory democracy entered the American mainstream. Businesses began introducing their own variations of it for staff coordination and problem-solving at various organizational levels throughout a production enterprise.[17] The "essence" that was picked up involved welcoming "expertise" from all levels of an enterprise, not just from the official leadership, and offering all participants some control over the actual operation of a venture on a day-to-day basis. Where participation was not spontaneous and voluntary—as in business and industry, and in governmental activities—the range of input and mutual decision-making that came into actual use varied widely. In bureaucratic or industrial settings, the use of local expertise often took precedence over "democracy," but the new practices recognized that persons most directly involved in an operation often make wiser tactical decisions than planners or "leaders" are able to do. Within health care, movements toward greater autonomy for nurses, the involvement of patients in treatment and management decisions about their own medical problems, and the movement of "healthcare consumers" to "take responsibility for their own health" when seeking medical treatment all reflect the same themes at work. Other social movements that spun off of these original New Left ventures helped make this organizational strategy directly relevant to health care.

Action Networks and Networking

In coordinating its various ventures, the New Left rejected the hierarchical, bureaucratic methods commonly used in the rest of the political economy, with its centralized control of resources and decision-making. Instead it used networking to coordinate common action.

Targets for moral confrontation were often chosen informally. A group of their "leaders" who had come to recognize one another during previous demonstrations would share collective judgment about how attractive a target would be to potential demonstrators, about the best timing for an action, and about how to make sure that the range of efforts going on at any one time did not compete unduly for participants, who could drop in and out of various ventures. A campaign could be announced by anyone; no one could veto an action; those that were ill-conceived or that lacked widespread support simply fizzled out. Once key ideological points about the target had been made, campaign strategies required relatively little coordination.[18]

Events were sponsored by shifting coalitions of groups, a loose network of individuals and organizations whose interests overlapped. The organizations themselves varied enormously in their own agendas. They also varied widely in terms of their own internal organizational structure. There were tightly disciplined political "cells," highly democratic and open public organizations, and "paper" organizations consisting of two or three people who invented an organizational name in order to participate in forming a particular coalition. Coordination from event to event occurred through informal meetings of "leaders." Ideology, slogans, and ritual confrontations provided the basis for unity among participants. These encounters thus involved a very different form of social coordination than was used in most American organizations.

Virginia Hines and Luther Gerlach, two anthropologists who studied New Left activism, suggested that the organizing principle used to coordinate them resembled one used in many tribal groups in the Middle East, Africa, and Asia. A variety of groups, with quite different organizational structures, sometimes led by archrivals, would coalesce and separate, depending upon which particular threat or common opportunity was involved. Many individuals would assume personal responsibility for innovative actions, gathering a group of people who were attracted to what they were saying or doing. Participation, withdrawal, and forms of cooperation and separate activity created constantly changing patterns, almost as in a kaleidoscope. The forms were deliberately temporary and everchanging. More important was the organizing principle behind them: egalitarian self-responsibility among cooperating groups, and coordination through information sharing rather than through resource centralization or control.

Hines and Gerlach, after studying these ventures and then a whole series of groups who seemed to be using a similar organizational form, called this common organizational strategy SP<I>N. Segments, consisting of organizations and groups, which are Poly-encephalous—or many headed in leadership—relate to one another through a common Ideology, forming overlapping Networks. These networks can be activated quickly in times of emergency or opportunity because some individuals belong to more than one segment at a time, and other individuals maintain informal communication with persons in other segments. The acronym itself, SP<I>N, appropriately suggests something that is not stationary or permanently "structural" but constantly whirling, in motion.[19]

This alternative to bureaucratic organizational structure, which is common to many resistance movements, can also can be seen at work, as Hines points out, among transnational corporations, national governments, and other bureaucratically organized entities, which are at times fiercely competitive and at other times strongly united in an effort to solve a common problem. The importance of this principle for contemporary social activity has prompted efforts to give it a non-academic name, and one that focuses attention on dynamic *process* instead of static *form*. I will use the terms *Action Network* and the more common *networking*—the process of identifying creative people who share a common enthusiasm for certain directions of change, develop informal consultation among themselves, and create new ventures together.

"Networking" can be used to mount protest movements and rebellions; but it also can be used to generate new activities within organizations or among ideological colleagues of many persuasions. Indeed, networking has become a part of coalition building and problem solving for many potential interests within the political economy, both nationally and internationally. Ideologically focused informal networks for consultation and planning have been part of the American scene at least since the time of the American Revolution. But the strategy for coordination, resource mobilization, and project initiation is historically new. It lets innovation arise from many sources and makes rapid response to changing situations simple.

The New Left political protest campaigns, therefore, did more than introduce a heightened dialectic tension that focused resistance to war and racial discrimination. They also introduced new strategies for social coordination to elite segments of a new social generation that was emerging. In addition, they introduced new frameworks for seeing relationships and for choosing points of influence on a problem.

Holistic and Ecological Frameworks

Members of this social generation made different connections among the problems they addressed. At the end of World War I, Jan Smuts, the South African philosopher and statesman who had urged the formation of a League of Nations to deal with political problems more globally, wrote about "holistic analysis," which he saw as a necessary complement and antidote to the narrowing of attention and particularistic focus that scientific and technological inquiry had introduced into thinking and problem-solving.[20] Members of the "new generation" often framed issues holistically when they engaged in social criticism. This could be seen, for example, in their discussion of common themes underlying American racial segregation and international power struggles. (Both were described as forms of "colonialism" in which people of color were kept in subjugation to others, systematically exploited to increase the wealth and power of "whites.")[21]

Before long this way of thinking about "the whole" spread into many areas. It had a profound effect on how scientists thought about the earth. Young geologists began thinking in literally global terms; soon "plate tectonics"—the explanation of geologic processes in terms of the movement of large "plates" beneath the surface of the earth—revolutionized our understanding of earthquakes, volcanoes, and the formation of mountain chains, as well as the movement of continents.[22] Younger biologists showed an increasing interest in ecology—understanding the behavior, growth and decline of species in terms of how an ecological setting is jointly created and sustained, and how it sets conditions for the survival of each species within it. By the mid-1970s the development of atmospheric sciences—in part a result of military developments that furthered knowledge about the earth and its surrounding layers, but also in part an extension of this kind of larger reframing of attention—directed scientific and political concern to environmental conditions in the stratosphere that affect health and illness, and to how industrial emissions affect them.

Thus long after the social movements of the 1960s had come and gone, and their ideological viewpoints were no longer popular even among former members of the New Left, a more global way of approaching problems and understanding relationships continued to be used.

"Holistic analysis," in practice, has both advantages and disadvantages. It lets one see commonalities underlying seemingly different patterns of activity and common causes for seemingly different results. When done well, it can identify an essence that underlies a variety of qualitatively different manifestations of some principle which is at work. However, its "global" focus is also its area of vulnerability. It can sometimes lead to simplifying assertions that do not do justice to the complex reality that is present. Rather than providing a replacement for the kinds of linear, reductive analysis that underlies much "scientific" analysis, it offers a corrective. Each works best in combination with the other.

Although the American New Left of the 1960s and early 1970s remained centrally focused on "peace and freedom" issues, it had three distinct wings that became visible as time went on. The main thrust of its activity went into massive moral confrontation campaigns, in which participants often "put their bodies on the line," physically disrupting "establishment" activities that furthered the war effort or discriminated against members of racial or ethnic minorities. But a second, more radical wing of the movement, influenced by theoretical arguments that social reality is constructed by those who participate in it,[23] wanted to form a counterculture—a new set of institutions to replace those now used in a morally "sick society." Finally, a third wing mobilized moral confrontations against threats to the environment—to the ecological whole—that came from military campaigns, from the search for new sources of energy, and from industrial activity. Parallel movements in Europe focused on peace issues (the international arms race, nuclear testing, disarmament), the creation of an international counterculture, and environmental concerns.

When the war in Vietnam ended and the civil rights movement headed off in separatist directions that left little welcome for white participants, former New Lefters put their energy into the three quite different social movements already set in motion by earlier New Left activity. These movements, of course, were only part of an evolving mix of influences on the direction of future change; and indeed, their contributions often came in response to developments originating in more mainstream activity. Their collective impact was strong enough, however, to deserve continuing attention in its own right. And because each had quite different implications for health-care reform, we shall look at each in turn.

Liberation Movements. The peace and freedom movement of the 1960s and early 1970s eventually succeeded in discrediting American military ventures in Southeast Asia. As the war in Southeast Asia wound down and the military draft was ended, war resistance ceased to be the center of dissident attention. A new kind of focus on "civil rights" emerged, as a splintering of activity into a series of U.S. "liberation" movements gained center stage. Black Power movements[24] (which tended to exclude white supporters) were soon joined by the American Indian Movement[25] and by efforts within the Hispanic-American community to improve their rights (notably, the farm workers movement to aid migrant laborers).[26] Other "liberation" movements arose among welfare mothers, the elderly, and renters seeking "tenants' rights."[27] All these movements adopted the dramatic confrontation tactics of their predecessors. The principle of direct moral confrontation in the name of "liberation" now became applicable to any group that faced discrimination—because of color, ethnicity, age, or other immutable characteristics, or because of economic vulnerability. This created a recognizable but clearly evolving character for the struggles.

This could be seen in the growth of movements resisting gender-based discrimination, most particularly the women's liberation movement and later the gay liberation movement among homosexuals.[28] Extending the earlier principle of resisting discrimination based on attributes with which one is born (such as one's gender)—a resistance fueled in part by the experience of male domination in the earlier protest movements—women's health collectives pioneered the idea of self-care, reacting against domination by male doctors. Deploring the excessive power of physicians, the women's health movement reasserted female authority in the area of childbirth and related fields of gynecological and obstetrical care. Women's collectively-run health services emphasized prevention, rejecting dehumanized approaches to service delivery and what they defined as dysfunctional relationships between patients and providers, including expectations of unquestioning patient compliance. They pointed out parallels between the character of the health delivery system and what they identified as exploitive social, economic, and political structures of society. The self-care book, *Our Bodies, Our Selves,* developed by a Boston-based women's health collective, influenced women across the country.[29] In addition, medicine men who were active in the American Indian Movement also began to teach other movement participants about the Indian cultures' understanding of health and how it is pursued in relation to Mother Earth.[30] Assertion of the right to dignity and self-determination, to ownership of one's own body, and the admonition to "take responsibility for your own health" emerged from these sources. The radical fringe was producing a health movement that made these concerns central in health care, as we shall see in the next chapter.

The liberation movements demanded respect for social differences, not simply a chance to be treated as part of the majority. "Freedom," "justice," and "equality" were slogans that had united Americans for generations. Now, groups who were organized around identities that separated them from other Americans were using these slogans to assert an equal right to privileges other Americans enjoyed.

Gradually these various movements began to pay attention to survival issues, and some developed a growing interest in questions related to health. Gay health clinics arose to serve the interests of a minority life-style, and women's health clinics offered alternatives to dominance by male doctors. A movement arose within mental health circles to respect the civil rights of the mentally ill, to release mental patients from long-term confinement in hospitals, and to provide community mental health clinics for outpatient services.[31]

Over time, activities of the various liberation movements had a variety of health consequences for their members. Sexual liberation and non-possessive sex became a two-edged sword for the international gay community, after the HIV virus began to spread in their midst with no effective pharmaceutical antidote. Conservatives used budget-balancing arguments to limit medical research into the problem in the early days of that epidemic.[32] Similarly, "freeing mental health patients" became a convenient way to limit inpatient facilities for the mentally ill, while providing few equivalents in the communities to which they returned, adding an additional component to a growing homeless population.[33] The gains that liberation movements won for subcommunities within America were quite real; but so were the costs that some of them were required to pay.

Consumer Rights. The New Left's earlier criticism of the policies of multinational corporations also began to produce spin-off movements. A consumer advocate movement emerged from the organizing initiative of Ralph Nader, who personally called corporations to account for unsafe products and stimulated wide imitation at the grassroots level.[34] Confrontation, often through the courts, and demands for justice again gave a recognizable identity to these ventures, applied now to "life" and "the pursuit of happiness." The same ethical imperative soon led to the extension of this concern beyond consumer products to corporation decisions that affect the third world. Particularly on college campuses, because universities are major institutional investors in corporation stocks, movements arose to mobilize stockholders to debate corporation policies in the third world and to vote their stock "in conscience."

One focus for activism which united women's concerns, consumer protection efforts, and international humanitarianism, was a campaign to stop the promotion of infant formula to replace breast feeding in countries where contaminated water supplies often meant that infant formula produced fatal diarrhea among babies. Students mobilized on college campuses across the country to urge trustees of their universities to raise the issue as stockholders at the annual shareholders' meetings of companies that manufactured and marketed infant formula.[35] At both an institutional and an individual level, these movements appraised health issues internationally and held large corporate interests accountable for the impact of their products, urging people to take responsibility for actions that affect the welfare of all. Moral confrontation was manifesting itself in a new arena.

The consumer movement gained particular attention for its lawsuits to protect the physical safety of American motorists. Beyond that, it focused attention on consumer rights, a theme some health movements would also develop. The mainstream of the American public was being drawn into engagement with issues of corporate responsibility for the public welfare. Within business circles, as noted in Chapter 3, these same themes were reworked as business leaders formed business health coalitions to further promote their interests as the funders of health-care consumption.

The evolution of social protest from civil rights to liberation movements and the consumer rights movements constantly extended moral confrontation with the broader society and its institutional practices into new areas, attracting new constituencies as the tactic was put to new uses. As all this was happening, a still more radical wing of social protest that developed in the 1960s and took new directions in the 1970s had even more striking implications for health care.

Emergence of a Counterculture

During the 1960s the most radical wing of the New Left, despairing that American institutions were reformable, had set up a self-conscious counterculture, which they hoped would demonstrate an alternative and superior way for people to live together. They experimented with food cooperatives, communal living arrangements, free medical clinics, and free universities with socially focused curricula. Countercultures sprang up simultaneously in the U.S., France, Great Britain, Germany, Japan, several Latin American countries, and even in the Soviet Union.[36]

For inspiration in their own effort to construct a more humane lifestyle, participants in the American counterculture looked to political movements in many parts of the world whose political, moral, and aesthetic stands they respected. From the Chinese revolution they took the idea of communes (propertyless relations in which all "served the people" for the common good without concern for personal wealth or profit), noting that even 19th century American utopian movements had often been communal. They took moral confrontation strategies from India, whose experience with non-violent resistance to domination they admired. They also took yoga as a route to consciousness of unity with the whole. From Japan, which had turned its back on the nuclear arms race, they looked to Zen for a moral aesthetic. Native American cultures, the admired underdogs of their own history, provided an understanding of how one can relate to Mother Earth and become her helper. This fit an emerging ecological perspective that was developing within the New Left more broadly as part of a horrified response to the American military's chemical defoliation policy in Vietnam. A protest of this military tactic gradually enlarged into a growing awareness within the New Left of the extent to which applications of modern technology were polluting the environment and endangering many species. For the counterculture, the need to rediscover preindustrial and Native American respect for the environment became urgent.

Not surprisingly, when they began to deal with health problems in their midst, many members of the counterculture looked for alternatives to the professional domination, bureaucratic medicalization, and concern for profit that characterized contemporary American health care. In cooperation with other New Left activists, they set up free medical clinics, staffed by student doctors and other volunteers. Since these innovative clinics primarily served a young, mobile population with its own unique lifestyle-related health problems (including venereal disease, pregnancy, and drug side effects), they did not become a widely imitated model for health care beyond New Left circles, especially since public health service clinics already provided many of these same services.[37] A more lasting impact on broader health-care practice came from their introduction of "patient advocates," people who knew the clinics well and who would help patients articulate and express to the medical staff any challenge they felt they needed to make in order to protect their own best interests. As noted already, with time, such a role became institutionalized not only in the free clinics but in many large, bureaucratic medical settings.[38]

Still more innovative was the counterculture's explorations of a mixed medical model. For health-care inspiration, as in other matters, many members of the counterculture began to turn to other cultures whose political stands seemed to resonate with their own. They also looked at earlier American medical traditions. Many began to use techniques from other health traditions, both to deal with issues of disease and for health building and to achieve altered states of consciousness.

Evolving Questions and Approaches to Health

The New Left counterculture had encouraged its members to explore altered states of consciousness as a way to transcend the materialism they believed was corrupting American society. Many had used psychedelic drugs as a route to higher consciousness; they had experienced states of being and nonsensory modes of communication and union with others that permanently altered their sense of reality.[39] Many others—especially the college-educated—quickly discovered that such states and modes of relating were part of the cultural "technologies" of many non-Western societies, where they were often acquired without using drugs. Soon many of the counterculture's avant-garde were journeying to India and other Asian countries where spiritual masters could teach them new routes to a higher consciousness.[40]

Just as a "youth market" had developed for rock music and unisex clothing styles, so a youth market developed for lectures, books, weekend workshops, and apprenticeships with those who offered Asian or "New Age" routes to personal and social transformation. Packaged to be available to the young elite who had entered the American business world as well as to counterculture dropouts and college students, the new programs were available on evenings and weekends, and could be used privately through books, records, and tapes. Many who had admired the New Left counterculture and dabbled in its recreational patterns now explored Eastern thought and practice. Soon many were exploring non-Western health approaches as well, ranging from acupuncture to yoga (approached as meditation, mind and body control, physical exercise, or any combination of these).[41]

Participants in this quest, abandoning old attitudes of cultural superiority, explored world views, alternatives to scientific frames of reference, new modes for relating to others, and different experiences with time and space. For many, this exploration took precedence over other concerns of the New Left. As they pursued Eastern understandings and adapted them for use in America and Europe, they attracted others who had not been part of the New Left's counterculture. This venture, called the Human Potential or New Age movement, directed attention away from the confrontational struggles that had characterized the New Left and the liberation movements, and sought in Asian and Native American traditions a new basis for inner peace and for individual and common activity. Its focus on "unity" rather than "confrontation," and "spirituality" rather than "social ethics," however, shifted the grounds that could be used for moral confrontation. Some saw this as a powerful deepening of the basis for engagement in the value issues of the time; others saw it as fundamentally undercutting the earlier clarity of protest movements.[42]

Holistic Health

The holistic (sometimes spelled wholistic) health movement emerged from the meeting of these various social liberation movements and the New Left and New Age countercultures, and was strongly influenced by the women's health movement. Its wildly eclectic health strategies, taken from many cultures and time periods in history, nevertheless had many common features: they focused attention on ways individual "consumers" could improve health and recover from disease; they encouraged individuals to "take responsibility for their own health" rather than remain passive "patients" in the hands of an expert; they avoided high-tech, invasive physical interventions, and strongly rejected impersonal, bureaucratic relationships in the provision of health services; and they emphasized the interaction of mind, body, and spirit in the health-disease process. Health traditions they introduced came for the most part from non-industrial cultures that the New Left and New Age countercultures were exploring: Indian, Chinese, and Japanese traditional medical systems; Native American health practices; and earlier American practices such as homeopathy and naturopathy. Besides a common respect for the interaction of mind, body, and spirit, in contrast to medical science's materialist commitment, these traditions shared a belief that health-disease interventions interact with a "life-force" principle which operates at a deeper level than biochemistry, though it often produces biochemical reactions. Thus the holistic health movement, by challenging the assumptions on which modern medical science and the health-care industry proceeded, reintroduced a mixed medical model into American life, an alternative to the monopoly enjoyed by medical science for a half century.[43]

To many, the New Age movement and its holistic health offshoot seemed an odd and regressive reaction to the political events of the period. Some social critics described the New Age counterculture as a withdrawal from political confrontation into self-absorption by pacified adults in the American middle class, many of whom had once been part of a major challenge to the American political establishment. They saw the holistic health movement as an abandonment of class issues involving health problems of the poor in favor of middle-class consumerism.[44] These charges were not completely inaccurate. The New Age and holistic health movements, and also much of the women's health movement, can also be understood, however, as a pendulum swing in counterculture forms of resistance to the dominant themes of modern technological society.

The holistic health movement took many concerns of the earlier social movements and refocused them to raise fundamental policy issues. For this reason it quickly began to attract the interest not only of countercultures but also of government planners, some industrial executives, and some of the policy elite who guide health-care planning in the nation.[45] It became a fringe medical movement that began to critique the health-care industry at a fundamental level and to define the parameters in which new health-care policy would be explored.

Preventive Health or Wellness

Business, industry, a few government health agencies, and philanthropic foundations, viewing the constantly escalating costs of high-tech medicine, listened with a special interest to the holistic health movement's emphasis on health promotion and on individual responsibility for health improvement. Picking up on themes that had been sounded by members of the public health movement for several decades, a variety of innovators began to ask new questions about the *sources* of disease, focusing attention on personal behaviors that lead to disease states and on the social influences that affect these behaviors. Government health agencies began to fund demonstration studies at worksites and in the community, identifying health risks and trying to change risk behaviors *before* people become ill.[46]

By the early 1990s, the baby-boom generation was almost 20 to 25 years into adulthood and its elite members now were occupying leadership roles in many organizations and institutions around the world. Many applied parts of their earlier New Left experience—or their ongoing exploration of New Age or Human Potential programs—to problem-solving in their work settings.

A "wellness movement" emerged, with considerable funding from government, business, and philanthropic sources. More innovative leaders in the health-care industry joined holistic health movement participants in creating worksite and community interventions designed to maintain and improve health rather than to control disease problems. The worksite wellness movement approached holistic health practices cautiously, wishing to maintain its acceptability within a larger health-care system. Many holistically oriented entrepreneurs, however, joined the new endeavors, adapting their approaches so that they would be acceptable in the new milieu. Chapter 8 discusses these developments in more depth.

Health and the Environment

Meanwhile, as the other social movements discussed above were moving in parallel, the global consciousness of the 1960s found concrete physical expression. Another social movement united New Left concerns with those of a much broader spectrum of the national and international community and came to be known as the environmental movement. Although the environmental movement received major support from radical social movements that had opposed U.S. policy in Southeast Asia during the Cold War, its concerns did not originate in those quarters and its support was not limited to those social networks. Instead, an international band of scientific researchers, academicians, physicians, politicians, military officials, and leaders from many religious traditions found themselves raising a set of questions that had much in common with those being raised by the radical Left. A new and quite surprising action network was emerging, one that regrouped older coalitions, as new questions brought into focus by a global perspective caught the attention of thoughtful people in many walks of life.

Concern for the environment did not emerge only in the 1960s. In the U.S., John Muir and Teddy Roosevelt had championed preservation of forests, lakes, and natural habitats at the beginning of the century. By mid-century, organizations like the Sierra Club were becoming important lobby groups within American politics. After World War II groups around the world—such as the Union of Atomic Scientists and various political movements arguing for a "sane nuclear policy"—expressed concern about the health implications of nuclear testing and threats to the environment posed by military strategies, the spread of various industrial technologies, and the development of various power sources for technological activity. The "new generation" may have responded with special fervor to environmental concerns, but they were introduced to them by many older sources.[47]

In 1962, Rachel Carson's best selling book *The Silent Spring* described how pesticide spraying for insect control in the U.S. was poisoning the bird population and disrupting the balance of nature. Popular outcry led to changes in pesticide spraying both in the U.S. and internationally, as people began to notice its larger ecological consequences. Carson's eloquent demonstration of how an ecological framework changes one's understanding of technological problem-solving was picked up a few years later by New Left opponents to the war in Vietnam and their allies, in ways that had an equally vivid impact on the public. At the time, North Vietnamese guerrillas fighting American troops were avoiding U.S. military air reconnaissance by hiding in the jungles and forests. The U.S. military responded with a "scorched earth" policy, using napalm, white phosphorus, and Agent Orange to kill the vegetation in disputed territory, coincidentally destroying the crops and livelihood of farmers, endangering the survival of non-human species in the area, and posing health hazards to humans. Eventually this policy defoliated between one-fourth and one-half of the Vietnamese land mass, decimated tropical forests and agricultural lands, and produced birth defects in the Vietnamese civilian population. The anti-war movement criticized this not only as a crime against humanity, but as a crime against nature, one that would have serious consequences for the health of the planet.[48]

After 1969, space exploration pictures beamed back from the moon began to provide the first photographic images of "planet earth." The anti-war movement took advantage of these images, and of public excitement about this new technological triumph, to make its own points about living in a "global village" where damage to one part of the environment affects us all.[49]

A variety of agendas and motivations prompted use of a more ecological frame of reference by Americans thereafter. In 1969 an oil slick off the coast of California, washing up on beaches near Santa Barbara, made pollution a matter of public concern to wealthy property owners as well as to young activists. That summer President Richard Nixon brought these various concerns together. After celebrating the landing of the first space team on the moon, Nixon urged NATO to use spy satellites to assess damage to the global environment coming from technological developments, and then to propose ways to address the problem. Nixon also called on the young people of America to direct their youthful idealism into "cleaning up the environment."[50] With these diverse sources of endorsement, an environmental movement quickly attracted broad support. Within a year Congress had passed legislation to protect the environment from technological pollution and had authorized the establishment of an Environmental Protection Agency (EPA).[51] Internationally, pressure built to halt atomic weapons testing and to address the global issues of an increasingly contaminated environment that seemed to be changing the conditions for global survival.

The momentum increased rapidly thereafter. In 1972, responding to the discovery of high levels of radioactive strontium 90 in milk supplies all over the world, the UN convened a first worldwide environmental summit conference in Stockholm, Sweden, and set up a new UN agency charged with the task of monitoring the health of the global environment and with convening international conferences to propose multi-national actions to lessen threats to the health of the world's population. These led to agreements to halt above-ground nuclear weapons testing.[52] Then, over the next 20 years, as scientific evidence began to accumulate regarding threats to the planet's surrounding atmosphere—from manufacturing processes, the spreading use of internal combustion engines in automobiles, and the thinning of forests—a new kind of pressure began to build for dealing with the sources of disease that lie in social practices which affect the global environment.

During the period when the American New Left was splintering, the European New Left had remained more clearly political and more peace-oriented, focusing on problems of economically disadvantaged population groups such as immigrant workers in expanding European industries. The motivating core of their activity, however, lay in more global issues: international arms testing, the armaments race, and—increasingly—environmental policy. In Germany the various New Left political interests regrouped as the Green Party, drawing various concerns together around the issue of a deteriorating national and global environment. Health issues became a graphic, easily graspable theme of the new Green movements that sprang up in many countries. By 1983 Swiss, Belgian, German, and Finnish Greens held seats in their respective parliaments, and Green parties were active in every European country, as well as in Canada, the U.S., Japan, Australia, New Zealand, Mexico, Costa Rica, Chile, and Brazil.[53] The extent to which Green political parties could set the agenda for national discussion varied from country to country, but it became not uncommon for Green candidates to get 15 percent or more of the popular vote. In parliamentary systems that divided legislative seats among parties on the basis of their percentage of the total popular vote, Greens became an important minority party able to affect day-to-day decision making by offering limited support to other political parties in return for support of their own positions on the environment. With time, the ecological perspective of the Green parties played a larger role in European political deliberations and helped bring a new dimension for health-care planning to the attention of world leaders.

Social movements concerned with environmental issues attracted participants from many backgrounds, not simply radical baby boomers. Committees working internationally for a "sane nuclear policy," Physicians for Social Responsibility, and international church and peace groups from the major faiths of the world worked together with scientists and politicians to confront the danger of a "nuclear winter" that could result if the arms race between the U.S. and the Soviet Union or the proliferation of nuclear weapons to smaller nations around the globe went awry.[54] Then, as evidence of the deteriorating atmosphere surrounding the planet came to light in the 1980s and early 1990s, new moral confrontation movements began to arise. Among the more dramatic of these movements was Greenpeace, an international environmental protest group which used moral confrontation tactics to pressure various political bodies around the world to examine policies that damage the ecological balance of nature, pollute the oceans, destroy forests through "acid rain" emissions from industrial smokestacks, threaten the Antarctic habitat, and so on.

Greenpeace "confronted the establishment" in classic New Left style, staging dramatic confrontations that attracted headlines around the world and helped set the agenda for political debate. Greenpeace attracted participation from young people around the world, and especially from those in nations whose electoral systems chose candidates district by district, making it difficult for "environmental parties" or other minority groups to hold seats in parliament or congress. While young people from these countries could not be part of day-to-day legislative processes, through their direct-action and moral confrontation they could raise issues that others would have to address.[55]

Greenpeace volunteers tackled many environmental issues—the slaughter of dolphins, whales, sea cubs and sea turtles; dangers involved in ocean pollution; threats to the environment from international competition to exploit Antarctica's resources; health dangers from nuclear wastes; problems of acid rain and the decimation of forests. Highly dramatic, direct-action campaigns alerted governments and private citizens to actions

Greenpeace believed threaten the health of the environment. Over the years, an increasingly sophisticated set of scientific researchers helped select critical issues for "moral initiative campaigns" and provided data regarding the nature of the environmental dangers to which Greenpeace volunteers call attention. Greenpeace's dramatic campaigns focused attention on environmental issues that were not being addressed effectively through more conventional channels.

Friends of the Earth, a London-based international environmental lobby founded by the former head of the American Sierra Club, and the World Wildlife Fund, a Swiss-based organization with leadership from the British scientific community and backing from the British royal family, began to work in concert with the Green parties, with other nongovernmental international lobbying groups, and the United Nations Environmental Programme (UNEP), which had been created at the time of the 1972 Stockholm conference. Together they created a new agenda for action.[56]

During the 1970s, UNEP sponsored a series of international conferences on the growing global environmental crisis. It played an important role in gaining international agreements to suspend nuclear tests in the atmosphere. In the 1980s, UNEP sponsored conferences which resulted in an international treaty obligating its signers to reduce industrial emissions that cause "acid rain" deposits that kill forests and pollute lakes and waterways in areas all over the world that are downwind from the industrial sites.[57] The U.S. government ceased to play a leading role in the global environmental movement after the 1980 election produced a conservative U.S. administration more concerned about the loss of U.S. manufacturing capacity than about environmental problems, but European nations and Japan proved much more responsive to environmental issues. Green party activity in many European parliaments helped move this along, as did leadership from the Queen in the Netherlands and occasional pro-environmental leadership from such international figures as Britain's Prime Minister Margaret Thatcher and French President Francois Mitterrand.[58]

By 1984, UN-coordinated scientific research was documenting serious changes in the earth's atmosphere that could threaten the health, safety, and wellbeing of most nations in the world. Hydrocarbon emissions from industrial manufacturing and from some industrial products were destroying the ozone layer in the earth's stratosphere, which shields the earth from dangerous radiation from the sun. Other threats to the balance of nature—from automobile smog, the destruction of forests and from energy uses that many scientists believe are increasing the temperature of the earth—became the subject of widespread study and debate. Global warming, it was argued, was affecting the food production for the world, and could eventually result in widespread flooding of coastal areas if the polar ice caps begin to melt. As evidence grew that the thinning of the ozone layer and global warming would reinforce each other and that their combined destructive action is now accelerating, such debates moved outside the halls of science and into the international political arena. By the beginning of the 1990s the environmental crisis had become a major concern for most of the nations in the world.[59]

In June of 1992, a second global environmental summit conference was called by the UN; it was held in Rio de Janeiro, Brazil, and attended by representatives of 178 nations and over 100 heads of state. (The Rio Conference will be discussed in more detail in Chapter 9.) By the 1990s the three streams of global awareness—coming from scientific research, from social protest movements, and from major organizations and institutions around the world—had joined. A new frame of reference was being used in many quarters, one that created a new priority for decision making and reorganized our sense of how different kinds of problems relate to one another.

The events briefly chronicled above point to a striking shift in emphasis that is emerging throughout the world, one likely to reorient much public policy thinking in the years ahead. It is becoming clear that unless health issues are addressed at a global level, demands for disease services will escalate rapidly, out of all proportion to demands now anticipated simply from the changing age structure of the population. Thus it forces us to move beyond the compartmentalized planning that treats health issues as distinct from other policy decisions. As several nations are beginning to recognize, that approach no longer is an adequate basis for policy planning.

Each of the next three chapters looks at health reform developments that emerged from the dynamics described in this chapter. Earlier tensions generated by an emerging global political economy produced a major shift in generational perspective which, a quarter century later, now is reorienting approaches to problem-solving at many institutional levels. New perspectives fundamentally regroup problems that need addressing, the coalitions that work on them, and the strategies used to address them. Each of these next three chapters identifies a different part of the puzzle that has to be solved if we are to move beyond the problems and dilemmas that currently confound the American health-care system. Each chapter identifies an area where more attention is needed, the circumstances which mobilized a particular interest group to tackle these problems, and the kinds of solutions they introduced. Then it identifies strengths and problems inherent in their strategy, as seen by advocates and critics. I will close each chapter with my own sense of the most important lessons to be taken from these current efforts to reform American health care.

7
Holistic Health

At the heart of the health-care industry's cost dilemma lies a commitment to making high-tech disease care the center-point for health interventions. Few would question the value of such interventions for certain kinds of medical emergencies, but many have come to question the value of making high-tech medicine the first line of defense. The most radical critiques of contemporary medical science and the health-care industry have come from individuals and organizations within the holistic health movement. They also have provided some of the most radical alternatives to current strategies for health care that are used within the contemporary health-care industry.

The holistic health movement introduced the following innovations into contemporary American health care: (1) It reintroduced a mixed medical model, using treatment and health-building strategies from many cultures, including pre-scientific medical systems. Thus it ended the monopoly of science-based strategies for health care. (2) Holistic health sees health as much more than the absence of disease. It focuses on health-building, even during treatment of disease, rather than making disease care the center of attention. By intervening earlier and differently in the health-disease process it minimizes reliance on high-tech diagnosis and care. (3) It directs attention to mind/body relationships in health and disease and to mobilizing an individual's own healing potential. (4) It reintroduces spiritual dimensions as part of health care, something medical science ignores. One consequence of this is a focus on the life/death process as a continuous evolution, an approach which provides different strategies for assisting with birth, aging and death. (5) It fundamentally reorganizes relationships within health care, challenging bureaucratic modes of interpersonal coordination and relationship and changing the nature of dependence and cooperation between care-receiver and care-giver.

Holistic health first emerged as part of New Left social protest of the 1960s and became strongly influenced by both the radical counterculture and the women's health movement. These approaches gradually made their way into the mainstream of American life. As this movement has evolved over a quarter century some serious limitations inherent in its approach also came to light. (These will be addressed shortly.) During the 1980s many social critics of health care focused on the holistic health movement's problems and predicted that although holistic health would find a niche within folk medicine, it would have little impact on the health-care system as a whole. To their surprise the 1990s saw Congress establish an Office of Alternative Medicine within the National Institutes of Health and other NIH budgets also began to include more evaluation of alternative medical treatment strategies. Centers for the study of Alternative Medicine were established in some of the leading American universities, and a few of the more innovative managed care organizations made plans to introduce a mixed model for health care as part of their treatment options. A third of the American public, it turned out, already were using these approaches and represented a potential market. A few health insurance companies also expressed willingness to reimburse for alternative treatments that proved to be more cost-effective.[1]

Some policy analysts considered holistic shifts in approach to health and disease an important way both to improve American health care and to make it more cost-effective. Others, not surprisingly, disagreed sharply. But a growing group of observers began to ask a different kind of question about holistic health: Whether or not it proved to be a model which could replace the present health-care system, what did holistic health have to teach us that could be used more generally?

Because its approach differs in important ways from that of the medical-science based health-care industry, our own examination of these developments should begin with a simple question:

What is Holistic Health?

The Preamble to the constitution for the United Nations World Health Organization provides this definition of health: "Health is a state of complete physical, mental, and social well-being and not merely the absence of disease or infirmity. The enjoyment of the highest standard of health is one of the basic rights of every human being, without distinction of race, religion, political belief, economic or social condition." Taking seriously the World Health Organization's understanding of the nature of health, the holistic health movement shifted its attention beyond the health-care system's previous focus on disease, its cure and prevention.

Earlier public health perspectives had focused on preventing disease by keeping disease-producing organisms out of the drinking water, by improving public and private sanitation, by encouraging low-income families to limit their childbearing so that more adequate nutrition can be available to family members, and by discouraging personal behaviors, such as smoking, that put health at risk. The central concern of holistic health, in contrast, was with active health-building, with encouraging a positive state of well-being, not simply the absence of disease. A person's state of health, participants believed, reflects the current balance that exists between his or her physical, mental, emotional, and spiritual processes—which cannot be addressed in isolation from one another. Nor, they insisted, is health improvement something others do for you; each person must play a major role in their own health development. This approach contrasts strikingly with medical science's reduction of health and disease to a series of biochemical processes and its advocacy of scientific interventions directed by experts.[2]

Holistic approaches start with the individual, recognize that one's state of health includes how one relates to other people and how one coexists with other species and with the larger environment. Health care must involve more than isolated individuals, participants insist, because we are all inescapably part of an ecosystem. The larger social and physical environment affects individual health processes, and that environment, in turn, is affected by the actions of individuals.[3] Because members of the movement understood health to be part of a larger cycle, they argued that health can be present throughout the continuing life-death process, and that death should be approached as a natural part of living. They tried to create conditions under which one can die well as that process runs its course. Health, in short, means optimal well-being at any stage of the life-death process rather than simply the prolongation of physical existence. Putting the promotion of health and well-being in place of the goal of conquering disease, of course, reorients health-care interventions quite basically.

Holism

Holism involves a particular way of seeing relationships. It contrasts with the "reductionism" that underlies science, bureaucracy, and technocratic management more generally. Reductionism breaks things down into their smallest component parts. Higher, more complex levels of organization are analyzed as if they were simply combinations of these simpler parts. In medicine, for example, "cracking the genetic code" involves discovering which of a multitude of possible combinations of four DNA elements are actually occurring to produce a specific, complex biochemical process. Reductionist analysis considers different levels of a system to be a series of increasingly complicated combinations of the same biochemical processes first seen at the simplest levels. For this reason it has difficulty explaining shifts in the *quality* of what is happening at different levels within a system, and in dealing with non-physical states and events.

Holism, in contrast, looks for a larger pattern that characterizes the entire system and that can explain the character of each system level, including the non-physical and most complex levels of interaction. It tries to understand each part in terms of its relation to the whole. When proceeding holistically, one looks for a larger principle that *integrates* a complex system, providing a simple way for highly differentiated parts to relate to one another.[4] Thus when holistic analysts see a problem in the healthy functioning of one part of a system, they look for reflections of that kind of problem at other system levels as well. For example, if a particular organ system (like the liver or gall bladder) is malfunctioning, holistic analysis looks for a reflection of that pattern in emotional states (such as anger or resentment) and in unresolved spiritual issues (such as difficulty in forgiving) that might be relevant. The holistic analyst also examines foods, drugs, exercise, and social behaviors that might be involved. Holistic intervention strategies then identify some currently accessible way to affect one or more levels where that larger pattern is being expressed. It is assumed that an intervention made at one level will affect all other levels as well.

Holistic practitioners typically make fairly simple interventions, intruding as little as possible into the normal functioning of the larger system. They draw attention to any larger pattern found, so that clients can continue to work on their own with the physical, mental, emotional, social, and spiritual issues that may emerge as the larger system adjusts to what has been happening. A physical symptom, for example, may be used as a clue that particular emotional issues may also need addressing. Persons in emotional trauma might be asked about their broader social relationships as well as about diet, exercise, and physical or spiritual changes that could be relevant to what is happening. Whenever practical, given the nature of the problem, holistic health interventions try to free a health-building, integrative process to do its work, rather than relying on an outside chemical agent to force the body into line. Practitioners encourage clients to take responsibility for their own health, in the sense of being an active part of the change process that is underway.

A number of medical systems popular before the triumph of medical science proceed holistically, in the sense just described. Classic Chinese medicine, of which acupuncture is a part, is an example. So are classic Indian medicine and the homeopathic tradition that was medical science's chief rival in America at the beginning of the twentieth century. Most of these traditions share two assumptions that distinguish them sharply from medical science. First, they do not view the separation of mind and body as "real"; instead, they maintain that the "mind-body" is a single continuous process. Some, in fact, have no separate concepts for "body" and "mind." Other holistic traditions believe that the body expresses what is happening in the mind and the spirit, and also that the body "learns" from its environment and teaches the mind and spirit. Second, they assume that a "life-force" principle, working at all levels of the self, provides the holistic integration of activity in humans. They see biochemical reactions not as the "root reality" of human functioning but as secondary by-products of this more basic phenomenon.

Holistic health practitioners and participants do not question the reality of biochemical processes nor do they deny that drugs have powerful effects. However, most of them consider the use of drugs a crude and drastic way to intervene in a subtle process. Drugs, they believe, affect not only the physical site to which they are directed but also more subtle health processes occurring at physical, mental, and spiritual levels. Because an intervention at any level affects the whole, they argue, drugs should be used primarily when a genetic defect is present or when there is not time to let a slower integrative process complete its course. In their view, drugs should be a last resort, rather than a preferred first option.

The analytic strategies of science, in contrast, describe a human system in terms of biochemical reactions. The analysis often becomes quite complex and difficult to grasp, requiring professional expertise of a high order. What is happening at higher levels within the human system—whether issues of personality, social interaction, or spiritual struggle—tends to be ignored, except when it can be described in terms of physics and chemistry. In contrast, when holistic strategies are used, the analysis often becomes quite simple; each subpart is described in terms of its unique expression of a common integrative principle at work throughout all levels of the system. People who are well-versed in the complexities of a reductionist, scientific analysis of health phenomena are often astonished and occasionally disturbed by the simplification of analysis that occurs when holistic perspectives are used. Sometimes earlier biochemical detail can be incorporated and rearranged in this new context. At other times the pattern presented by a holistic analyst largely ignores the kinds of physiological processes that are the focus for medical science.

Types of Holistic Interventions. The holistic health movement, in borrowing from the healing traditions of other cultures, reintroduced a mixed medical model into American health care. In addition to Chinese and Indian healing traditions, health methods that came from North America were embraced, including shamanistic Native American practices, nineteenth-century uses of homeopathy, naturopathy, the chiropractic, and Edgar Cayce's late nineteenth-century approaches to psychic healing. More contemporary practices—jogging (with yoga stretches), weight lifting and body-building, holistic forms of psychotherapy, vegetarian diets, organically grown foods, and herb teas—became popular, as did all-cotton clothing to let the body's natural energy flow unimpeded. So did affirmations to direct the mind's attention to health improvements, along with affirmations of sexuality and the use of sexual energy for health-building. The use of healing crystals, palmistry, and astrology, even the ancient tradition of alchemy—there seemed to be no end to the range of methods and traditions members of the holistic health movement were willing to explore. Most, in fact, combined these more esoteric approaches with use of the American medical system for urgent emergencies (such as broken bones or life-threatening illnesses, where the gentler rhythms of natural healing might take too long). This was indeed a mixed medical model.[5]

Holistic practitioners often begin by specializing in one particular healing method and later adapt their practice to include elements from many healing traditions. Many, in fact, came to specialize in the training of lay clients to do health maintenance work with one another. A number of the health-building techniques popular within the movement can be learned fairly simply and practiced without immediate supervision. Many involve the use of special forms of breathing, meditation, or "body work" to create altered states of consciousness in which mind and body can interact in a different way.

In this approach, what works and what does not work must be determined through direct experience, which means trial and error. The holistic health movement focuses not on diseases, for which some standard treatment exists, but on restoring an individual's internal "balance" so that he or she can deal effectively with other organisms in the environment, thus avoiding illness or recovering quickly when it develops. Holistic practitioners often quote the eminent biologist, René DuBois, who noted that even in the most severe epidemics only about a third of the persons exposed to the "causative agent" succumb to it. If the central problem for health and disease is to improve one's internal balance and external relation with the larger ecological system, they argue, corrections for problems must be fine-tuned to each person.[6] Participants are therefore taught to approach themselves as unique entities; what works most effectively for one person may be inappropriate for another.

This more individualized approach to cause and effect has bothered many medically trained observers, who argue that the methods being used by the holistic health movement are simply placebos, mental suggestions that produce a health improvement. Holistic health enthusiasts reply that the "placebo effect" is precisely what they hope to achieve: a signal to the mind to correct whatever imbalances have been occurring in physical, mental, or emotional functioning. Holistic health enthusiasts for the most part are unwilling to write off their results as "only a placebo effect", but are happy to mobilize suggestion as part of their own health-building.

Such a strategy created chaos for scientific verification, by making double-blind studies and other assessment strategies of medical science impractical to use. To many participants in the holistic health movement, who claimed they had made major improvements in their own ability to remain free of disease, such problems of verification seemed unimportant. Many physicians, however, worry that holistic practices may lead some people to ignore serious illnesses for which effective medical interventions are available, or to try useless remedies during the time period when a cancer or other life-threatening disease is still amenable to scientific treatment. From anecdotal reports, it seems clear that this sometimes happens. Believers in the movement, however, note that medical science itself has a documented rate of problems and failures, from its use of drugs and surgery. The real question, they argue, is not whether problems and failures occur (which happens in any medical system) but the comparative rate of success both in turning disease around and in promoting higher levels of health in the total self. Unfortunately, the movement has not yet developed a way to keep large-scale, systematic records of health outcomes for the people who have used its methods. In consequence, the debate goes on.[7]

In 1984, a Coalition of Holistic Health Organizations, representing about 65 groups from across the country, met in Washington, D.C., and identified eight principles that underlay their approach to health and disease (lefthand column, Table 7.1). These principles present a striking alternative to the outlook and practices that have guided more conventional health care. This becomes clear immediately when one compares each of them to a correspondingly numbered statement in the righthand column, which gives traditional views in found textbooks and classic writings used by medical schools throughout America.

The assumptions and procedures of the "wellness model" and the "disease model" for health care at many levels are mirror opposites. Yet the two systems can be used together, as many consumers began to demonstrate in the 1970s and as a growing number of physicians encouraged patients to do, thereafter.

Holism offered a new approach to psychosomatic problems. Rather than seeing psychosomatic illness as "not quite real" because a mental or emotional component was involved, holistic approaches look for simple, direct ways that unresolved stress manifests itself physically. For example, holistically oriented researchers have mapped circadian rhythms in the body that affect blood pressure and the functioning of the immune system.[8] They have noted how stress interferes with these rhythms, leaving one susceptible to illness. Holistic health advocates argue that several of the major unsolved health problems of the nation—including heart disease, cancer, and alcoholism—are diseases in which stress plays a major role and for which lifestyle choices become critical.[9] "Ease" and "dis-ease" became important concepts for holistic practitioners, and alternations between the "fight-flight" and the "relaxation" response became an important focus for holistic thinking about health processes. Individuals are encouraged to recognize the ways they use stress in their own lives, and to develop health-building alternatives for habits that lead to "dis-ease." When dealing with disease itself, holistic health participants emphasize health-building at every stage of response to illness.

TABLE 7.1 Comparing Holistic Health and Medical Science

Underlying Principles	
Holistic Health[10]	*Medical Science*[11]
1. A human being is a living energy system rather than an arrangement of parts. Any disturbance in body, mind or spirit reflects a disturbance in the whole system.	1. The body is a machine that operates according to the principles of physics, chemistry, and biology. It is, in fact, best described as a biochemical machine (and can be understood by observing how these principles operate at the level of the individual cell).[12]
2. Holistic health recognizes the spiritual dimension of healing as well as the power of the body to heal the mind and the power of the mind to heal the body.	2. Medical science eschews superstition, basing its operations on clinically observable physical events and laboratory experiments. "Spiritual healing," if it exists, has little to do with "medical science."[13]
3. The most sensible approach to health and illness is to seek our physical, mental, and spiritual potential.	3. The task of medicine is to diagnose and cure disease.[14]
4. Holistic health recognizes the mutually responsive relationship between the person, human society, and the natural universe in which both exist. The healing response is a shared concern of the individual and society.	4. Disease appears when there is a genetic defect in biological coding for the cells, when degeneration occurs as part of the aging process (or from accidents), or when other organisms invade the body. Medical science intervenes to minimize damage, to stop invasive or degenerative activity when possible, and to provide drugs that will correct improper biochemical reactions.[15]

(continues)

TABLE 7.1 *(continued)*

Underlying Principles	
Holistic Health	*Medical Science*

5. The practitioner is a facilitator for the individual to find optimal health in a societal and natural context, by providing the conditions under which the person's natural healing ability is strengthened.

6. Practitioners use the resources of others and all means for completing health care for the individual, relating illness symptoms in all cases to a whole person perspective.

7. Natural, low-risk methods which mobilize the individual's healing resources take precedence whenever possible.

8. Self-help and self-care are fundamental principles of holistic health. The holistic approach minimizes dependence on the practitioner and recognizes that each person is unique, while providing information to help the individual find his or her own way to optimal health.

5. The ideal doctor-patient relationship involves a competent doctor who diagnoses disease and provides the most up-to-date treatment strategies, and a cooperative, compliant patient who follows the doctor's orders faithfully and intelligently.[16]

6. Medical practitioners refer their patients to competent specialists who are trained to deal with the more technical aspects of those disease states whose treatment falls outside their own expertise.[17]

7. Medical researchers search for more powerful drugs, for innovative surgical procedures, and for equipment that can take over when parts of the human body malfunction.[18]

8. Patients should use good judgment about when to seek medical attention. While some self-care is appropriate, the intelligent patient will not attempt to take treatment into his/her own hands, but will seek the advice of a competent professional.[19]

Transformation

Participants in the holistic health movement frequently talk about "transformation," a term borrowed from the human potential movement; there it referred to a natural evolution that supposedly unfolds as one attunes more clearly to "root reality." In holistic health circles, "holistic transformation" refers to a health-building process in which the "life-force" principle guides a larger evolution of the self. The well person maintains health through exercise, diet, meditation, and physical touch designed to maximize the flow of life-force energies. As blocks to the flow of one's own integrative principle are overcome, it is expected to work more freely, improving one's sense of well-being as life processes come into better balance and aiding one's continuing personal development. The pursuit of high-level wellness thus includes an expectation that individuals will continue to grow and change as their total health improves.[20] Participants in the movement have sometimes spelled "holistic" with a "w," to emphasize the importance of dealing with the whole person.

The movement's simple slogan, "Take responsibility for your own health," captures the importance it places on life-style choices and on one's active involvement in the health-building process. To critics who focus on social and environmental sources of disease, this sounds narcissistic, neglectful of responsibility for others or for the larger environment.[21] Advocates reply that what is involved is less individual self-centeredness than a demedicalization of health processes.

The movement's effort to demedicalize health can be seen in its promotion of home birth and midwifery and its support for the hospice movement, which enables people to die at home with dignity.[22] It can also be seen in the small health food stores that members of the movement opened, challenging the monopoly of medical pharmacies and calling foods "your best medicine." It is most strikingly apparent, however, in its reliance on "healers," individuals who have demonstrated a personal capacity for helping with the health-building process in others. While some training programs in "healing" take as long to complete as Western medical school, many holistic health treatment methods can be learned in six weeks to a year, and some, indeed, in a weekend. Thus many approaches taught lay people how to work with each other on health-building.

Alternatives to Patriarchy and Hierarchical Control

In place of patriarchal or bureaucratic relationships, the holistic health movement accented equalitarian, emotionally supportive interactions, with practitioners offering resources to be used by clients rather than taking control of the health process. (Some physicians, of course, already emphasized this style of interaction with patients, but the holistic health movement made this central in the process of health-building.) Organizational procedures used within the movement encouraged both men and women to be entrepreneurial and to assume leadership positions. In addition, people were encouraged to work directly with what participants described as male and female energy principles at work within each person. Given its strong emphasis on touch, intuition, nurturing roles for the therapist, and on self-effacement by the professional who works to enable clients to do their own work, this venture did more than open its ranks to women. It required serious male participants to develop traits normally associated in western cultures with women, such as intuition and emotional sensitivity, and it sought to avoid subservient power contexts for either the provider or the recipient of services. In this latter effort, it did not always succeed: stereotypic patterns of gender interaction continued to appear among holistic health participants, and formal organizations often had a preponderance of male leaders.[23]

Participants in the holistic health movement eschewed professional roles with one another and avoided the creation of bureaucratic organizations. In fact, their formal organizations tended to be short-lived, with few lasting longer than two or three years.[24] In place of bureaucratic organizations and forms of coordination, they relied on action networks that developed as loose-knit collections of people without permanent leadership or "heads" consulted each other. Projects were undertaken on the initiative of creative individuals and groups. If someone came up with an attractive new approach others joined in or replicated it quickly, or perhaps introduced their own original strategies for proceeding with the common agenda. This organizing strategy encouraged flexibility and organizational creativity, but it is too chaotic to produce organizational "staying power" over time.

Holistic endeavors often included individuals and organizations that differed widely in their own personal outlooks, agendas, and forms of internal organization, and who sometimes were suspicious of one another or competed for leadership roles. Nevertheless, the fact that an action network was holistic affected how it proceeded. For example, holistic rituals used to bond members together often involved establishing "energy" connections between participants. Holistic action networks used other bonding strategies as well, such as ideology, or the establishment of a common emotional identity. However, the non-verbal, more nearly "psychic" bonding used within many holistic health networks had an especially powerful impact on many participants.

Growth of the Movement. The new health magazines that began to spring up in the 1960s trace the growth of new themes for health care expressed in the New Left's free clinics, the women's health movement, and increasingly, holistic health: an interest in bringing "medical problems" back to the people, in de-medicalizing life experiences, and in humanizing health encounters.[25] Between 1960 and 1975, some 66 new publications that gave some special attention to holistic health themes made their debut, almost half of them after 1970. They were published in 14 states, and over time had made their way from university towns and adjacent neighborhoods to rural addresses of communes and back-to-nature enterprises, and then by 1975 to a locus in major metropolitan areas across the country.

Meanwhile, in San Diego, California, a group of holistic health enthusiasts in touch with the activities of the psychologist-entrepreneur David Harris had founded the Mandala Institute, which began to sponsor major conferences on holistic health. They also founded the American Holistic Health Association in 1975, the first national organization of people who made their living by providing holistic health services. Although they attracted only a portion of their target group and did not begin to tap the range of people who were using holistic health approaches or offering services to others on a non-professional basis, they quickly gained a membership of 1,000.[26]

Within another 10 years a number of magazines featuring holistic health themes were selling 100,000 copies per issue. Some did far better than this: *American Health: Fitness of Body and Mind* sold a half-million copies of each issue, and *Prevention Magazine*, with a circulation of over two and a half million, rivaled the *Reader's Digest*. Holistic health had moved beyond its counterculture origins into the mainstream.[27]

Holistic health was not simply a lay movement, or a revolt against science and professionalism. The American Holistic Health Association had been joined by organizations for medical professionals, including the American Holistic Medical Association and the American Holistic Nursing Association, the Therapeutic Touch Nurses Association, and others. A past-president of the American Medical Association was speaking at Holistic Health conferences. Within a few more years a number of agencies within the federal health bureaucracy would co-sponsor conferences on holistic health as a possible new public policy, and foundations and government agencies would provide funds to encourage further development of some of these approaches.

Holistic Health Comes to the Attention of National Policy Makers

The ideas and organizational approaches of the holistic health movement, born in the counterculture, were in the beginning controversial. The speed with which they spread beyond the cultural fringes and came to the attention of bureaucrats and the policy elite demonstrates both their resonance with other questions being asked by policy makers and the power of entrepreneurial "networking" activity. In describing this activity, it will be useful to focus on the roles played by two innovators, Rick Carlson and Effie Chow.

In 1968, Rick Carlson abandoned corporation law to join the staff of the Institute for Interdisciplinary Studies (later renamed Interstudy) in

Minneapolis. For the next four years he participated in an interdisciplinary team exploring the implications of a proposed public policy initiative to create health maintenance organizations (HMOs). He eventually became convinced that HMOs would not solve the real health-care problems of the country. They could hold down some of the cost for conventional health-care services, but they provided no way to address the really large creators of health-care costs—the disease categories against which conventional medicine was making little headway at the time, namely cardiovascular disease, cancer, and chronic illnesses. The reason, he concluded, was that each of these diseases had at least part of its origin in environmental conditions or in the results of life-style choices like smoking, over-eating, drinking, and living under persistent stress. Extending government-sponsored health insurance in the Medicare style was even less likely to solve these problems, he believed, because it would simply be used for hospital costs *after* health had broken down.[28]

Convinced that the push toward HMOs was irrelevant, Carlson left Minneapolis for a position as Visiting Fellow at Robert Maynard Hutchins' Center for the Study of Democratic Institutions in Santa Barbara, California. He shared ideas with another visiting scholar, Ivan Illich, who was also formulating a critique of American health care. Whereas Illich's book, *Medical Nemesis*, was written for the general public and became a best-seller, Carlson's book, *The End of Medicine*, was aimed at policy makers. The controversy aroused by reviews of these books brought them to the attention of major figures in the world of health policy. Walt McNerney, who headed Blue Cross-Blue Shield nationally, found Carlson's analysis intriguing. So did Kerr White, an epidemiologist at Johns Hopkins University who was on an Institute of Medicine Task Force for the National Academy of Science; he called Carlson's book to the attention of John Knowles, then head of the Rockefeller Foundation. When his tenure at Santa Barbara ended, Carlson decided to become a freelance policy specialist and offered to set up private, off-the-record, invitation-only conferences for policy makers. Knowles and McNerney agreed to help him raise funds for a conference and to provide contacts to other key leaders, provided they were not presented as endorsing his proposals.[29]

Thus in early 1976, Carlson hosted an off-the-record conference at Airlie House in Washington D.C., attended by 200 key figures in government, business, and health care. There Carlson presented his analysis of why current health-care proposals could not solve the nation's health problems. At the conference he introduced them to innovators from Harvard and the University of California medical schools who were developing new approaches to stress control, to innovators developing new approaches to health problems of the elderly, and to policy analysts discussed ways to transform the medical care system.[30] Positive responses to this conference encouraged its sponsors to hold a follow-up invitational meeting, to include another layer of influential persons. In late November 1976, some 300 people came to a conference at the Waldorf-Astoria Hotel in New York City, called "The Limits of Medicine: The Promise of Holistic Health." The conference repeated what had happened at Airlie House a few months earlier, but the sponsoring group had expanded to include Don Frederickson, who headed the National Institutes of Health (NIH), and Phil Lee of the University of California San Francisco Medical School. With this sponsorship and word of the Airlie House conference circulating, the 300 places were oversubscribed.

In 1976, legislation was passed to create a consumer education unit within the office of the Assistant Secretary for Health. The new Office of Health Information and Health Promotion was headed by Jane Fullerton, an experienced health bureaucrat in Washington. She attended the Waldorf-Astoria conference and then brought aboard as a key administrative assistant Alice McGill, who had expressed some interest in the holistic health movement and who had worked in NIH with Ted Cooper, now the Assistant Secretary for Health. During the first two years of its existence, the Office of Health Information and Health Promotion spent much of its time trying to bring together potential constituencies across the country and to get single-health-issue groups to cooperate with one another in a larger approach to health and wellness.

A few months later, in the spring of 1977, the Institute of Medicine of the National Academy of Science joined the earlier sponsoring group in presenting "The Limits of Medicine: The Promise of Holistic Health: II," once again to an invitational list of 300 new participants at the Waldorf-Astoria. The proceedings of this conference were published under the title, *Future Directions in Health Care: A New Public Policy.*

In 1977, John Knowles edited a special edition of *Daedelus, Journal of the National Academy Of Arts and Sciences,* entitled "Doing Better and Feeling Worse: The Health Care Crisis in America." His editorial made it clear that he was not personally using this arena to advocate holistic health policies, nor endorsing Carlson's indictment of the present health-care system. But the publication dealt with a wide range of issues raised by conventional health care, and Knowles's editorial noted that 80 percent of current illnesses are caused by human behavior choices that affect proneness to disease. The conferences seem to have affected the questions being asked by "the establishment," whether or not all of the answers were being endorsed.[31]

Carlson's initiative in setting up the Airlie House and Waldorf-Astoria conferences picked up on a momentum that had already started to gather. Senator Edward Kennedy was investigating the "health-care crisis" in Congress, where there was general agreement that the cost of health care was spiraling upward at an alarming rate. A number of innovators within government were already suggesting that a disease-prevention and health-promotion approach was needed, and the invitational conferences for policy advisers added a coherent overview of the situation, as well as introducing radically different possibilities for addressing the problems. While communication was developing between the health-care policy elite and would-be shapers of policy within the federal bureaucracy, other innovators, unaware of these events, were exploring their own routes to policy influence. One of the more interesting of these was a San Francisco nurse named Effie Poy Yew Chow.[32]

Effie Chow, a Canadian with nursing experience in Asia as well as in Canada, had moved to the San Francisco Bay area in the mid-1960s after establishing ties to researchers at the Stanford Medical School. A highly innovative nurse who could work effectively with the minority community, she established the first family planning and sex education program for the Chinese in the United States. She was soon working with the state legislature to legalize planned parenthood programs in sex education, sterilization, and abortion. At the same time, her links to the Chinese community had led her to continue a study of acupuncture, which she had begun on an exchange visit to China a few years before.

When American physicians started expressing interest in acupuncture, following Dr. Paul Dudley White's well-publicized visit to China as part of the Nixon-era détente efforts, Effie Chow helped the Academy of Parapsychology and Medicine, in Palo Alto, set up the first U.S. training program in acupuncture for MDs. It brought in French and English doctors who were experts in the technique, and offered programs across the country from 1972 to 1975. In 1973 Chow formed the East-West Academy of the Healing Arts, a non-profit educational venture. In 1974, when the federal government set up regional Health System Agencies (HSA) to help coordinate local approaches to health care (as described in Chapter 2), she was asked to direct the San Francisco effort, one of 17 programs in California. Most HSA programs focused on health facility planning or on staff training needs. Chow, however, proposed an alternative approach for San Francisco, focusing on the special needs of minority groups and exploring how to integrate cultural aspects of their own health practices into the larger medical care system. These programs brought her to the attention of federal health-care administrators in Washington. She was recruited to join the American Nursing Association's Council for Minority Doctoral Programs in mental health, which worked with NIMH to recruit minority members and fund their Ph.D. training. She became Vice-Chairman of the Ad Hoc Committee on Hypertension in Minority Populations, which had been set up in the NIMH's National Heart, Lung, and Blood Institute as part of the response to minority pressures for government services. Then in 1976 she was appointed to the National Advisory Council to the Secretary of HEW on Health Professions Education, where she chaired a subcommittee on Disease Prevention and Health Promotion.

Meanwhile Chow's East-West Academy of the Healing Arts, was playing an increasingly public role in the programs she was heading for San Francisco's HSA. Starting in 1975, the East-West Academy began sponsoring two to three major conferences each year on the West Coast, attracting up to 4,000 participants each time. In 1977, Chow decided it was time to use her Washington network in the interests of holistic health.

The new president of the U.S., Jimmy Carter, had brought physicians who were interested in Chinese medicine onto his health advisory team. Moreover, the president's sister, Ruth Carter Stapleton, was a faith healer. All this suggested that Washington might be receptive to holistic approaches. The way to get Washington's attention, Chow believed, was to organize a conference around topics currently exciting widespread interest, for which holistic health had significant new inputs. Using network contacts, she drew in a wide variety of agency people in Washington who had similar interests. In September of 1977, Effie Chow held her first Washington conference at the Shoreham Americana Hotel. The theme was "Stress Without Distress: Cancer, Death, and Dying." Major addresses were given by international figures who re-enforced the holistic concerns of the conference organizers. The real coup, however, was getting Ruth Carter Stapleton to address the conference. Over 2,000 people attended, and enthusiasm quickly developed for a follow-up conference focused on holistic health.

The second Shoreham conference took place in Washington, D.C., on April 21-25, 1978, with the theme "Holistic Health: A Public Policy?"[33] The Second Congress of Nurse-Healers, also sponsored by the East-West Academy of the Healing Arts, was held simultaneously. More significantly, the Shoreham conference on holistic health was co-sponsored by five government agencies and five private organizations, in addition to the East-West Academy of the Healing Arts. In organizing it Effie Chow involved additional people with whom she became involved through the earlier conference on stress. She encouraged each collaborator to work through his or her own networks to make sponsorship as widespread as possible. Critically important assistance came from other minority members of the federal bureaucracy with whom she had worked earlier. They made sure that a variety of federal agencies not only endorsed the conference but provided the funding to underwrite it. Chow also had Rick Carlson on the planning committee, along with Alice McGill of the Office of Health Information and Health Promotion and a number of other people who were active in the Washington area. Networking, as Chow's example demonstrates, could be used to mobilize bureaucratic resources, not simply to resist bureaucracy.

The conference itself emphasized indigenous healing traditions present in American minority communities, as well as the new holistic modalities. Major conference presentations were followed with workshops, in which participants could experience alternative healing approaches. There was something for everyone, during the four days. Unlike Carlson's carefully selected, academically respectable roster of holistic health interpreters and advocates, Chow's conference presented the full range of holistic health enthusiasts. Politicians, religious leaders, minority spokespeople, sensational healers, academics, and public policy analysts spoke. In addition to the people who attended representing hospitals, public health planning agencies, and other government agencies, the well-publicized program drew members of the holistic health movement from many parts of the country.

When interviewed later, Effie Chow stated her intent simply and directly: She wanted to influence policy by drawing out people within the establishment who were interested in holistic health, demonstrating the extent of interest in these approaches and creating an arena in which a wide range of policy-makers could begin to examine other approaches to health, thus influencing how the government thinks about alternative health care. At least three of the Washington-area planners for this conference told me while I was attending the conference that their own hidden agenda was to create a climate in which mid-level bureaucrats would receive permission to begin funding education projects and demonstration grants in holistic health.

Rick Carlson's conferences had helped create a climate of openness among elite decision-makers in government and in the private sphere. Effie Chow's conferences, which followed almost immediately, produced an informal friendship network across government bureaucracies, one based on a common new agenda for health care. This new network let mid-level bureaucrats cooperate with each other, also off-the-record, to encourage the creation of wellness policies within their various agencies. Some of them actually began to implement this through their control of the administration of government grants.

Developing a Base at the State Level

Carlson's next major innovation was the creation of a state-level agency to encourage innovative holistic health projects. This state agency also stimulated the creation of holistic health coalitions made up of holistic innovators, business and education leaders, and the more progressive-minded health-care professionals in local communities. With this move he began to create an ongoing structural base for continuing health-care innovation.[34]

In the late 1970s, after he had established himself as a freelance health policy consultant and scheduled the conferences in Washington and New York, Rick Carlson moved to Marin County, California. Soon he was invited to join a group of people who were meeting with Jerry Brown to assess what had gone wrong in his 1976 presidential nomination race and how he could use "new politics" to increase his viability on the national scene. Out of that two and a half day meeting at the home of Brown's friend, Paul Hawken, came the suggestion that Brown should use his governorship to demonstrate new initiatives to resolve the growing health-care crisis. If California could lead the way in approaching this national issue, Jerry Brown would have enhanced political stature and would gain support from new constituencies. Brown decided to use a device created during the Kennedy administration in the early 1960s—Governors' Councils on Physical Fitness—as the vehicle for this effort. It would be renamed the California Governor's Council on Wellness and Physical Fitness and expand its mandate to include innovations in risk reduction and health promotion activities in the state. Brown asked Rick Carlson to head the council. As he developed a working relationship with Brown, Carlson became the unofficial liaison between Brown, the California health bureaucracy, and the state legislature.

The California Governor's Council on Wellness and Physical Fitness was set up in 1979. Brown was interested in having the Council develop precedent-setting demonstration projects and created a demonstration-grant budget for the Council. Carlson, however, wanted to use the Council to make sure that the initiatives it set in motion would not end when Brown was no longer governor. He therefore worked to generate an institutionalized process for generating wellness activities that could continue without a governor's personal sponsorship. The Council had 26 prominent Californians on it.

People active in physical fitness, business leaders, and political supporters of the Governor were included in the Council which focused on three major tasks. First, it worked to stimulate the formation of local and regional councils that would bring together business leaders, school district officials, and other community representatives to collaborate on developing wellness initiatives at the local level.

Second, the Council set up a grant program. For example, it offered an annual, competitive, $50,000 award to a public employee agency at the state or local level which developed a particularly effective proposal for using its employees to help with community health promotion. The first award went to a southern California community to develop training programs to teach firefighters, the police, and other public employees who have regular contact with the public how to do health promotion work in their community.

Third, the Council sponsored a series of demonstration projects to introduce new risk reduction and health promotion approaches. The Council sponsored a Senior Olympics program to encourage fitness activities among the aging population. They also set up community health fairs.

Other activities of the Council had clear political implications. For example, it sponsored a project in toxic waste mapping, locating toxic waste sites throughout the state and developing a series of overlay maps which traced the incidence of various health problems in concentric rings around each waste site. Materials and counsel were offered to local groups interested in working on this problem.

A school nutrition program encouraged local communities to develop materials to provide direct experience with nutritional effects and how they were created in their own community. Grade school children were encouraged to have a sugar-binge day and a sugar-free day to discover for themselves how their bodies felt when they consumed junk foods. High school students were sent out into local grocery stores to do price comparisons and also food supply comparisons. These projects were designed to show students how stores of the same chain offered products of different types and quality to different economic and ethnic neighborhoods, and to show them that food-stamp necessity items were priced higher in the poor communities than in stores catering to more affluent customers who used only their own cash. The students were then encouraged to try to discover why these practices occurred, which engaged them in direct questioning of people who put these policies into practice.

The most ambitious project involved school districts, the state legislature, and the state bureaucracy. Two school districts in California began experimenting with incentive plans to encourage employees to improve their own health status. Blue Shield of California cooperated with them, allowing the districts to pay health insurance premiums once a year instead of monthly, and in the meantime to put the interest gained on the money into a pool for the employee's own use. The employees could spend their share of this money in any way they chose to improve their own health, and there would be a "profit sharing" feature for employees if health expenditures for the district went down over a period of years because of decreased need for hospitalization. Health self-care materials were developed at Stanford University to use with those who participated in the plan.

When the two school districts reported high enthusiasm for the plan and an early drop in health-care expenditures, the state legislature allocated $750,000 for demonstration projects to be set up among employees in the state government and in industry. The funds were voted in 1982, but the new Governor elected in that year, Republican George Dukemejian, vetoed the appropriation and abolished the Governor's Council. The legislature then absorbed the Council and created a non-profit action arm to continue the projects. The state agency demonstration project could not go forward, but Blue Shield and the Hartford Insurance Company sponsored a study that included a controlled "health incentive" experiment using one of the original school districts and Bank of America employees who lived in comparable communities.³⁵

Rick Carlson had already taken steps to make sure activities would continue without Brown's direct sponsorship. (He had resigned as Chairman of the Council in late 1982 so that Assemblyman John Vasconcellos could succeed him as chairman and pave the way for the legislature to take over responsibility for the venture.) During the four years the Governor's Council operated, he served as official consultant to the American Hospital Association, encouraging them to revamp their structure and redirect efforts toward wellness. And he worked closely with the Washington Business Group on Health, a spin-off from the Business Roundtable, which brings together many of the Fortune 500 firms and represents their interests in Washington.

Looking back, we can see that from 1975 to 1980 the different frame of reference, organizing principles, and specific problem-solving strategies of the radical counterculture had found their way into mainstream health-care thinking and planning. The funders of health-care services were starting to ask some of the same questions that were coming from grassroots critics, and a new model for health-care services had become a serious contender on the national scene. The innovations did not take over, but they became an important source of ferment and provided criteria against which to evaluate other developments within the health-care industry. New approaches to health care were no longer fringe phenomena, but were being sponsored by established interest groups too powerful to be ignored by opponents within the health-care establishment.

The 1980 election brought a conservative political administration to Washington, with an agenda pledged to reducing health and welfare budgets and to strengthening military spending. Not only were holistic health agendas low on the priority list for new heads of governmental agencies, but conservative religious constituencies of the now-dominant political coalition were attacking New Age movements and the holistic health movement as "dangerous." Official government sponsorship disappeared, though Effie Chow continued to get sponsorship of her approach from government agencies in Canada. In the U.S., government innovation now encouraged the corporatization of health-care services, as discussed in Chapter 3. Innovators who were interested in a new health-care model increasingly turned to businesses and to foundations for an institutional base of support. As they did so, the thrust of a new model for health-care changed directions once again, as it adjusted to the concerns of new sponsoring groups.

In short, as the 1980s progressed, the holistic health movement lost its ability to set the health policy agenda. The movement itself, and the mixed model for health care that it advocated, continued to be popular with the public, as subscription rates for holistic health magazines attest. Holistic outlooks, moreover, began to inform research agendas. Selected aspects of holistic health practice, notably biofeedback and the analysis of stress factors in illness, made their way more widely into general health care. But it seemed clear that holistic health was not the wave of the future in America. Critics had noted some glaring weaknesses in the movement, seen from the vantage point of the health-care needs of the nation as a whole.

Problems with Holistic Health

The holistic health movement's radical reconceptualization of issues and strategies for health care was criticized from many perspectives, once it was being taken seriously by important institutional interests. Beginning with the mid-seventies, and continuing thereafter, the critics on the left, the right, and in the center took issue with core approaches of the new movement, and critics from within the movement itself voiced concerns. From the plethora of responses—ranging from editorials in the *Journal of the American Medical Association (JAMA)* to critiques from Marxist scholars, and from within the holistic health movement itself—came a small set of themes that emphasized vulnerabilities and distortions to which the movement seemed prone.

First, many critics—particularly Marxists and other academics on the left—were outraged by the movement's admonition to "take responsibility for your own health," especially when it was coupled with an emphasis on mind-body relations which suggested that internal stress was a central factor in many disease states. This approach, they felt, amounted to "blaming the victim."[36] Some also worried that right-wing policy-makers would use the self-help perspective to justify withholding medical services from the poor.[37] Editorials in *JAMA*, and a number of clinicians (and some holistic health practitioners) expressed concern that cancer victims would have their suffering compounded if holistic practitioners encouraged them to feel guilty about being susceptible to disease—or worse yet, to avoid seeking chemotherapy.

Second, other critics—particularly those from the public health arena—felt that the holistic health movement was repeating the fundamental error of medical science—focusing on the individual to the neglect of social and environmental influences on health and disease.[38] Despite such additional slogans as "think globally, act locally," or some of the demonstration projects of the California Governor's Commission on Wellness and Physical Fitness, the movement as a whole made individual health its central concern. To the extent that its social and environmental concerns were limited to protesting the use of pesticides and drugs in foods, it failed to provide a corrective to the myopic focus of medical science on individuals and their diseases. Given the movement's origins in an amalgam of social movements, including those concerned with the ecology of the planet, this individual focus was particularly ironic.

Third, political radicals argued that holistic health not only perpetuated but intensified the class divisions of the mainstream health-care system. Most holistic health practitioners were college-educated, middle-class men and women who provided services—and workshops and training seminars—to others like themselves; and their fees, largely uncovered by third-party payers, put their services beyond the reach of persons of limited income. Thus the over-serviced sector of the population received still more services, while those most in need of basic health care remained unserved.[39]

Still other critics, both within medicine and within the holistic health movement itself, noted that the movement offered the public little consumer protection from poorly trained or incompetent care-givers; because practitioners were not licensed, the only guideline for potential clients was *caveat emptor,* "let the buyer beware." While members of the movement acknowledged the problem, they diverged in their sense of what to do about it. Some felt this lack of regulation was an asset; it prevented special interests from establishing a monopoly and gave consumers a wider choice. Others longed for the equivalent of AMA licensing control over entry into the ranks of holistic practitioners, and some proposed training certification as an intermediate control strategy: Consumers could discover whether a holistic tradition's trainers had certified a practitioner as competent; this would alert consumers to competency judgments made within the field, while preventing practitioners already on the scene from excluding new competitors from the field. The holistic health movement, in short, raised once again the questions that had engaged medical scientists at the turn of the twentieth century. The difference was that they were exploring a wider range of policy options.[40]

Critics loyal to the canons of medical science were concerned less about certification of practitioners than about verification of treatment results. They noted that holistic health had no equivalent to the skepticism built into scientific investigation, and no objective method of assessing outcomes, whether scientific or not.

Defenders answered each of those attacks. In response to the charge that urging people to take responsibility for their own health was blaming the victim, holistic health defenders answered that such attacks misunderstood what the movement meant by its slogan. It encouraged individuals to take responsibility for their own part of the health process, by discovering what their own mind-body systems can and cannot do and by actively considering what kinds of health interventions work best for them.[41] It seemed clear, however, that some holistic practitioners and many persons who were themselves wrestling with a life-threatening or debilitating disease used this kind of approach in ways that heightened guilt rather than empowered the person with the disease to proceed in new ways. If understood at its deepest level, nonetheless, the admonition opened profound areas for exploration.

In response to charges that they were focused on individuals to the neglect of the environment, defenders argued that a deeper understanding of holistic health requires a sense of the whole, including the social and environmental web of which individuals are part. Critics responded that the main thrust of holistic health practice was much more individualistic.

Responding to criticisms that its fees made services unavailable to the poor, holistic practitioners sometimes protested that fee-for-service was the only practical way to remain independent of bureaucratic control and protect the special quality of person-to-person encounters. They argued that their incomes were far lower than those of physicians; that when they charged individual clients the equivalent of a physician's office visit fee, it was for an hour or more of service, rather than 10 minutes; and that they often worked out barter arrangements with clients who could not afford to pay in cash. Finally, they pointed out that a number of practitioners teach self-care classes through adult education programs, thereby helping the public become less dependent on services by health-care professionals (either inside or outside the holistic health movement). It seemed clear, however, that neither mutual self-help nor barter arrangements would find the widespread acceptance needed to correct the class bias inherent in a system of uninsured fee-for-service funding. No matter how effective its individual interventions might prove to be, unless the movement found an alternative source of funding it would remain irrelevant for the health problems of the nation as a whole.

Responding to criticisms that they lacked verification of treatment results, defenders of holistic health pointed out that many classic medical traditions, such as acupuncture or Indian yoga and ayurveda, have evolved over centuries; observation over time can substitute for scientific appraisals of effectiveness. Critics could answer, however, that holistic practitioners rarely limited themselves to the use of a classic medical tradition from a single culture, and that many also used contemporary approaches that had not stood the test of time. They rejected the belief that "you should let your body tell you what works for it and what doesn't," finding this an inadequate basis for assessing many health states and outcomes.[42]

In assessing evidence that is mixed or incomplete, as it usually is in situations concerning health and disease, two types of error are common. One can too readily reject a claim that something is having an effect, thereby ignoring some of its real relevance to what is happening. Or, at the opposite extreme, one can accept a causal claim too readily, before there is sufficient evidence to substantiate it. Medical science, with its orientation toward doubt and skepticism, is prone to the first type of error; holistic health, with its willingness to suspend doubt and to believe in multiple forms of cause and effect, is prone to the second type. Statisticians argue that if one cannot avoid the possibility of an error in judgment, it is important to decide whether a Type 1 or Type 2 error would be preferable.[43]

In real life, of course, decision-making often requires deciding which kind of error to risk. For example, if a cancer is spreading slowly, one might prefer to try to strengthen the immune system's functioning through changes in nutrition and the use of biofeedback meditative imaging, for example (even if the outcome from these approaches were not certain), before deciding to try chemotherapy which damages the immune system as it tries to destroy a tumor. But if the cancer turns out to be spreading rapidly, relying on a less invasive but "unproven" therapy could put one's life at risk. In short, the concern of critics that mixed model medical treatments may not be effective is a valid one. All one can say is that there are times when decision logic would lead one to try relatively benign interventions first, and other times when uncertainty regarding the outcome of such treatment should lead one to be cautious about choosing them. But which time is which?

Given the kinds of problems outlined above, it seems clear that holistic health, whatever its successes in certain areas, had not developed the broader social vision or environmental thrust needed to become an adequate replacement for the health-care industry. Nonetheless, it has made important contributions toward an evolving health-care strategy, and still provides a useful vantage point from which to critique other developments.

A New Look at Alternative Medicine

In the early 1990s, alternative medicine reappeared on the Washington scene. Senator Tom Harkins, the Iowa Democrat who headed the Senate Appropriations Committee, put through Congress an additional appropriation for NIH of $2 million for the fiscal year 1992, earmarked to "more adequately explore...unconventional medical practices." The congressional appropriations language commented that Congress was not satisfied that "NIH has fully explored the potential that exists in unconventional medical practices" and directed NIH to "convene and establish an advisory panel to screen and select the procedures for investigation and to recommend a research program to fully test the most promising unconventional medical practices."[44]

Harkins had been approached by Fred Wiewel, an Iowan who had organized People Against Cancer, and by his friend and former Iowa Congressman Berkley Bedell. Wiewel was convinced that both AIDS and cancer patients need to be free to explore unconventional routes of treatment, and that the federal government should help evaluate the effectiveness of these treatments. Bedell agreed. He had left Congress because of serious health problems that had disappeared after using alternative medicine. Convinced that the treatment he received had been beneficial, he joined Wiewel in approaching Tom Harkins. Impressed by their argument, Harkins, who was using unconventional treatments for his allergy problems, sponsored the amendment to the Senate Appropriations bill, and shepherded it through Congress.[45]

Once Congress made the appropriation, an Office of Alternative Medicine was set up within NIH, and an ad hoc advisory panel on unconventional medical practices was established, made up of 20 advisers—MDs, PhDs, and representatives from the Brooklyn AIDS Task Force, People Against Cancer, innovative cancer treatment programs, and former congressman Bedell. At their first meeting in June 1992, the advisory panel encouraged the acting director of the new office to seek advice from practitioners of unconventional therapies as well as from researchers. They identified six areas of unconventional medical practice that should be explored (see Table 7.2). Three months later, a workshop convened to advise the Office of Alternative Medicine on next steps invited 120 participants from these varied backgrounds, and made it clear that others were welcome to attend.[46]

The September 1992 Chantilly conference included members of the original advisory panel, practitioners from all the fields listed in the table, medical researchers and government agency personnel who were personally interested in the problems. A few academics interested in health-care policy and innovation also attended, as did some members of the public who learned about the workshop and decided to come. NIH officials welcomed participants and described types of research already underway that might provide models for evaluating the promise of unconventional medical practices. Evaluation methods need to respect key assumptions underlying unconventional treatments while still providing a rigorous assessment of outcomes. Participants gave advice about the health problems that various unconventional medical approaches tackle most successfully, kinds of documentation and data currently available about how these approaches work, and criteria that should be used for evaluating them. They recommended the office have its own peer review committees to judge research proposals, and that these committees include practitioners as well as researchers, in order to make sure study designs do not violate basic assumptions underlying treatment methods. At the end of the workshop, Jay Moskowitz, Associate Director for Science Policy and Legislation at NIH, announced that NIH would fund six research projects studying unconventional medical practice in the coming year. The appropriation was increased the following year and the Office of Alternative Medicine set, as its first priority, identifying specific therapies and therapists outside the mainstream of medical science reported to be producing documentable clinical improvements, and gathering evidence which evaluates their effectiveness.[47] If this became clearly documented, the Office would fund research exploring *how* such effects occur.

TABLE 7.2 Areas of Unconventional Medicine Recommended for Further Study

Areas of Treatment	*Examples of What This Includes*
1. Diet, nutrition, and lifestyle	Macrobiotic diets, vegetarian diets, use of mega-vitamins
2. Mind-body control	Biofeedback, counseling & prayer therapies, guided imagery, hypnotherapy, art therapy, sound or music therapy
3. Traditional medicine and ethno-medicine	Accupuncture, ayurveda, herbal medicine, homeopathic medicine, Native American healing, natural products, oriental medicine
4. Structural manipulation therapies and "energy" medicine	Osteopathy, chiropractic medicine, accupressure, massage therapy, polarity therapy, chi gong, Rolfing, therapeutic touch
5. Unconventional pharmacological biological treatments	Cell treatment, chelation therapy, metabolic therapy, use of oxidizing and anti-oxidizing agents (e.g., ozone, hydrogen peroxide)
6. Electro-magnetic applications with exposure to electro-magnetic fields	Treatment of broken bones

It was not simple for NIH to absorb an office devoted to the scientific study of alternative medicine, nor to understand the priorities and concerns of its advisory committee. Some of the most respected canons of medical research seem inappropriate for studying alternative medicine. (Double-blind studies, mentioned earlier, where neither subjects nor evaluators know who has had what treatment, do not work well when "the placebo effect" is being cultivated rather than avoided. More conventionally trained members of peer-review committees within NIH do not always consider these problems when evaluating research designs.) Some members of the Advisory Committee were determined not to be co-opted into using too narrow a scientific research model, one that might distort evidence relevant to alternative medicine. More suspicious advisers worried that NIH might be using its own bureaucratic procedures to prevent challenges to conventional scientific thinking. But other advisory committee members were unconcerned about NIH motives. They noted that NIH itself was allocating $12 million from budgets outside the Office of Alternative Medicine to investigate alternative treatments. Tensions that occasionally arose between NIH leadership and the advisory committee, they believed, came because of NIH's effort to provide quick response to requests, while not understanding fully some of the issues that were involved in studying alternative medicine. The more politically active members of the advisory committee had additional concerns, however. They argued that the Congressional mandate to the new office called for quick identification of promising approaches to AIDS and cancer. They sometimes expressed impatience with the slow pace of scientific research, wanting field studies of promising treatments and clinical evaluation of health outcomes from potentially promising treatments to take precedence over more usual NIH research strategies.

Consequently, the first three years of the new Office of Alternative Medicine were chaotic. There were frequent changes of staff, considerable tension between staff and members of the advisory committee and within the staff itself. The program did, however, begin field evaluations of a few, controversial treatment strategies that had come to the attention of members of the Advisory Committee or members of Congress. It also established two research centers with responsibility to evaluate alternative treatments for HIV and AIDS. In 1995, NIH appointed Wayne Jonas to head the office. He had been heading medical research evaluation training at the U.S. Army's Walter Reed Hospital and had studied homeopathy in Europe and used it with some of his patients. It seemed clear that NIH was serious in its commitment to the new venture, and recognized the importance of giving the office leadership that was both methodologically sophisticated and had some understanding of alternative medical approaches. Jonas replaced former staff and asked the advisory committee to help him identify strategic research areas that would move the field forward systematically. At Jonas' recommendation, 12 academic research centers were funded to coordinate the investigation of specific uses of alternative medicine. The various academic research centers were given grants to study alternative approaches to the treatment of AIDS and HIV, drug addiction, cancer, stroke and neurological conditions, asthma, allergy and immunology, women's health issues, aging, the use of alternative treatments for pain control, and its use in general medicine. Some of the grants were made jointly with other NIH programs.[48] A particular treatment modality (such as acupuncture) might be evaluated at several centers. Following NIH tradition, each center was disease-focused. None examined health-*improvement* as a central research concern.

A study appearing in the *New England Journal of Medicine* reported that a third of the American public makes use of alternative medicine. Clearly alternative medicine is alive and well in America, and is now getting attention from researchers.[49]

A few health insurance companies began to reimburse for alternative treatments that have both a clinically demonstrated success rate and lower cost than conventional medical treatment for the same problem.[50] And a few health maintenance organizations announced plans to include alternative medicine as part of their treatment options.[51] Their motives may have been mixed. Some seemed genuinely intrigued by the health benefits possible through a mixed medical model; others seemed motivated most strongly by an opportunity to capture a demonstrated market segment. Alternative medicine clearly was entering a new arena as the twenty-first century appeared on the horizon.

These signs of new life for holistic health did little, however, to settle the range of challenges and questions that critics of holistic health had been raising. These deserve attention.

Holistic health cannot replace the conventional medical system. Nonetheless it has important lessons to teach. This chapter will close, as will Chapters 8 and 9, with a summary of its implications for broader health planning.

Lessons from the Holistic Health Movement That are Useful for Current Health Planning

Lessons offered by the holistic health movement might be summarized as follows:

1. Low-tech health improvement methods from many cultures, which focus on strengthening or restoring the body's self-regulatory ability, can play a significant role in any health-care system.

2. A focus on mutual help, self-care, and the demedicalization of basic life events can offer humane alternatives to invasive, high-tech approaches to birth, aging, and dying—which now consume a disproportionate share of our health budgets.

3. An emphasis on non-bureaucratic encounters and the deprofessionalization of many health services opens up a wider range of possibilities for finding personnel to deal with currently medicalized health problems and life transitions.

4. Research into mind-body interactions and the role of stress in disease, now pursued within psychoneuroimmunology (a new research specialty that crosses the boundaries of psychology and medicine), can help evaluate potentially significant new strategies for disease prevention and health-building.

5. We need a *health-care* system, not simply a system for disease management. Holistic health's strategies for health improvement show ways to move in that direction.

8

Prevention and Health Promotion: Industry, the Government and Foundations Innovate

In parallel with the more radical reforms introduced by the holistic health movement came demonstrations of how to create a different focus for *health* care within the American mainstream. Using more conventional understandings of disease and disease-care than were seen in holistic health, the prevention movement focused on early interventions in the health-disease process. It changed the health-care model so that it was proactive rather than reactive, reaching people where they live and work, actively intervening before disease develops.

Since the 1970s, reform-minded innovators in industry, the government, private health organizations, and philanthropic foundations have undertaken various ventures in preventive health-care efforts that fall between and sometimes overlap those of the holistic health movement at one extreme and the health-care industry at the other.

Both the conventional health-care industry and the holistic health movement focus on how the health-disease process works within the individual person, though the former focuses on biochemistry and the latter on interactions between body, mind, and spirit. In contrast, preventive health, drawing on its earlier public health heritage, is primarily concerned with how features of the social and physical environment directly affect health and disease in individuals.

Some preventive health approaches resembled those found in the holistic health and women's health movements. All of these approaches, for example, paid attention to lifestyle behaviors and choices that affect susceptibility to disease. Each advocated using self-help procedures whenever possible, though the prevention movement's recommendations were more congruent with a medical science perspective. Both noted the role that stress plays in making one susceptible to behaviors that put health at risk, and in the actual development of various disease states. Both encouraged the use of support groups; that is, they advocated taking advantage of the experience of others and finding emotional support when dealing with stressful situations in one's life. These areas of similarity made it possible for many holistic health participants to adapt their approaches sufficiently to be hired as staff or consultants to prevention-focused programs sponsored by industry, the government, or foundations.

Indeed, a number of people who sponsored prevention-oriented health initiatives were also personally involved in activities of the holistic health or human potential movements. Recognizing that their efforts went beyond earlier public health strategies, they often referred to themselves as participants in "the wellness movement," a term that bridged the two ventures and made it easy for practitioners to go back and forth between them, shifting their emphasis when working within one arena or the other. Thus the preventive health ventures of the 1970s and 1980s were by no means always distinct or isolated from those of the holistic health movement. Nevertheless they had a different point of origin, related differently to science, bureaucracy, and established interests, and—most significantly—proceeded from a different understanding of where to intervene in the health-disease process.

Early Prevention Efforts

The preventive health movement represents a regrouping of interests that have been part of American health care for generations. When the Rockefeller Foundation began to underwrite health-care reform efforts in the first two decades of the twentieth century, they tried to encourage broad planning for health-care needs. In 1914, for example, the Rockefeller-funded General Education Board convened a conference to discuss changes occurring in public health and needs for the future. From about 1840 to 1890 members of the sanitation movement, reformers who came from the ranks of civil engineers and city planners, had worked to eliminate the impact of dirt and filth on the modern environment, seeing these as the source of disease. Their efforts had resulted in the creation of clean water supplies and sanitary sewage systems for American towns and cities, as well as elsewhere in the world.[1] Then after 1890, as modern medical science embraced the germ theory of disease, their concerns combined with those of the American Medical Association (AMA) and other groups to create a public health movement focusing on germ control: Tuberculosis sanitariums to isolate carriers of that airborne disease and fumigation of infected houses became favorite strategies.

In 1906, Congress passed the Food and Drug Act which initiated controls on the manufacture, labeling, and sale of food. In 1912 the U.S. Public Health Service (PHS) was established, along with the Children's Bureau, and in 1914 the General Education Board's conference tried to build a consensus regarding the public institutions needed to train public health workers for the future.[2]

From the 1914 conference came a decision to draw up plans for institutes of hygiene to train workers who dealt with hygiene, sanitary science, public health, and preventive medicine. A report to the Rockefeller Foundation, growing out of that conference, recommended that an institute of hygiene should be separate from a medical school, though closely affiliated with it, and that both should be part of a larger university, in order to take full advantage of scientific discoveries being made. Eventually eight graduate schools of public health were established: at Johns Hopkins, Harvard, Yale, and Columbia, and at four state universities—in Michigan, Minnesota, North Carolina, and California (at Berkeley).[3] The U.S. Public Health Service was given increasing responsibility for handling diseases that might threaten the larger public, and for providing services to the indigent. It established a leprosy colony in 1917 and a division of venereal diseases in 1918, and became responsible for maternal and child health service coordination with a further reorganization in 1922. As time went on, public health funding and planning increasingly adopted medical science's focus on individuals and their diseases. Tuberculosis control, for example, became focused on use of chest X-rays and skin tests to diagnose diseased individuals. In 1938, the U.S. PHS was given responsibility for administering federal medical research, coordinated through the newly created National Institutes of Health.[4] After World War II, as federal funding for medical research increased rapidly, NIH became responsible for channeling federal health research moneys to researchers across the country. Public health's focus became increasingly directed toward disease-oriented research. A few new schools of public health were established, broadening health-care training beyond that found in medical schools to include training biostatistical experts who could help evaluate medical research results, epidemiological researchers who could track the spread of disease patterns within the population, professionals who could work with birth control programs and maternal and child health problems, specialists in industrial medicine, persons trained in health administration, and public health policy analysts and advisers.[5]

In short, public health problems had become redefined during the half century following the establishment of the U.S. PHS and the 1914 conference that established standards for training public health workers. With few exceptions (such as some of the medical service programs for native Americans and the indigent), the concerns of contemporary public health fit easily within the emerging health-care industry's model for providing disease-focused health services.

Renewed Efforts

As noted in Chapter 2, Congress had established the John E. Fogarty International Center for Advanced Study in the Health Sciences in 1968 as part of the NIH complex. It sponsored conferences and study reports on medical education, environmental health, societal factors influencing health and disease, geographic health problems, international health and research, and preventive medicine. As this list of topics suggests, many of the concerns that had taken a particular form within the holistic health movement were in fact part of a larger orientation that was gaining broader support within academic and policy planning circles within the country. John Knowles of the Rockefeller Foundation and Walt McNerney of Blue Cross/Blue Shield, both active with the Fogarty Center, felt strongly that something had to be done to lower the utilization rate for hospital services and for medical services more generally and became interested in the possibility of encouraging Americans to do more self-care.[6] Responding to these themes, Nixon appointed a presidential commission on health education that held regional hearings across the country during 1970 and 1971. Public health professionals in academia, the Health Maintenance Organization movement, and community health education councils gave testimony and helped generate enthusiasm for preventive health programs.[7]

In 1970, the National Heart, Lung, and Blood Institute (NHLBI) in the NIH sponsored a Multiple Risk Factor Intervention Trial (with the catchy acronym MRFIT), a study of the impact that several lifestyle behaviors make on long-term health risks.[8] Ted Cooper, the director of the NHLBI, was a participant in the informal groups discussing the need for new national policy. MRFIT's focus for study reinforced the Fogarty Center's interest in preventive medicine and helped extend discussion of policy alternatives beyond self-care to preventive health measures: It began to seem clear that if Americans could be persuaded to stop smoking, get their blood pressure under control, and lose weight, demand for medical services would drop significantly.

Focusing on Worksites

By 1972, recommendations from the President's Commission on Health Education and related discussions within the health policy elite had created enough momentum in Congress to pass legislation setting up a program in Health Education and Disease Prevention as part of PHS's Centers for Disease Control (CDC) in Atlanta. Clarence Pearson of Metropolitan Life Insurance Company, who approached policy issues from the vantage point of the business community, immediately saw the potential of worksites as the locale in which preventive health programs should work.

Believing that parallel thrusts should be developed by government and the business community, he helped organize the National Center for Health Education, a private sector program to work with the American business community. Dr. Monty Duvall, Assistant Secretary for Health during this period, played a key role in securing the new federal health promotion center in Atlanta. After he left public office he headed the National Center for Health Education, moving it from its early home in New York to San Francisco, where the most widespread interest in health promotion seemed to be centered.[9]

Three years later a coalition of health policy advocates in academia sponsored a conference that produced a 1975 Fogarty Center Report focusing on consumer choices and the role of the media in health promotion. This led in 1976 to congressional legislation creating the Office of Health Information and Health Promotion, put under the direct supervision of Ted Cooper, who had become the Assistant Secretary of Health.[10]

Meanwhile informal, health-oriented action networks emerged in Washington, D.C., within the civil service system's health bureaucracy. Participants in these networks not only cooperated among themselves but developed common wellness-agenda ties with businessmen, politicians, and staff members of such organizations as the American Hospital Association. Particularly effective was an informal network of women who held positions in several federal and private agencies, or were married to influential leaders in health care and politics, or had close ties to minority congressmen or well-organized special interest groups. As one member of this informal group remarked, "The best thing about our work is that no one can ever see where the political pressure to support our projects came from." They succeeded in shifting an increasing proportion of funds they administered toward wellness-promoting efforts, many of which were outside the control of the more conventional parts of the health-care industry.[11]

Other health-oriented action networks developed among business leaders who cooperated to set up worksite wellness programs in their corporations. These "wellness" networks also cooperated with more formal coalitions of businessmen in local areas to introduce into their communities such health-care organizational innovations as HMOs and Preferred Provider Organizations (PPOs) and to set up data pools for keeping track of the performance record of various health-care providers.[12] At the same time institutional interests in business and philanthropic foundations were beginning to provide a structural base for a new kind of health-care system. For example, the National Center for Health Education sponsored conferences that encouraged business leaders to refocus their health-care benefits programs toward wellness promotion rather than conventional disease care, with its constantly spiraling costs.

In 1976, the same year that HEW was setting up its new office for health promotion, it sponsored the Secretary's Conference on High Blood Pressure Control in the Work Setting. This conference brought providers and academics together to discuss the possibilities of using worksites as the place to deliver preventive health-care services. The National Heart, Lung, and Blood Institute of NIH then sponsored demonstration projects examining the clinical and cost implications of delivering hypertension control at the worksite. For the next 10 years, the office set up to supervise these projects brought risk reduction and health promotion strategies to the attention of government and business leaders.[13]

In 1984, the national media found it newsworthy that a new contract between the United Auto Workers and General Motors stressed job security over pay increases and included "wellness benefits." In fact, other corporate giants had pioneered worksite wellness programs since the mid-1970s. Johnson & Johnson and Xerox had been selling their programs to other companies, and industrial operations as diverse as IBM, AT&T, Pepsico, General Foods, and the Shaklee Corporation, as well as various national insurance companies, had seen their wellness programs featured in national news magazines.[14]

In 1985, the U.S. Department of Health and Human Services directed the U.S. Public Health Service's Office of Disease Prevention and Health Promotion to conduct a national survey of worksite wellness programs. It was guided by an advisory committee composed of prominent university researchers involved in public health, in the holistic health and wellness movements, innovative officials in the federal health bureaucracies, and representatives from major corporations and business health groups. Sampling from Dun & Bradstreet listings, the project surveyed business operations where 50 or more employees were working. The results surprised even enthusiasts of the worksite wellness movement. Over 87 percent of the larger worksites, with 750 employees or more, reported some kind of health promotion activity in their plant or business operation. Over 70 percent of worksites employing between 100 and 250 employees had such activity, and 55 percent of the worksites with fewer than 100 employees also were doing something about health promotion. Clearly, the idea of keeping people healthy had caught on among American businesses.[15]

Health promotion activities reported by these businesses—listed in order of popularity—included stop-smoking programs, health risk assessments, programs for back care, stress management, physical fitness and exercise, off-the-job accident prevention, nutrition education, high blood-pressure control, and weight control. Over 35 percent of all businesses interviewed had some kind of stop-smoking program; less than 15 percent offered weight control programs. Employees in business locations with 750 or more employees were at least twice as likely to have each type of health promotion activity listed above as were people in worksites having less than 100 employees.

The vast majority of worksites provided company-paid health promotion activities, and 60 to 80 percent of the worksites provided them on company time. The widespread provision of time off for these activities, coupled with the fact that very few businesses had bothered to collect data on actual savings realized from their programs, suggests that corporate interest in worksite health promotion programs in 1985 was not based primarily on a desire to cut the costs of health expenditures. It apparently made sense to corporate officers independent of evidence that it worked for cost control.

Business and government health policy groups, however, argued that if the worksite wellness movement was to survive, it would eventually have to demonstrate its cost-effectiveness: The constant escalation of costs for disease-oriented health services was so great that it squeezed other service-oriented budgets. Health promotion activities, in consequence, would have to demonstrate that they save money that otherwise would go into higher health insurance costs. Soon a number of reviews were attempting to assess the effectiveness of worksite health promotion programs.[16]

Most of the initial reviews were disquieting to health policy planners who favored worksite wellness activities. Many programs made no attempt to keep track of how many employees participated in them. Where records were kept, a disturbing pattern began to emerge. Although tens of millions of American employees now had health promotion services available at their worksites, usually only about 8 to 15 percent of the employees for whom a particular health promotion program was relevant took part in it. In most companies, participation was heavily skewed toward management employees, and participation from the rank and file was minimal. Critics suggested that participants were mostly persons already oriented toward a wellness model, who would be taking care of themselves even without an on-site wellness program.[17] Even more disquieting was the track record of many programs. Among those who joined programs to stop smoking or to lose weight, for example, recidivism rates were high. If a quarter or more of those who attempted such behavior change were successful at the end of a year's time, programs were considered a success. Given low participation rates to begin with, the impact of worksite wellness programs on the health of a plant as a whole was often small.

Searching for A Workable Strategy

When General Motors and the United Auto Workers signed their 1984 contract guaranteeing "wellness benefits" in addition to sickness care, both the promise and the problems of worksite health promotion were clearly in view. General Motors had six years' experience with blood pressure control efforts, with some good results. Company and union health executives, however, recognized the problems other corporations were having in getting widespread participation in other health promotion activities. Consequently their joint task force for health promotion decided to commission experimental studies in a group of General Motors plants, to discover what worksite health promotion activities would be most effective with their employees. The NHLBI of the NIH was also interested in evaluating the impact of different worksite wellness programs. These agencies jointly sponsored an experimental study to be conducted by the University of Michigan's Worker Health Program.[18]

Four GM worksites in the Detroit metropolitan area which were similar in size and had comparable demographic profiles for their employee populations, were chosen for this quasi-experiment. Each site used a different strategy to encourage behavior changes relevant to cardiovascular disease prevention. The first site provided plant-wide health screenings and immediate health counseling for all participants. Site two also did this, then followed up with a three-year health education program similar to that offered more widely in industry, using some of the better-known worksite wellness programs. A local plant wellness committee sponsored special health events and encouraged employees to take part in health improvement classes. By comparing health changes at sites one and two after three years, the study team could determine whether health screening and counseling actually affect health behavior over time, and also see how much is gained by adding local sponsorship of health activities and on-site health education classes.

Site three, building on the experience of blood pressure control programs introduced at a few Ford and GM plants, emphasized personal follow-up of employees who had health risks. Besides conducting the wellness activities seen at site two, wellness counselors personally contacted the employees who had cardiovascular risk factors—68 percent of the employees, it turned out—and kept in contact with them over a three-year period.

Site four added an additional strategy to those used at site three. Here wellness counselors worked with the entire employee population, encouraging all employees to actively improve their present level of health and well-being. Counselors helped employees replace behaviors that increased their cardiovascular risk, like smoking, overeating, drinking alcohol excessively, or getting little exercise when off the job, replacing these with health-building alternatives. Recognizing that these "risky behaviors" are pleasurable, and that they can reduce personal stress in the short run, counselors encouraged employees to form buddy systems and social support groups when trying to make health changes. Plant-wide contests and other events helped keep attention focused on health improvements. The plant's wellness committee also worked on improving the health of the plant as a whole, introducing "heart-healthy" menu choices in the cafeteria, monitoring blood pressure changes as work conditions changed, and helping design stress management classes that could give people skills for coping with or for changing stressful situations they faced on the job as well as in their private lives.

Researchers made four predictions as the study began. First, because each site added one additional approach to those used at the preceding site, program impact should increase at each successive site. Second, blood pressure control should be the most successful specific outcome, since it could be controlled by medication, whereas other cardiovascular risk factors (such as smoking and weight) require major lifestyle changes. Third, if one-to-one outreach and follow-up of employees is critical for health behavior change, the most dramatic difference in outcome should occur between sites two and three (since sites three and four used wellness counselors, whereas sites one and two did not). Finally, recidivism should be lowest at site four, because of its social organization to focus attention on wellness issues and its efforts to substitute health-building behaviors for those that temporarily reduce stress while *increasing* other health risks.

When employees were rescreened three years later, in 1988, all four predictions proved to be correct. Results at sites one and two were similar to those seen nationally at worksites around the country. However, sites three and four had high participation rates in wellness programs, with 59 percent of at-risk employees participating in various health change efforts. They were successful: 50 percent of the risk factors identified three years earlier had improved markedly.[19]

As the GM study began producing positive results, Ford and the UAW negotiated to use the site three approach among Ford employees, and introduced a similar program, more narrowly focused on blood pressure and cholesterol control, in its 84 plants across the nation. Over a three year period it produced results comparable to those seen in the GM study. This partial replication throughout a large corporate setting demonstrated that the enthusiasm for health promotion now being seen throughout American business and industry could lead to real health improvement among a wide range of rank and file employees. It also showed, however, that success requires the use of appropriate health promotion "technologies" that are labor-intensive: one-to-one engagement; follow-up of employees that encourages them to personalize health promotion strategies; and social organization of the worksite that helps employees support each other in developing health-building behaviors.[20] Service delivery vendors who used the approach with smaller businesses were able to get participation rates of 90 to 95 percent, measurable health improvements for 75 percent of these participants, and the elimination of earlier cardiovascular risks in over half the workforce.[21]

Estimates for the cost of this program (in 1995 dollars), with full participation from a workforce, came to about $150-$175 per employee per year. If participation were lower, of course, the cost also would be lower. Given the clear reduction in health risks, such figures put the approach within reach for many businesses, [22]

Meanwhile, health officers in Burlington Industries had become concerned about the high rate of hysterectomies being performed on their women employees in the southern states. They contracted with free-lance medical staff to develop a system of counseling about surgical choices and alternative ways to handle the same problems. Options & Choices, the contracting service supplier, trained nurses in worksite counseling, instructing them not to lead people to a particular choice, but to help them evaluate the advantages and disadvantages of alternative strategies for handling their health problems. Most people, it turned out, prefer to avoid surgery if they can. The cost savings to Burlington Industries and to other companies that used this service was substantial.

Learning of this success, Federal Express hired Options & Choices to manage their total health benefits program. Dealing with a nationwide company whose employees live in remote rural areas and central city ghettos as well as in locales with more readily available health services, Options & Choices adopted an individualized counseling and follow-up strategy similar to that tested in the University of Michigan model. Each year they identified a "pareto group" of employees who had made the highest use of health benefits in the preceding year: 19 percent of the employees generate about 80 percent of health benefits spending each year. These employees were targeted for special attention. Rather than trying to stop their use of benefits or eliminate them from the payroll, Options & Choices provided individual counseling—often by phone—that dealt with the health-building needs of the whole person. Over an eight year period from 1984 to 1992 they were able to hold health expenditures "flat": Federal Express' health-care spending increased no faster than the general inflation rate. This result was achieved despite Federal Express' acquisition of the Flying Tigers Airline during this period, which required absorbing new employees with higher than average health risks.[23] Both the Ford and Federal Express experience demonstrate that these approaches can be used nationwide, and with populations living in areas that differ widely in the availability of conventional medical services.

When working with a widely scattered workforce, Options & Choices found that this program costs about $175 annually per employee reached. But if only the "pareto group" of employees is targeted for attention, the service can be paid for by budgeting about $25 per employee for the entire workforce. Gradually extending services to other at-risk employees, Options & Choices discovered that per-employee expenditures of up to $150 annually produced demonstrable cost-benefits.[24]

In short, industry's enthusiasm for a worksite wellness model during the 1970s and 1980s led to the widespread adoption of health promotion programs across the country within a short span of years. As more sophisticated organizational approaches to health promotion produced higher participation and more measurable health improvements, these efforts gained new relevance for those who hoped to change the country's health-care model.

By the mid 1990s these approaches to disease prevention and health promotion were becoming institutionalized. National funding through state health departments offered worksite wellness services to small businesses as well as to larger employers. The NHLBI of the NIH published a manual giving detailed instructions on how to introduce such risk-reduction technology at large and small worksites.[25]

Meanwhile, WELCOA (the Wellness Council of America) began a program to encourage businesses across the United States to develop worksite wellness programs of increasing quality. Their bronze, silver, and gold awards were given to companies who reported differing levels of health promotion activity at the worksite.[26] At the same time, the Health Project began to work with CEOs and government administrators, identifying and publicizing cost-effective innovations in health benefits management and health promotion that were making measurable improvements in health status and measurable reductions in the cost of health-care services.[27] On a variety of fronts, worksite health promotion was being moved toward setting clear standards and developing outcome accountability.

A number of corporations across the country began introducing proactive wellness outreach programs at their worksites, and a few HMOs and community primary care clinics were beginning to experiment with variations on the University of Michigan Model in community settings. Moreover, in California, Blue Shield agreed to make worksite wellness services reimbursable as part of company health insurance policies. Two pharmaceutical companies were recommending its use, nationwide.[28]

The few available cost-benefit studies suggested that the strategy was cost-effective in the relatively short-run, providing notable savings in expenditures for disease care after a three- to five-year period. Such savings, it appeared, could be expected to continue so long as proactive outreach to the target population was maintained. When one-to-one outreach and social reinforcement is abandoned, however, many people revert to earlier risk-producing behaviors.[29]

Worksite Prevention and Health-Care Insurance Reform

In 1993, many advocates of worksite prevention programs were dismayed to discover that the Clinton Health Insurance Reform Task Force ignored this area in its proposals for reform. Its prevention plans dealt only with physician-focused services—e.g., inoculations, well baby and pediatric clinic services, and early cancer detection. Moreover, its proposed insurance rate-setting procedures, they feared, might destroy the burgeoning worksite wellness "industry". The Clinton plan provided no reimbursement for worksite prevention services and would have established a single community rate for general health insurance, prohibiting insurance companies from offering discounts to employers whose employees had lower health-care costs than the community at-large. Thus, employers who paid for prevention services at their worksites would have higher operating costs than competitors who did not, and they would lose current financial benefits from lower insurance rates given to companies whose employees require less disease care than others in the community. The Clinton Task Force version of a single "community rating" for insurance premiums was designed to give small businesses cheaper health insurance rates and to prevent discrimination against persons with pre-existing health problems, but it inadvertently would have destroyed much of the funding base—and a strong employer motivation—for worksite-based health promotion and disease prevention.

Once it was clear that Congress intended to rewrite the Clinton health insurance reform plan, advocates of worksite wellness programs began to organize. In early 1994, they formed the Worksite Health Promotion Alliance, made up of employers, organizations that provided worksite prevention services, and relevant professional organizations dealing with occupational health issues. Hiring a former key staff member in Congress as their lobbyist, they recommended necessary services that should be provided by approved worksite health promotion programs, proposed insurance rebates or discounts as a means to help fund these programs, and levels of achievement that would let programs qualify for such funding. They gained strong bipartisan support in Congress for their proposals. The final bills which reached the floor of the House and Senate contained extensive language favorable to worksite health promotion. Although health insurance reform did not come to a vote in 1994 (because of a Republican strategy to withhold action until after the fall elections, which they swept), the strong bipartisan support for these measures augured well for future legislative action, either as part of comprehensive insurance reform or as its own proposal. By mid-1995, five of the six bills regarding health-care reform introduced into the new Congress contained provisions that would allow health promotion incentives. The 1996 health insurance reform bill included language that guaranteed access to insurance discounts for worksite health promotion programs, regardless of what more general premium-setting strategies might be devised to pay for the increased insurance coverage required by the new law.[30]

In the 1994 legislative proposals, which became the basis for later bills, worksite health promotion program elements would cover seven areas, which are summarized in Table 8.1.

TABLE 8.1   The Content of Worksite Health Promotion Programs

Service	*To Deal With*
1. Education, screening, counseling, and followup treatment or referral to reduce lifestyle or other modifiable risk factors	Cholesterol, nutrition, weight management, exercise manage- smoking cessation, cancer prevention
2. Management of chronic health risks or problems	High blood pressure, diabetes
3. Exercise and fitness programs	Inactivity risks
4. Employee assistance programs for areas of personal concern that affect job performance	Substance abuse, stress, parenting concerns
5. Workplace health and safety prevention programs	Injury prevention
6. Prenatal counseling and education	The number of premature births, low birth-weight infants, or birth defects
7. Development of living wills	End-of-life autonomy issues

In order to qualify for funding, worksite health promotion programs would have to achieve a specified annual employee participation rate. Some recommendations to Congress also required evaluation of outcomes and gave a federal certifying agency authority to set performance standards that would qualify for additional insurance premium rebates. Outcome accountability was seen as a prerequisite for securing institutionalized funding for any redirection of health-care services.[31]

In 1995, the Worksite Health Promotion Alliance convened a meeting of major national professional and vendor organizations whose members would be affected by proposed legislation. More than 18 national organizations took part, and agreed to develop national guidelines for health promotion or wellness programs and for certifying those who provided the services.[32] The relatively new area of worksite health promotion was developing its own internal standards for content, professional training, and performance outcomes. These seemed likely to upgrade program standards across the nation, and to provide more consistent outcomes from worksite prevention efforts. When national legislation gets passed, prevention programs would provide an enlarged range of services to promote and maintain health, many of which had been offered previously, if at all, primarily in doctor's offices. These would now would be offered proactively, taken to where people live and work.

Community Health Initiatives

Meanwhile, health policy planners were turning their attention to the 37 million Americans who have no health insurance and are unlikely to get health services through an employer. This vast group includes many members of racial and ethnic minorities who live in low-income neighborhoods, retired and unemployed persons who do not meet Medicare or Medicaid qualifying conditions in their community (either because they are not yet 65 or because local requirements for Medicaid preclude them), and people residing in small communities or rural areas where there are few doctors. Planners interested in preventive health also directed attention to teenagers just forming their lifestyle habits, who may be especially vulnerable to use of alcohol, harmful drugs including nicotine, or unprotected sex—pleasurable activities that may put their health seriously at risk in the long run.

Foundation Efforts

Over a dozen philanthropic foundations targeted specific unsolved problems of the health-care system. By the end of the 1980s the Metropolitan Life Foundation, the Pew Charitable Trusts (set up by the Sun Oil Company heirs), and the Harris Foundation were funding prevention programs aimed at discouraging teenage pregnancies and substance abuse among minority populations. The W. G. Kellogg, Nathan Cummings, and Johnson Controls Foundations were helping fund health center programs that would work with underserved populations and give them a role in defining the health needs of their own communities. The Ruth Mott, Skillman, and Kraft Foundations were also funding projects that involved health promotion activities.[33]

One of the Ruth Mott Fund grants went to a coastal North Carolina project that provided programs in nutrition, stress management, exercise and physical fitness for low-income populations, working through more than a hundred religious congregations in 10 counties. Altogether, about 25 percent of the Mott grants went for community-based health promotion efforts. The Kraft Foundation funded projects that introduced self-help, nutrition, and physical fitness. The Skillman Foundation's grants directed preventive health programs to the elderly; a program in rural Alabama, for example, provided "holistic" care for the elderly, including not only health services but also home repairs and other practical assistance. In addition, the Milbank family's J.M. Foundation supported studies of the effectiveness of prevention and early-intervention projects being sponsored by other foundations.

In the 1980s the Robert Wood Johnson Foundation, the nation's largest private foundation devoted exclusively to health, began to target an increasing proportion of its funds to public policy issues and to major health crises. In the spring of 1990, for example, it announced a $26.8 million national initiative to encourage comprehensive, community-wide efforts to deal with drug and alcohol abuse in cities with populations between 100,000 and 250,000; selecting 15 cities from 300 who applied for aid, the foundation funded programs of drug and alcohol treatment, and after-care and relapse prevention. In cooperation with the federal Health Resources and Service Administration (HRSA), it funded a community-based AIDS care program and various AIDS prevention projects, and also paid for publication of *AIDS Quarterly*, a journal focusing on the AIDS epidemic, key research, and public policy issues relevant to it. In addition to its own programs, the Foundation urged a consortium of philanthropic foundations interested in health care to plan initiatives in common and to jointly fund ventures that could help move American health care in new directions. The appointment of Steven Schroeder as its president in 1990 further underscored these directions for funding policy: Schroeder was an MD known for his advocacy of preventive medicine, community-oriented health care, and effective delivery of services to underserved populations.

A New Look at Sources of Disease. One of the most interesting foundation agendas was the one developed during the 1980s by the Henry J. Kaiser Family Foundation. It will be discussed in some detail, because its vision for a new health-care strategy provided a more integrated approach to preventive health than could be seen in the programs of other philanthropic foundations.[34]

When Henry Kaiser established the Kaiser Family Foundation in Menlo Park, California, in 1948, Kaiser industries already had sponsored the development of the Kaiser-Permanente Health Plan, providing prepaid total health care, not simply prepaid hospitalization insurance. For the first 15 years of its existence the Kaiser Family Foundation promoted interest in comprehensive, prepaid health care as a broader public policy. It gradually added programs to improve the education of physicians who would go into general medicine or internal medicine rather than into more esoteric specialties, and it began to give grants for research and analysis in health-care policy. By 1984, the Kaiser Family Foundation Board expanded its mission in redirecting *goals* for health care in the U.S., and encouraging innovation in the provision of services. The new mandate included five action areas: reshaping health public policy; creating supportive environments for health building; strengthening community action; developing personal skills relevant to health; and reorienting the focus for conventional health services.

In 1980, the Kaiser Family Foundation estimated that if direct medical costs and lost work time were added together, the U.S. spent at least $455 billion dealing with health problems that were preventable. A third of that cost was due to health problems that result from smoking, drinking alcohol, or misusing drugs. Almost half of the cost came from poor nutrition and other behaviors that encourage a series of chronic illnesses. Most of the rest of the cost was attributable to alcohol-related accidents. Looking more conventionally at causes of illness and death, the Foundation identified five major preventable problems: cardiovascular disease, substance misuse, adolescent pregnancy, injuries, and cancer—30 percent of cancers are attributable to tobacco use, about 30 to 35 percent to diet (including cancers of the colon, prostate, and perhaps breast), and a smaller proportion to chemicals in the workplace and the environment.

Kaiser began working with government officials, philanthropic foundations, the National Advertising Council, and other groups to promote a new public definition of the "real" health issues confronting the country. Kaiser's literature directed attention to conditions that create susceptibility to disease; beyond fixed genetic factors, these fell into two categories—behavioral patterns, and social or environmental influences.

The Foundation argued that changing health-relevant behaviors involves more than informing the public about the consequences of individual behavior choices. Norms of behavior in one's peer groups, advertising, and media content affect what people see as desirable and possible. The quality of one's physical environment also affects the attractiveness of health-risk behaviors like smoking, which may help one adjust to an immediate situation at the cost of longer-range health problems. Legislation and various regulations also affect individual behavior choices. Prevalence of the smoking habit, for example, is influenced by advertising and the marketing of tobacco products, by tax laws that influence the price and sale of cigarettes, and by local ordinances that restrict smoking. Thus when social and environmental influences on health behavior become part of the analysis of health problems, a variety of potential strategies for affecting health behaviors begin to appear.

With these tasks in mind, the Foundation began to create a nationwide health promotion network. It sponsored social reconnaissance studies to identify creative and imaginative people who shared a similar vision of the health tasks that need addressing and who had specific, locally relevant ideas about how to proceed. Once these people were identified, the Foundation encouraged the creation of state and local health coalitions. It urged government officials to redefine the place of prevention programs in state health priorities, and it offered demonstration-project grants to groups that would tackle the disease prevention problems most salient in their local communities. To get a Kaiser grant, local communities had to create a coalition of business and community interests that would help direct other resources, beyond those coming from the Kaiser Foundation, to address these health problems. Then, with the cooperation of the Advertising Council and other media sources, the Foundation planned to direct the attention of the general public to behavior changes that might improve health.

The Foundation encouraged the development of an integrated national nutrition policy and funded programs to heighten public awareness of good nutrition. It encouraged the advertising media to do "social marketing" to increase consumer demand for food products that would be beneficial rather than deleterious to health. As consumer demand was stimulated, the Foundation planned to develop programs to enlist the support of food producers, distributors, and retailers to develop and market products that would be nutritionally beneficial. Because poor nutrition, poor health, and premature mortality are particularly acute in low-income and minority communities, the Foundation often gave them funding priority.

In addition to giving grants to state and local community projects, the Kaiser Family Foundation's Health Promotion program funded regional technical assistance centers for health promotion. These centers, affiliated with area universities, worked with grantees in developing their community health programs. Stanford University and Morehouse School of Medicine in Atlanta received the first of these grants.

The Foundation hoped to create persistent social influences that could help motivate and then reinforce health behavior changes. To mount its nationwide effort, it divided the U.S. into four regions. Each region contained between nine and 16 states and had a population ranging from roughly 50 million to 80 million persons. The program began in 1986 in the thirteen-state Western region of the country.

Seven of the first 11 Kaiser health promotion grants in the Western communities, which ranged from $370,000 to $450,000, went to programs geared toward adolescents, and especially those from impoverished and minority backgrounds. One, to Kaiser-Permanente of the Northwest, funded organizing efforts to recruit local businesses in four northwestern communities to adopt secondary schools in their area, jointly pledging funds and working with the community to develop health promotion activities for adolescents. Other grants went for substance abuse prevention programs, recognizing the health threat that was emerging strongly among America's teenagers. The demonstration programs that the Kaiser Family Foundation funded in the West were directed to Alaskan Eskimo adolescents, to Native American reservation-dwelling adolescents, and to adolescents in mountain area communities in Utah and California. The strategies for working on the substance abuse problem differed widely in these sites, reflecting differences in local culture and points of access to young people.

Teenage pregnancy prevention programs for Black adolescents in San Diego, California, and for a statewide program in Montana also were funded, as was a San Francisco program to help prevent injuries among senior citizens. In addition, nutrition programs aimed at reducing the risk of cancer and cardiovascular disease through education programs at worksites, at schools, and through Spanish language newspapers and other media sources within the San Diego Hispanic community received initial grants. So did a statewide health promotion program for the state of Colorado.

The Foundation adopted a ten-year plan for reaching all four regions of the country, moving progressively from the West to the South, the Northeast, and the Midwest. Social reconnaissance would be used in each area to identify effective health innovators and community support sources in each area. During the second year of the program the Kaiser Family Foundation awarded an additional 37 grants, placing half of them beyond the original Western region. Early health promotion grants also went to national organizations, including a grant to the National Academy of Sciences to develop national diet and health guidelines, and grants to the U.S. Public Health Service and the U.S. Department of Health and Human Services for publications dealing with health promotion and aging. Other grants were made to private organizations like the Advocacy Institute, the Center for Science and the Public Interest, the National Council on Alcoholism, and the Girls Clubs of America, as well as to organizations of health professionals, to encourage greater emphasis on disease prevention and active health promotion.

During the next two years the Health Promotion program made 21 more grants, totaling $5.5 million. These supported work on health issues for low-income white and Black residents in both the Deep South and Appalachia, funded programs for young people of junior high age in low-income neighborhoods of Boston and New York, funded Health Promotion Resource Centers in California, Georgia, and Tennessee, encouraged the development of state-sponsored community programs in West Virginia,

Georgia, New Mexico, and Colorado, and sponsored a variety of prevention programs that national organizations would introduce across the country. Grants were also given to university researchers to develop methods to assess the effectiveness of the various programs.

By 1989, 12 other foundations and several federal agencies had become participating partners in its health promotion efforts.[35] By the time a consortium of health-oriented philanthropic foundations scheduled its national meeting at the Kaiser Family Foundation's national headquarters in 1990, it seemed clear that a redefinition of health issues and ways to approach them was getting a national hearing.

Business corporations and private foundations had shown that they can often innovate in ways not possible for politically vulnerable governmental agencies or a health-care industry committed to its financial investments in conventional medical care. On the other hand, foundation agendas and innovative corporate programs are vulnerable to the whims of boards of directors. That is precisely what happened with Kaiser's new national health initiative. In 1989, the Kaiser Family Foundation, rotated off its board Kaiser family members and others who had endorsed the new initiative, inadvertently replacing them with people who had a different agenda. In 1990, when Kaiser's national campaign was nearing the end of its Southern outreach phase, a new majority on the board voted to suspend the program, except for outcome assessment programs already underway. Most of the Foundation's leadership was replaced.[36]

The vision of what was possible for reorienting American health care did not die, but funding for it and the coordinating energy of a major philanthropic foundation had been withdrawn. A strategy for circumventing the health-care industry's focus on disease care and for creating new coalitions of local, regional, state and national interests who would tackle the social sources of illness had been set in motion, only to be set aside. However, networks and visions of a new agenda, once created, do not disappear when central coordinating and funding are no longer forthcoming. They remain available for use by other public policy planners in the future.

Centers for Disease Control (CDC) Initiatives

The federal government, in fact, took on much of that role. In 1988, the Centers for Disease Control reorganized its Center for Health Promotion and Education as the National Center for Chronic Disease Prevention and Health Promotion (NCCDPHP), with the following Mission:

To prevent death and disability from chronic diseases
To promote maternal, infant, and adolescent health
To promote healthy personal behaviors

To accomplish these goals in partnership with health and education agencies, major voluntary associations, the private sector, and other federal agencies.[37]

The federal agency adopted three major strategies to accomplish these goals. First, it developed strategies to help the public begin to think about health, disease, and cause of death in simple but sophisticated terms. Earlier public health messages had identified disease states which are the leading causes of death in the United States—heart disease, cancer, stroke, bronchitis/emphysema, injuries, pneumonia/influenza, diabetes, AIDS, suicide, and homicide (in that order). Now these were presented alongside lists of the actual *causes* of death, ranked in terms of their contribution to total deaths: first, tobacco (implicated in 20 percent of the illnesses leading to death); second, poor diet and lack of exercise (a factor in about 15 percent of illnesses leading to death); third, alcohol abuse; fourth, infectious agents; fifth, pollutants and toxic substances; sixth, firearms; seventh, sexual behavior; eighth, motor vehicles; and ninth, illicit drug use. This redirection of attention from consequence to cause of ill health, identified in terms of modifiable behaviors, creates a different agenda for action.

Second, CDC set a series of goals for health improvement for the U.S. population within a ten-year period. In 1990, the National Center for Chronic Disease Prevention and Health Promotion published *Healthy People 2000*, a compendium which James O. Mason, Assistant Secretary for Health at the time, described as "a national strategy for significantly improving the health of the nation over the coming decade." *Healthy People 2000* set three broad health goals for the nation: (1) to increase the span of healthy life for Americans, decreasing both infant mortality and deaths before the age of 75; (2) to reduce health disparities among Americans because of race or income; and (3) to achieve access to preventive services for all Americans, leading to the birth of healthy babies because of improved prenatal care and counseling; and to major decreases in toxic exposures, in use of tobacco, alcohol, and other drugs, and in exposure to sexually transmitted diseases, including HIV. Starting with an assessment of current health practices and behaviors in the United States, *Healthy People 2000* established a series of priorities for Health Promotion, for Health Protection, and for improvement of Preventive Services, setting what were believed to be achievable target goals for health improvement in each area. Quite specific target goals were set for health improvement in each area, including the goal of eliminating financial barriers to provision and use of clinical prevention services.

Third, it created a coordinated national data system to track changes in health status that were recommended as national goals by *Healthy People*

2000. The analysis would include calculation of benefits-to-cost ratios involved in achieving these health improvements.

Healthy People 2000 invited a wide sector of the public to assume responsibility for health improvement, beginning with individual and family choices and actions by local health officials to make appropriate prevention and health promotion services available. Voluntary organizations were asked to work together on common health promotion target goals. Schools and churches were requested to improve their health education and health promotion activities. Business, community leaders, and labor were urged to cosponsor health promotion and employee assistance projects. Health professionals were encouraged to offer more health screenings, immunizations, health education and counseling. Cable TV, radio, and regional magazines were invited to cooperate with community groups providing health education and publicity about health projects. State and federal agencies were asked to encourage local initiatives and to provide backup support. *Healthy People 2000* also noted a wide range of legislative action areas that have impact on the health of the population.[38]

While quite specific targets were set, noticeably lacking from the CDC document were specific guidelines or protocols for achieving its objectives. Instead, *Healthy People 2000* called for the creation of partnerships between federal, state, and local health agencies, with federal grants providing incentives for innovative health improvement efforts at each level. It called, as well, for developing common health status indicators for use by federal, state, and local health agencies and for surveillance and data systems that could monitor progress toward each of the specified goals. The NCCDPPH's staff of more than 500 federal employees was given responsibility for developing collaborative relations with state health departments and for administering grant programs for HIV prevention evaluation.[39] Not surprisingly, a large number of local efforts began in response to this call for collective action and problem solving, with federal grants available to help pay for some of the costs.

In addition, the Centers for Disease Control and Prevention which had begun funding Sexually Transmitted Disease (STD) Prevention/Training (P/T) Centers, in cooperation with state and local health departments and medical schools in 1979, gave the Prevention/Training Centers special responsibility for helping achieve the AIDS and STD reduction goals established by *Healthy People 2000.* CDC noted that only one in five medical schools offers any STD clinical training, that state and local STD training efforts are usually non-recurrent seminars, workshops or special presentations by hospitals, professional societies, or voluntary groups, and urged more systematic health education in this area.[40]

In contrast to the Kaiser Family Foundation strategy of identifying effective innovators in the community or state, funding them, and encouraging the development of local support coalitions to work with the innovators on health promotion, the CDC programs more often dispersed funds through existing public channels, attempting to shift the emphasis of existing governmental programs at the state and local level. Not surprisingly, the results were mixed.

One example is seen in the block grants CDC gave state health departments to encourage worksite health promotion. Some states built their programs on lessons learned through the NIH Heart Lung and Blood demonstration projects at worksites, setting protocols for performance, standards for achievement, and allocating sizable funding to a few demonstration projects in the state that could show how to do programs which impact both health risks and costs. Other states allocated a fixed amount (e.g., $25 per employee) that could be spent for health promotion, without specifying what target outcomes had to be achieved in a work force to qualify for funding. Where a state health department allocated small, across-the-board, per capita spending little more could be accomplished than an initial health screening and the kind of education-information offerings that previously had been demonstrated to have little impact on the health behaviors of a workforce. Quite impressive improvements in health risks among an employee population were achieved, in contrast, where the state programs used the funds more creatively, locating innovative health delivery provider groups, educating them about state-of-the-art worksite health promotion, sometimes creating partnerships with business sponsors, and providing sufficient funds for them to make an impact. In Ohio, where this was done, the state health department evaluated both health outcomes and cost effectiveness of programs, then co-sponsored conferences, partnering with Bristol-Myers Squibb, to highlight the more successful demonstrations and interest other local health departments and businesses in trying the recommended strategies.[41]

The CDC program's benefits-to-cost analysis highlighted the savings possible when chronic disease prevention, health promotion, and prevention-oriented clinical services are carried out effectively. Smoking cessation in pregnancy programs, for example, "can save over $6 for each dollar spent to implement the program. Each dollar spent on diabetes outpatient education saves $2 to $3 in hospitalization costs. Cervical cancer screening among low-income elderly women yields a net savings of at least $1,600 per person." The CDC benefits-to-cost projections predicted that "for every dollar spent on school-based tobacco, drug and alcohol, and sexuality education $14 are saved in avoided health-care costs."[42]

Because *Healthy People 2000* has such a wide-ranging agenda, there is insufficient space here to discuss each of the CDC health promotion, health protection, and prevention service programs in detail. Some were highly successful, others less so. The reasons for uneven performance were many, including differences in public *commitment* to meet various goals, the relative difficulty of achieving specific target goals, and *availability of protocols and resources* for accomplishing the recommended outcomes. It should be noted, moreover, that setting target goals, then dispersing funds through established agencies that have not met those goals in the past and often have not set high priorities for achieving those goals is an invitation to uneven performance—especially so if implementation of programs is left to the discretion of these state and local agencies. Where creative innovators are given local responsibility, making funds available through existing agency routes can produce the results intended. Under those circumstances local people are given sufficient initiative to creatively address local problems. The lack of required protocols can have the opposite effect, however, when funds are channeled through agencies that lack the knowledge, vision, or autonomy to proceed innovatively, with clear outcome goals in mind.

At midpoint of the ten-year initiative, in 1995, many of the *Healthy People 2000* target goals were far from being achieved.[43] Simply having target goals, and ways of measuring how close the nation was coming to meeting them, represented some progress. That should not be confused, however, with clear progress toward targeted outcomes. Initial experience with this initiative suggested that if existing agencies are to be held accountable for achieving health promotion goals, clearer protocols may need to be given and enforced. If the intent, in contrast, is to encourage greater local initiative for problem-solving in these areas, a more reliable strategy might be to channel funds to known innovators who have produced the kinds of results desired. Ideally some combination of the two strategies might be adopted, such as identifying effective innovators who demonstrate what is possible to achieve and who then work with existing agencies to set standards, goals, and protocols for action and accountability.

Strategies that emerged in the mid-1990s for addressing tobacco issues demonstrated the value of combining public and private initiatives when addressing controversial prevention issues. CDC encouraged the creation of a tobacco-control coalition of state representatives and national groups and helped provide them with information about current developments, assisted in the creation of data bases of tobacco-intervention programs and policies, collaborated in planning workshops, conferences and other professional gatherings and provided speakers for meetings that were national in scope, as well as analytical expertise and assistance in preparing materials for publication, and technical assistance to States and the national coordinating groups regarding tobacco control programs and policies. In funding grant efforts in this area, however, CDC prohibited using its funds to try to influence legislation. Thus it was necessary to have other major players in order to deal with tobacco issues more fundamentally. The struggle to change tobacco policy has been a long one, running concurrently with the broad range of CDC efforts. It represents quite a different approach to prevention issues.

Taking on the Tobacco Industry

In 1980, Matthew Myers, a public interest lawyer, was hired by the Federal Trade Commission to do an analysis of tobacco marketing's effects on public health. The report he wrote, recommending tougher warning labels on cigarette packs, came out a year later, shortly after the Reagan administration had changed some of the health priorities being pursued by the federal government. Myers left the FTC and in 1982 organized the Coalition on Smoking or Health, a venture sponsored by the American Cancer Society, the American Heart Association and the American Lung Association, which lobbied Congress to double the cigarette tax. Their effort succeeded after Myer enlisted Senator Al Gore, from Tennessee, to help persuade members of Congress that price increases for cigarettes could help discourage teenage smoking. (This was the first successful increase in tobacco tax in thirty-one years.) For more than a decade Matthew Myers fought the tobacco industry as a private lobbyist, helping create larger coalitions and becoming one of the best informed Americans on all aspects of the industry's activity, its marketing and advertising strategies. As he learned about decision making within the tobacco industry, Myers charged its leadership with being "responsible for the premature deaths of more Americans than any other group of individuals who have ever lived."[44] After Al Gore became vice president in 1992, Myers' access to the White House helped create a sharpened focus on the role of nicotine addiction in health problems of the nation. This, in turn strengthened the hand of Dr. David A. Kessler, who had been appointed to head the Food and Drug Administration.

Kessler mounted a campaign in Congress to secure tighter regulation of the tobacco industry. In June, of 1994, he testified before the Subcommittee on Health and the Environment of the House Energy and Commerce Committee. Kessler reported that the Brown and Williamson Tobacco Company had deliberately developed a more addicting, gene-altered form of tobacco with a higher nicotine content. Soon tobacco company reports were "leaked" to the press, reports which showed conclusively that despite their denial of this, the companies have had research evidence for years demonstrating that nicotine is addictive, that they were deliberately increasing its dosage, and that they were planning marketing campaigns aimed at the children's and teenage market. By July of 1995, Kessler's testimony was calling nicotine addiction a pediatric disease. With editorial support from Barry M. Goldwater, the former Arizona senator and Republican presidential candidate, Kessler called for a war on children's smoking, to be waged by requiring photo identification to purchase cigarettes. He suggested that it might be appropriate for the Food and Drug Administration to declare tobacco a drug and regulate its manufacture and use. Great controversy surrounded his tenure as FDA chief thereafter. By November of 1996 Kessler had resigned, but the proposal to have the FDA regulate tobacco as an addicting drug continued to gain momentum.[45]

The anti-tobacco forces grew stronger and more coordinated in 1996, when the Robert Wood Johnson Foundation and the American Cancer Society gave Matthew Myers a total of $30 million to create the National Center for Tobacco-Free Kids, which began to wage an aggressive anti-tobacco advertising campaign, publicizing the tobacco company's targeting of children and adolescents for cigarette marketing. Soon, various state governments began suing the tobacco companies to seek reimbursement for Medicaid spending on smoking-related illnesses. First Florida, Massachusetts, Mississippi, Louisiana and West Virginia filed law suits. By June of 1997, 44 states had done so.[46]

The tobacco companies at first banded together to resist both the proposal that the FDA regulate their products and to try to quash lawsuits against them being brought by individuals whose health had been ruined by smoking, all class action suits on behalf of smokers, or lawsuits by states for Medicaid costs due to smoking. FDA regulation of smoking became an issue in the 1996 Presidential election. The Republican candidate, Bob Dole, suffered a serious loss of public credibility when he claimed that he was unsure that tobacco was addicting.[47] Meanwhile efforts to get Congress to intervene on behalf of the tobacco companies faltered, despite the companies' retention of the Washington law firm that included George J. Mitchell, the former Senate majority leader. The anti-tobacco coalition publicized tobacco marketing practices that clearly were aimed at inducing children to smoke, creating a deep sense of revulsion both in Congress and among the public.[48] The Centers for Disease Control released a study predicting that five million children currently under eighteen years of age would die from the effects of smoking, based on current surveys of smoking among children. They also released data showing that tobacco was the leading actual cause of death in the United States, in 1990, when one calculates its contribution to heart disease, cancer, stroke, and emphysema, the four leading immediate causes of death in the U.S.[49] The Justice Department conducted a wide-ranging investigation into tobacco marketing and the conduct of tobacco industry executives and lawyers, including the truthfulness of testimony given in previous court cases.

A series of court decisions began to put the tobacco companies at a major disadvantage, and the courts began to play a role analogous to that played by the Warren Court during the Civil Rights movement of the 1950s and 1960s. In March of 1997, the Liggett Group settled a lawsuit brought by 22 states, agreeing to turn over potentially damaging internal documents spelling out the industry's knowledge of tobacco's harmful health effects. In April 1997, a North Carolina Federal Court ruled that the FDA has the right to curb tobacco as a drug (but also ruled that tobacco companies have a right to target advertising toward juveniles). Other court decisions established the right of cities to ban tobacco advertising on billboards. (Meanwhile, the tobacco companies began sophisticated cultivation of the youth market through advertising targeting juveniles on the Internet.)[50]

Other court decisions established the right of states and of private citizens to bring individual and class action lawsuits against the tobacco companies claiming damages from tobacco, and July 1997, was set for the first state suit for recovery of Medicaid costs for treating smoking-related illnesses. The stock market price for tobacco shares dropped sharply. The Liggett Group began negotiating with state attorney generals of five states, with talks led by Mississippi's attorney general, Michael Moore. By April of 1997, all of the tobacco companies, including their top executives, the attorney generals from 30 states, and Matthew Myers of the National Center for Tobacco-Free Kids began closed-door negotiation of the issues in dispute. By June 20th the negotiations had produced a 68-page settlement agreement in which the tobacco companies offered to pay $368.5 billion in compensation to states over the next 25 years for damages to health from use of tobacco, as their total payment to cover all liability for expenses of treating tobacco-related illnesses. The tobacco companies also agreed to far-reaching restrictions on marketing, stark warnings on cigarette packages, and money for state and local tobacco control initiative aimed at lowering smoking among youths. They agreed to pay up to $2 billion in fines if targeted reductions in levels of smoking among youths are not reached. In exchange, the companies demanded Congressional legislation granting them near-total immunity from smoking-related lawsuits and punitive damages. Fines for failing to reach targeted reductions in smoking levels among youths were to be treated as a tax-deductible business expense. The tobacco companies also demanded freedom from federal regulation of the nicotine content level of cigarettes, unless the government could prove that reducing the nicotine level would not create a black market for full-strength products.[51]

It seemed clear that the tobacco companies were willing to pay over $10 billion a year, plus additional funds for public health campaigns for 25 years, in order to limit further liability, thus stabilizing the value of their stock. Analysts argued that the tobacco companies were willing to forego some potential profits from the American market, where smoking is clearly on the decline, in order to concentrate on gaining access to the market in China, which was opening trading opportunities for foreign companies and whose vast population has high smoking rates. New markets in Asia would more than compensate the tobacco companies for lessened markets and damage payments in the United States.

The public health community, outraged by the terms offered, by the international ambitions of what they saw as a death-dealing business, and sensing the possibility of a greater victory, mobilized rapidly to oppose the compromise offered by the tobacco companies. A broad coalition of voluntary health and medical organizations released a statement of core principles which they believed should guide any resolution of tobacco litigation, in the courts, in Congress, or elsewhere:

1. The FDA must have the authority to regulate the manufacture, sale, labeling, distribution and marketing of tobacco products.
2. Current FDA requirements governing youth access and tobacco marketing are essential minimum components of any public policy initiative. The agency's ability to augment these requirements should not be curtailed.
3. The rights of victims of the tobacco industry to seek compensation for the injuries they have suffered should not be abridged and the tobacco industry should not be immunized from accountability for its wrongdoing.
4. A well-funded, effective sustained public education and tobacco control campaign that is protected from political pressure is critical to reducing tobacco use.
5. Congress should not preempt state or local laws that are stronger than federal laws, nor should the FDA be preempted from revising the form, content, and placement of the warnings on cigarette packages.
6. The tobacco industry must disclose its research and studies about the effects of its products, including nicotine, on the human body and the marketing of tobacco to children.

The coalition also recommended that an overall tobacco control plan include attention to increased tobacco taxes, protection of nonsmokers from environmental tobacco smoke, and the role of the American tobacco industry in international tobacco sales.[52]

Meanwhile, the U.S. Congress set up a tobacco control advisory panel chaired by former US Surgeon General Dr. C. Everett Koop, and including David A. Kessler (formerly FDA chief), Matthew Myers, and officials of the cancer, heart, and medical associations. The White House also created its own advisory panel of 50 officials including the Secretary for Health and Human Services, and representatives from the Food and Drug Administration, the Centers for Disease Control, and the Treasury and Justice Departments.[53]

When Mississippi unilaterally accepted the tobacco companies' proposal, settling out of court, the White House, Koop and Kessler all declared the negotiations an unacceptable compromise, demanding federal regulation of nicotine as an addicting drug. Congress increased the tobacco tax.[54]

It is clear that the prevention movement has entered a new stage. Not only private businesses which pay health benefits, but the states which pay Medicaid costs, public health organizations, Congress, and the courts are jointly seeking ways to change the health risks facing future generations. The earlier failure of laws prohibiting the sale of alcohol constrained the range of choices considered by the opponents of tobacco, and the tobacco industry was clearly planning internationally as it attempted to limit its liability in the US and protect its business growth opportunities elsewhere in the world. Whatever the outcome of this case would prove to be, it was clear that health policy analysts were learning the importance of prevention and the possibilities of a multi-pronged approach when developing new strategies.

Public Response to Preventive Health Themes

For two decades, government and private initiatives had emphasized the importance of preserving health rather than simply managing disease. To what extent had the American public, and not simply policy planners, begun to adopt a wellness or "prevention" perspective? In December of 1985, the Gallup Poll asked a nationwide sample of 1,500 households about their participation in leisure time activities. Their answers can be compared with Gallup polls conducted earlier. Between 1961 and 1985, for example, there was a twofold increase in the number of adult Americans who reported that they exercise daily; by 1985, they made up almost 60 percent of adult respondents. Over 40 percent of these adults said they swam, one-third said they rode bicycles, a quarter said they jogged, a fifth that they lifted weights, a similar number said they did aerobic exercises, and one out of six reported doing calisthenics. Applied nationally, that would translate into 40 million joggers and 32 million people doing aerobics. Much of the change had occurred since 1975, when only one person in 20 claimed to engage in jogging, one person in 25 reported doing aerobics, and one person in 10 claimed to ride a bicycle. The Gallup polls also showed that a sizable number of Americans were pursuing types of exercise encouraged by the holistic health movement.[55]

In profiles drawn from health screenings at various worksites during 1985, however, no more than 15 to 30 percent of employees reported exercising as often as three times a week.[56] In 1992, the federal government's Centers for Disease Control released a study indicating that 59 percent of Americans do little or no exercise.[57] Opinion polls suggest a new sense of "appropriate" health behaviors that is emerging and expressed in convenient exaggerations of memory; the belief that one *ought* to exercise regularly has taken hold with the public, whether or not people actually put it into practice.

Certain other indicators of health-relevant behaviors are less subject to memory distortion, however. Americans seem to have genuinely changed their nutritional habits. In 1960 about 40 percent of food commodities sold to Americans were high-cholesterol products; by 1985, however, high-cholesterol products had dropped to 27 percent of food purchases. Fish, grains, skim milk products and yogurt made up 12.5 percent of food consumption in 1960 but 20 percent in 1985. Whereas red meat outsold fish, poultry, and cheese by a ratio of three to one in 1960, the ratio had dropped to two to one by 1985. Fat consumption was still much higher than desired for optimal health, but there was a clear move toward cholesterol-reducing fats. Moreover, consumption of rice had increased 50 percent, and consumption of fresh fruits and vegetables also had risen markedly.[58] One everyday indication of these changing food preferences was the appearance of salad bars at many fast food restaurants.

Smoking had also decreased noticeably, particularly among men. In 1967 almost half of American men smoked, and another fifth were former smokers. By 1987 less than 30 percent were still smoking and another 30 percent had become former smokers. Over the same 20 years, the figures for women smokers were less dramatic but pointed in the same direction, dropping from about 30 percent to just under 24 percent. The percent who were former smokers had doubled during that time, however, amounting to over 19 percent of the total adult female population.[59] By 1992 over 500 communities in the U.S. had passed ordinances restricting or banning smoking in public places. Meanwhile federal health officials announced a national anti-smoking program, targeting 17 states and budgeting $115 million over a seven year period to counter the "sinister marketing strategies" of tobacco companies.[60] These were encouraging trends. However, the *Healthy People 2000* goals for the 1990s were not being met.

Self Help. Self-help had taken hold in a major way. Throughout the 1980s self-help groups grew in numbers and in their impact on the public's conception of how to deal with personal health issues. Frank Reissman and Thomas J. Powell, while independently assessing self-help ventures, have listed several types of self-help groups that have emerged as national organizations. Most of the major chronic diseases have self-help organization. There are groups that deal with issues faced at particular points in the life cycle (e.g., Alateen, La Leche League for expectant parents, the Gray Panthers among the retired). Groups like Alcoholics Anonymous and Smokestoppers deal with chemical addictions. Other groups, such as Take Off Pounds Sensibly (TOPS), Emotions Anonymous, and Sexual Addicts Anonymous, let people with emotion-based behavioral problems support and learn from one another. There are lifestyle support organizations (e.g., Parents without Partners, gay support organizations), and support groups for families and friends dealing with chemical dependency in their midst (e.g., Alanon, Families Anonymous, Tough Love). Though dealing with a wide range of problems, these groups had in common a determination to turn to persons with similar experience to solve problems in their lives, rather than depending primarily on health-care professionals.[61]

Estimating how many Americans participated in such groups is difficult. In 1978, however, the Task Panel of the President's Commission on Mental Health identified over 180 self-help organizations, with thousands of chapters and an estimated membership of at least 10 million. By 1982, social scientists were estimating a current self-help organizational membership of at least 15 million, meeting in approximately 750,000 face-to-face groups throughout the U.S. and Canada. In 1984, Alcoholics Anonymous alone counted more than half a million members in the U.S. and almost 70,000 in Canada. While surveys have not been updated, observation suggests a continuing increase in the 1990s.[62]

Besides joining mutual support groups for dealing with what often are called health problems, many Americans were demedicalizing the experience of birth and death. In 1970 in America 5,306 births were assisted by midwives rather than doctors and took place outside of hospitals. In 1986, there were 105,208 midwife-assisted births and almost 90,000 of them took place *in hospitals*, with the blessing of the health-care system. About the same number of midwife-assisted home births occurred, but the number of births outside the hospital at which physicians assisted had almost doubled, from 5,178 in 1970 to 9,400 in 1986.[63]

By 1986, there were also 1,356 hospice programs in American communities. These programs approached death as a natural part of the life process; they helped individuals die free of pain and provided practical assistance to families during the period when dying family members were helpless and dependent upon them. About a quarter of these programs were set up specifically to allow terminally ill people to die at home. All of them shared a determination to make "dying well" take precedence over prolonging life so long as medically possible.[64]

Whether one looks at changing habits of food consumption, habits of exercise, the use of self-help groups for dealing with health problems, or the demedicalization of basic life experiences like birth and death, there is growing evidence that a "wellness model for health care," in which participants play an active part, has been taking hold at the grassroots.

Criticisms of the Prevention Model

While few critics have challenged the argument that preventing disease is preferable to treating problems after health has broken down, many have asked whether the "prevention" or wellness movement has found viable answers for the problems it tries to address. They have made the following critiques.

First, by focusing on "lifestyle" behaviors, the movement largely ignores other sources of disease. The circumstances under which many people live or work can create physical, environmental, or social hazards to health that are independent of their own behaviors. Dealing with the sources of disease must include attention to such matters as occupational health and safety requirements and neighborhood living conditions. To emphasize taking personal responsibility for one's health through "lifestyle choices," say these critics, can be naive at best, and can become another way of "blaming the victim." Even worse, keeping track of employees' health risks could lead to prejudicial personnel policies by employers trying to avoid higher-cost health-care liability.[65]

Second, the movement's strategies for influencing individual behavior often ignore the fact that many powerful economic interests benefit directly from unhealthy lifestyle choices, such as the use of tobacco, alcohol, and "junk food." Changing the social climate for behavior choices must deal with this reality.[66]

Third, the wellness movement needs to develop more effective strategies for motivating personal behavior changes. It has a poor track record in terms of overall results achieved. Wellness programs engage too small a percentage of their target populations in prevention or health improvement efforts, and often reach only the people who least need their services. Moreover, the recidivism rate among the few who try to make lifestyle behavior changes is much too high.[67]

Fourth, say some critics, unless wellness programs reach a greater proportion of their target populations and lower the present relapse rates among persons who do try to change earlier, unhealthy behaviors, wellness programs will simply increase overall health-care expenditures while making little impact on the health problems of the nation.[68]

Finally, even if wellness programs were to become more successful at reaching their target populations, thereby decreasing the demand for disease-care services, some critics believe they would not lower overall health-care expenditures. The efforts of HMOs to keep their enrollees out of hospitals, and the success of Medicare DRG reimbursement policies in encouraging hospitals to release patients as rapidly as possible, may have succeeded in lowering the occupancy rate in hospitals across the country. But hospital per-day charges per person have risen steeply to make up for lost numbers of patients; and if wellness programs lessen total demand for expensive disease-oriented treatments, charges for disease services will simply go up to compensate for the loss in volume. Moreover, if older people do better self-care and live longer, each person will require services over a longer time period than otherwise would be the case. Thus, it is argued, adding wellness programs to the range of available options should increase overall health-care costs.[69]

Defenders of the wellness movement have countered each of these charges, as follows.

First, while lifestyle behaviors are not the only sources of disease, they do contribute significantly to the disease process. Even if all other physical, social and environmental sources of disease problems were corrected, lifestyle choices would continue to endanger individual health. In 1980, the cost for medical services and the value of work time lost because of health problems that could have been prevented by better lifestyle choices was approximately $455 billion.[70] In view of this cost, the wellness movement's focus, though incomplete, can hardly be called irrelevant. However, wellness records need to be confidential, not shared with personnel departments, so that there can be no possibility of them being used punitively. Reputable firms make this a firm policy. The right of confidentiality within the company should be protected by law, many wellness professionals agree.

Second, it simply is not true that the prevention movement ignores economic and political obstacles to implementation of a health agenda. Recognizing the power of tobacco interests, for example, the movement has supported the warnings of the U.S. Surgeon General, the laws restricting tobacco advertising, and the steps taken by local governments, airlines and workplaces to prohibit smoking in public areas where "secondhand" smoke can be a health hazard. In 1997, it began a more concerted attack on the tobacco industry itself. The struggle to eliminate consumer items that are harmful to health will be a long one, given the complex ownership patterns that now unite tobacco, liquor, and junk food companies in huge economic conglomerates with great political power. But this is all the more reason to alert the public to individual choices that can protect their health. The movement advocates working on sources of illness in any ways that seem likely to produce results; these include working within business organizations and with government officials, as well as helping to build coalitions of interests that will pursue a preventive health agenda.[71]

Business and government leaders who participate in the preventive health agenda have a joint reply to the third and fourth critiques. They agree that the wellness movement must find ways to reach a larger proportion of its target population and to reduce its recidivism rates. But it has done so, advocates argue. Proactive outreach—keeping in touch with a group of clients rather than waiting for them to return—works, as research has documented. It gets a high proportion of people to begin making personal health changes; and if a health professional keeps in touch with their clients when a relapse occurs, most clients eventually discover a strategy that works for them. Given the record-keeping and scheduling potential of sophisticated computer systems that are available, it is now practical for a health professional to maintain personal contact with a large number of clients. The step-by-step manual published by the NHLBI of NIH makes the technology of proactive strategies advocated in this model easily accessible to wellness professionals across the country.[72] This approach, some argue, if combined with Options & Choices' strategy of targeting the highest users of health services first, then gradually reaching out to the rest of a workforce as cost savings make this practical within budget constraints, could produce improved health and lower spending for disease services with no reduction in services.

But, reply some critics, counseling about lifestyle behaviors can amount to "blaming the victim," thus causing counterproductive stress. Many "lifestyle behavior choices" that are long-term health risks—such as smoking, drinking alcohol excessively, overeating or eating "junk food"—are pleasurable in themselves and reduce the immediate experience of stress in difficult work or life situations. Doesn't pressure to abandon these behaviors simply increase the stress that people have to live with, and add its own long-run dangers to health?[73]

There is no question that "boomerang dieting"—constantly losing a great deal of weight and then regaining it—or failing to achieve a goal like stopping smoking can increase the experience of personal stress at a time when the stress of living in one's immediate environment has led to the relapse in the first place. But advocates of wellness programs insist this is not an argument against providing such services; rather it underscores the importance of providing a wider range of them. Services must include helping people discover new and equally pleasurable stress relief methods; helping them find social support for their change efforts from peers as well as health professionals; and helping people work on the health of their organizations or their neighborhoods. Changing a corporate or neighborhood culture in ways that reduce stress and encourage health-building can be important to the long-term success of any wellness program, as research underlying preventive health care demonstrates.[74]

In short, say advocates of prevention, the movement has now discovered key ingredients that make prevention work, methods shown to be effective with all socioeconomic groups. In order to have greater impact, the wellness movement needs to disseminate prevention technologies that research has already validated, especially the tactics for social organization that make prevention efforts effective.[75]

It is not that easy, reply some critics. Despite research findings that proactive worksite wellness programs can be cost effective, many corporations, even when convinced they should move in this direction, cannot finance such programs. The three-to-five year period needed to recover the cost of new labor-intensive health services, when added to the rapidly expanding cost of providing conventional health-care coverage, becomes unbearable. Advocates of wellness programs agree that some new source for funding health-care innovations must be found if corporations, and especially smaller businesses, are to adopt them. That source, they argue, could be either tax incentives for businesses and health-maintenance providers, health insurance policies that include reimbursement for prevention costs as part of their benefits, or, alternatively, mandatory discounts on insurance premiums available to those who provide or participate in wellness programs.[76]

How can this become relevant to the people who are not employed? It is one thing to work intensively with individuals at their worksites but quite another to work with people in more scattered locations who have no regular contact with health professionals. The answer given by prevention advocates is that research and demonstration projects show people can be effectively reached through a variety of social networks beyond the workplace, such as schools, churches, social clubs, and health clinics working with Medicaid and Medicare enrollees. The question is not whether these people are reachable, but which routes are most effective. That is a research question, not an insurmountable obstacle to developing a universal prevention strategy.[77]

Will prevention really save money? Critics point out that the reduced use of hospitals, created by the expansion of HMOs and reimbursement policies for Medicare, has simply resulted in higher daily per-person charges for hospital services, thereby increasing rather than decreasing total health-care expenditures. Why should an additional impetus to lowered use of disease-care services not simply inflate the per-person costs of disease services, rather than lower the overall level of expenditures for health-care services? Moreover, if the preventive system is actually effective and people live longer, will that not increase costs even more?

Advocates of the wellness approach counter this objection in two ways. First, they point out that previous cost increases have come without comparable improvements in the health status of the population; with prevention, even if the skeptics' predictions turned out to be correct, we would be getting our money's worth for increased expenditures. But the objection is misguided, they insist, because demographic changes occurring in the population make that outcome unlikely. The demand for hospital and other disease-focused services will increase sharply in the next few years, as the baby-boom cohorts move into later middle age. Demand for services to the elderly will skyrocket a few years later. Thus the problem to be solved concerns how to accommodate this increased demand without having to enlarge existing facilities. Wellness-oriented services would be part of the answer. Furthermore, the time needed for American business and industry to convert to a proactive worksite wellness policy makes it unlikely that wellness investments of this type would increase per-person disease-service costs elsewhere. By 1995, the first baby boomers will be 50 years old, and the ranks of the elderly will increase rapidly. Thus a rapid expansion of proactive wellness services, for workers and retirees alike, will be necessary if the use of disease-care services is to remain anywhere near its present levels.[78]

Second, they continue, it is a fallacy to assume that health costs for the system as a whole will automatically increase as more people live longer. The health expenses of elderly persons vary enormously. What we need are more people who age well and require fewer expensive services as they near the end of their lives, rather than a growing number who require expensive high-tech efforts to undo the consequences of their earlier lifestyle. Improving the health-building potential of the population, including the elderly, is likely to be cost-effective in the long run, as well as more humane.[79]

In short, prevention advocates argue, although preventive health efforts will never replace the health-care industry, they can lessen demand for disease-focused services by dealing directly with some important sources of disease. A greater emphasis on preventive health, they insist, must be part of any rethinking of health-care policy.

Lessons from the Preventive Health or Wellness Movement for Current Health-Care Planning

The movement toward preventive health care, sometimes called the wellness movement, offers four contributions to rethinking health-care policy:

1. To be more effective, health care must place greater emphasis on addressing the sources of illness. Environmental hazards, social marketing practices that increase health risks, and personal behavior choices all are sources of illness that need attention. Addressing the sources of illness also will mean offering health-care services to individuals at an earlier point,

before health problems disrupt their lives and bring them to service providers. It will involve ongoing, personalized, *proactive* efforts to motivate people to act in ways that preserve health.

2. By directing more attention to social influences on individual health behaviors, we can incorporate the biochemical model of the health-disease process into a broader social model that describes how disease occurs and therefore suggests earlier and more effective interventions.

3. There are organizational strategies that can work well at the social level of health and disease dynamics. These include ongoing, proactive, one-to-one outreach by health professionals to people who are still healthy; counseling help in adapting lifestyles to health needs; the teaching of stress-management skills to replace individual behaviors that create health risks; the creation of social support networks to deal with stress and help maintain health improvements; and the organization of activities that promote the health of a worksite or a neighborhood as a whole, in addition to individual health efforts.

4. The wellness movement has begun to create new action networks, uniting people with a common preventive health agenda who work within different organizations and population groups, alerting them to ways they might mobilize resources to reinforce each other's efforts. Foundation grants have helped create important institutional resources: university-based centers that can assist grassroots efforts to create new prevention initiatives in local, state, or regional communities, and nationally coordinated efforts to influence social support for healthier lifestyle behaviors. These action networks and the institutional resources that help sustain them should be included in any health planning for the future.

9

Understanding the Ecology of
Health and Disease

While the developments chronicled in Chapters 6 and 7 were taking place, ecologically focused approaches to health and disease also were gaining momentum. As an ecological perspective—on what happens inside humans as well as how humans fit into a larger ecosystem—gained adherents, new questions and intervention strategies for improving health emerged from many interest groups. Physicians and medical researchers, public health advocates, atmospheric scientists, the military, radical political movements, and United Nations agencies all were involved. Some aspects of this emerging perspective became widely accepted; others remained deeply controversial. As ecological perspectives came into wider use, however, they began to restructure the medical community's understanding of the germ theory of disease, and the relation of biological processes to other levels of causation. Then, as an ecological perspective began to reorient some medical research and practice, the agendas of some political parties and nation-states began to change, as did priorities for addressing health problems that confront the entire global community. This evolving perspective and its relation to health policy will be described in this chapter.

The shift to a more ecological focus for understanding health and disease has been accelerated by social and political realities that currently affect opportunities for scientific inquiry. Scientific emphases on cancer and heart disease, which political realities of research funding brought to the fore in the first three decades following World War II, now have been joined by attention to the immune system, research stimulated by the AIDS pandemic. In addition, research responding to problems of drug addiction has brought attention to the processes by which the human system as a whole regulates itself. As attention has focused on health processes that underlie health and disease more generally, a more ecological framework for broader scientific inquiry has also grown apace. Atmospheric and oceanic research has demonstrated the deleterious effects that some global industrial and military activity is having on the health prospects of many species, including humans. Many nations now understand that national health policy cannot ignore international health issues—and that health policy cannot be isolated from other areas of social and economic decision-making. During the past 15 years the United Nations and various international agencies and organizations have taken the lead in identifying health problems and proposing new kinds of international policy that could affect the health of the planet.

New Directions in Medical Science—the Ecology of the Human Body

A revolution in our understanding of health processes began in the 1950s with discovery of the basic components of DNA, the molecular "blueprint" for all cellular components and processes. Research scientists began to think of biological processes as involving the transfer of information (which resides structurally in DNA) that then activates or inhibits various biochemical reactions. With the discovery of DNA came hopes of deciphering the genetic code, of discovering, in other words, the "language" and "instructions" that get passed on from one generation to another through physical inheritance.[1] In the 1970s a new laboratory technique based on understanding recombinant DNA methodology opened up the possibility of mapping the genes or codes that control physiological processes.[2] Thereafter, the National Institutes of Health made research aimed at "cracking the genetic code" a high priority.

Meanwhile, during the intervening years, researchers who were studying viruses had demonstrated that some genetic sequences of DNA can be altered by viral activity: a virus which has entered a cell may override that cell's own coded instructions by inserting a viral DNA or RNA sequence of information. The information sequence it transfers to a more complex organism then produces the chemical reactions the virus needs in order to reproduce itself.[3] This discovery turned the germ theory of disease in new directions. Researchers began to identify which micro-organisms are able to enter specific cells of the human body, how they enter, and what sequences of DNA or RNA they substitute for the original human genetic information coding.[4] Researchers also discovered that some of the organisms coexisting within the human body create a symbiotic relationship that is essential for human survival, as well as their own: They trigger basic biochemical reactions that the human body does not know how to produce for itself.[5] In fact, the number of non-human organisms within our body is greater than the number of human cells.[6] We are, indeed, an ecosystem, not an independent entity occasionally bombarded by foreign invaders, as the germ theory of disease taught us to view ourselves. A more ecological understanding of human health processes, in terms of their inter relations with the environment, has begun to emerge from this joining of DNA and viral research.

This general strategy for biochemical research also opened the way to understand how the larger inanimate environment affects health processes: chemical pollutants breathed into the body, food additives and even various nutritional combinations, as well as viral activity—all influence information transfer, the consequent chemical activity and even the mutation of individual cells, thereby affecting the development of cancer and other diseases. Besides learning to think about the human body in more ecological terms, scientists were also beginning to understand how it is affected by its immediate environment, and this led to a more "social" formulation of certain research questions. For example, researchers trying to understand lung cancer paid attention not only to the impact that inhaled chemicals (tobacco smoke) have on the lungs of smokers, but some began doing epidemiological studies of the incidence of lung cancer among non-smokers who share housing with heavy smokers, demonstrating that these people have a higher risk of developing lung cancer than is true for other non-smokers. This, in turn, directed attention to public policies to protect non-smokers from injury that might come because of other persons' smoking habits.[7]

Research on cardiovascular disease, a health problem that only occasionally can be traced to the work of infectious agents, also helped move medical understanding in a more 'ecological' direction. The first steps were modest—the discovery that while genetic factors predispose some individuals to develop cardiovascular disease, chemical and emotional inputs play an important role in the creation of susceptibility to cardiovascular problems. Tobacco and alcohol, when used for several years, decrease the cardiovascular system's flexibility when responding to external demands from the environment.[8] Nutrition, exercise habits and pronounced or prolonged emotional stress all affect both blood pressure and the HDL/LDL cholesterol ratio, thereby affecting susceptibility to heart attack and stroke.[9]

Concurrent cancer research reinforced these discoveries. Nutrition's role in cancer susceptibility and recovery, and the correlation of periods of prolonged emotional stress to subsequent development of cancer alerted medical researchers to the need to think in broader terms about how an individual human's relationship to a larger social and physical environment affects the development of health and disease.[10]

The work on heart disease and cancer seemed to be expanding the model for health and disease beyond biochemistry, and beyond simply biochemical interventions. Then the challenge brought by the AIDS pandemic and the spreading use of addicting drugs produced discoveries of how the human system solves problems and regulates itself, discoveries that challenged the more inert, simply reactive biochemical models that had guided earlier medical thinking.

Because the human immuno deficiency virus (HIV) specifically destroys cells in the immune system, persons infected with HIV become susceptible to a wide range of infectious diseases. As research funding became available in the 1980s (in response to the AIDS epidemic) to study the immune system more thoroughly, new understandings of the human body emerged. It was no longer seen simply as a passive recipient of inputs from genetic inheritance, chemicals taken into the body, and the activity of other organisms, but as an active problem-solver. Besides discovering the retrovirus that disables the immune system, and the particular kinds of immune system cells it invades and destroys as it reproduces, AIDS researchers found that other kinds of cells in the immune system monitor potentially dangerous activity and signal still other cells to act—either to attack an organism or to ignore it.[11] Other researchers identified the chemical route by which the activity of the immune system is turned on and off, and how psychological stress produces chemical reactions that alter the body's normal rhythms for immune system activity.[12] The image of the body as machine was being replaced with something more nearly akin to the body as mind, operating actively within a larger ecological context.

As this was happening, researchers who were trying to understand how narcotics affect the body located specific brain cell receptor sites where particular narcotics connect with a cell and stimulate its chemical activity. Reasoning that these receptor sites must be there for some more beneficial reason, they began to look for naturally produced chemicals in the body that have a chemical structure similar to that of narcotics. Researchers discovered neuropeptides—endorphins, the body's own "natural narcotics"—that affect many receptor sites within the body and block the experience of pain, producing instead a sense of euphoria. These discoveries stimulated the identification of more than 50 other kinds of neuropeptides, along with the biochemical reactions that they turn on and off.[13]

A larger picture is unfolding of how humans interact with their macro and micro environments. Collective human activity helps shape larger environmental conditions. Then, as individuals respond to that larger environment, their own cognitive, emotional, and behavioral responses become important, affecting how frequently particular micro-biochemical processes and interactions occur. A micro ecology gets created within each person, one that interacts with the macro ecology of the larger environment with greater or lesser effectiveness.

These various discoveries force medical science to do more complex analysis of the processes that produce health and disease. A hundred years ago, medical science made major headway in its fight with infectious diseases by insisting that one should seek a single cause for an observed effect. That, in turn, had led to the strategy of introducing a single pharmaceutical agent to destroy an invading organism or to correct some malfunction of an organ system. We now realize that such thinking is over-simplified. While some specific condition may be necessary for a disease to occur, it rarely is sufficient to cause the disease all by itself. A larger ecological context within the body determines what happens. Targeting a particular cell or "visitor" within the body for treatment will have wider effects than are intended: Chemical inputs affect many receptor sites throughout the body, affecting the way a variety of processes work. Awareness that chemical agents affect the more complex rhythm and sequencing of the body's chemistry, as well as the body's interaction with the flora and fauna of its own internal ecological environment, draws attention to second-, third-, and fourth-order effects from pharmaceutical interventions. For example, colitis can occur as a side-effect from antibiotics that change the balance of flora and fauna in the intestinal track.[14] Cancer therapists have to monitor side-effects from chemotherapy closely, including destructive effects on the immune system. These sometimes threaten survival of the patient. Indeed, unintended side-effects from medications are a more general problem. Currently about ten percent of hospital admissions occur in order to treat side-effects from prescription drugs.[15]

Other developments also force us to think more ecologically. Shortly after World War II, public health campaigns in many parts of the world used airplanes to spray insecticides in an effort to control malaria by killing mosquitoes. It took scientists a while to realize that we were also poisoning birds and other species needed for a healthy environment, that they were lessening rice production because DDT actually increased the incidence of the Brown Plant Hopper pest. It took longer still to discover that insects are more resistant to chemical poisons than other species, so that a stronger strain of mosquitoes, able to resist DDT, eventually brought the original health problem back to its earlier levels. DDT residues remain in the environment and become concentrated in human, bird, and animal cells, affecting how various health processes work.[16] In addition, now, 50 years after the widespread introduction of antibiotics, we face a resurgence of once-conquered diseases, including tuberculosis and pneumonia, as time has allowed viruses and other species to mutate in ways that make earlier antibiotics less effective.[17] We are now seeing the limits of biochemical intervention strategies that we thought had triumphed over infectious disease.

Recent research trying to understand who will develop cancer under varying environmental conditions begins to put all this together. We now know that enzymes which are found in the liver and other tissues metabolize carcinogens found in food, the air, cigarette smoke, and other sources. When a chemical comes into contact with a cell membrane, it is met by enzymes that make the chemical more or less water soluble. If the entire chemical molecule becomes transformed in this way, it is excreted completely from the body. Sometimes, however, chemicals become altered in a way that makes it easier for them to bind to protein or DNA, potentially altering how genetically programmed health processes function within the human body. There are genetic differences among individuals in how quickly their bodies are able to detoxify chemicals. Slow detoxifiers have a greater chance of getting cancer, because more of their cells are likely to become contaminated by having carcinogenic chemicals bound up with their DNA or proteins, thus setting cancerous processes in motion. It is not entirely a matter of genetics, however. Foundry workers in Poland, for example, as well as people living in the polluted air of large cities, and those who are exposed to polyaromatic hydrocarbons from the burning of fossil fuels and other industrial chemicals all show higher levels of "adducts," cells in which chemicals have become bound to DNA or protein. However persons who are slow detoxifiers will develop more adducts than the rest of the population of an area.[18]

The addition of environmental chemicals to the blood stream or other systems of the body can speed the mutation of cells, including the p53 gene that helps suppress tumor formation in the body. Other mutations speed up the normal genetic coding sequences that influence cell division, while still other environmentally-stimulated mutations affect the ability of the immune system to isolate and destroy aberrant cells that develop within the body.[19]

To give one example, research has shown that for most people, an inversion of the DNA sequence on chromosome 7 occurs in one out of 5,000 to 50,000 white blood cells. At this level it apparently has no overall ill effect. When the inversion occurs at 100 times that rate, however, leukemia or lymphoma develops 100 times more often than in the general population. This inversion can develop as a genetically triggered mutation, or in response to exposure to chemicals. For example, in summer farmers who are exposed to pesticides, herbicides and fungicides show a marked increase in inversions of the DNA sequence on chromosome 7. Not every farmer exposed to these chemicals will develop leukemia or lymphoma, however; those with unusually heavy exposure and those whose genetic DNA is less stable, more prone to invert, are more at risk for these forms of cancer. The combination of environmental threat and genetic susceptibility puts a person much more at risk than either does alone.[20]

Adducts, gene and chromosome mutations, alterations in DNA repair enzymes, various forms of enzymes for metabolizing foreign chemicals and levels of nutrients in the blood stream, all affect susceptibility to cancer. Environmental pollution starts a process that then interacts with our own genetic inheritance. When chemical pollutants are present in the environment the body must work harder to function normally. In people who are slow chemical detoxifiers, exposure to environmental pollution levels that their neighbors are able to tolerate leads step by step to the development of cancer. The path of transmission is complex and fascinating, but there is a larger lesson to be learned, which the new genetic information reinforces: Health care increasingly must try to limit exposure to environmental risks, rather than wait until the damage has been done.[21]

Unfortunately, many current health-care strategies rely primarily on after-the-fact medical responses to environmentally produced changes in the body, rather than dealing with the environmental source of the problem. However there are limits to what we can correct after-the-fact. We are discovering this in the treatment of low birth-weight infants, lead poisoning in children, AIDS, recovery from substance abuse, and increasingly in the treatment of environmentally stimulated cancers and breathing difficulties. Social and larger environmental factors shape the parameters within which the individual's own disease processes occur, and these factors determine whether or not medical treatment strategies will be effective. Ecologically-sophisticated policy analysts argue that health policy, consequently, must begin to pay greater attention to the environmental context which shapes many current disease problems.

Changes in the Biological and Social Environment that Affect Health

During the past half-century, the biological and social environments have been changing in ways that affect health. Both viral evolution, already mentioned, and changing rates of HIV infection in humans are fundamentally altering the nature of infectious disease problems that have to be faced worldwide. Mutations among the infectious agents that trigger once-conquered diseases, are allowing them to survive medicine's "magic bullets" and reappear as serious health problems.

More recently, retroviruses that wipe out human defenses against infection have been passed from person to person around the globe. For 15 years, the fast-mutating HIV retrovirus outwitted all attempts to conquer it pharmacologically. By 1995, worldwide, an estimated 21.8 million people were living with HIV/AIDS. That was almost surely an underestimate, given record-keeping procedures in many parts of the world. In the U.S. alone there were an estimated 600,000 to 900,000 carriers of the virus. When hope of a cure finally came, with the discovery that a combination of protease inhibitor drugs could outwit the virus' reproduction at least for periods of time, the cost of these drugs and the clinical requirements for using them effectively gave little hope that AIDS would cease to be a scourge throughout the world.

There is little hope that continued research will produce a simpler, less costly cure. The rapid mutation of this retrovirus precludes one-shot cures.

Preventing initial infection, thus, becomes even more important than for infectious diseases where a universally usable and affordable cure is known.

Countries faced with the threat of AIDS have tried quite different strategies for containing it: restricting foreigner's entrance to the country; quarantining known carriers; physically destroying persons known to be infected; as well as the more humane strategies of educating persons who might be at risk about how to avoid getting the disease or passing it on to others; and advocating monogamy, sexual abstinence, and avoidance of possible exposure to contaminated blood, since blood and semen are major routes of transmission.[22] AIDS' spread worldwide, despite these various measures, has made it clear that, although the steps which prevent the spread of HIV from person to person are simple, the prevention of AIDS—in practice—is much more difficult. Many humans have more than one sexual partner during their lifetime. As military, economic and social factors create pressures for population movement around the world, opportunities for sexual interaction increase.

The global challenge of AIDS, both to find a cure and to prevent its spread, forces us to rethink health-care strategies rather fundamentally. HIV is spreading within the general population of all countries. It creates enormous demand for disease care services, and particularly for assistance with other infectious diseases of all kinds. Preventing the spread of AIDS becomes particularly difficult because infected persons apparently are most highly infectious in early stages of their infection, before they are aware that they are carriers. In the U.S., HIV-infection currently is spreading among adolescents—heterosexuals more likely to have multiple partners. It also is now spreading, although more slowly, among heterosexual adults.[23]

The social character of health risks is underscored not only by AIDS but also by the use of addicting drugs, and by the international economic interests that continue to develop and market these products despite efforts by various governments to discourage or prohibit their use. Investigations of American tobacco companies and efforts to quash the Colombian "crack" cocaine cartels illuminate the enormous profits that are available to those who are willing to provide products for which there is demand, without regard to the health implications of their activity. The use of recombinant DNA to develop more addicting strains of tobacco, their growth on Latin American plantations and importation into the U.S.[24] as well as the establishment of "crack" processing operations in the jungles of Mexico to take advantage of NAFTA free trade agreements that reduce border inspections,[25] make it clear that the international trading and law enforcement environment is part of the evolving ecology of health.

The spread of AIDS and the use of addicting drugs, both legal and illegal, increases the need for health-care services and escalates the costs of health care when the system responds to these problems. Their costs, even when the problems are ignored, are far from trivial. They are measured in terms of lost human productivity, the disruption of families and neighborhoods, increased crime and violence, and the cost of responding to the disruption or breakdown of the social order. At present they exact a heavy toll from some population groups and neighborhoods, while leaving others little affected. In contrast, concurrent changes that have occurred in the global physical environment affect the entire population of an area, and sometimes of the entire world.

Changes in the Global Physical Environment that Affect Health

Since World War II, the global physical and atmospheric environment has changed in ways that have important implications for the health of humans in various parts of the world, including persons living in the United States. These changes have come because of nuclear weapons testing and the development of atomic power sources, followed by an increasing level of industrial activity worldwide. The development of atomic warfare during World War II, the atomic testing that has been part of the arms race over the ensuing half-century, and the more recent proliferation of atomic weapons in political states around the world introduced both immediate and longer-range health challenges throughout the planet. The discovery of strontium-90 radiation in milk throughout the world, for example, in the wake of nuclear developments in the 1960s started UN monitoring of environmental health problems.[26]

In the 1990s, the collapse of the Soviet political economy and the emergence of environmental concerns as a new focus for international discussion reinforced each other. As *glasnost* encouraged open discussion of problems in the Soviet system and as new political leaders tried to discredit their predecessors, the Soviet contributions to an endangered environment have received strong attention. The health dangers created by the Soviet atomic energy program can now be grasped from tours of Russian atomic facilities. The 1986 Chernobyl disaster, first monitored abroad, released 50 million curies of radioactive energy.[27] Its import has since been reinforced by disclosures of earlier Soviet nuclear accidents and nuclear waste disposal policies, which contaminated the Tech, Tom, and Yenisey rivers, numerous lakes, and shallower portions of the Barents and Kara seas. A nuclear accident near the Urals town of Chelyabinsk in 1957, and continued negligence in the disposal of wastes since then, contaminated nearly 11,000 square miles and subjected 437,000 people to above-normal radiation. During the 1950s and 1960s, Soviet above-ground nuclear weapons tests contaminated rich farmlands of the Altai region and exposed up to 500,000 people to dangerous radiation. After international treaties took nuclear testing underground, caverns near the Volga River became sources of contamination after geological shifts released radioactive gases from the caverns. In addition, more than 100 nuclear devices were exploded in the Soviet Union in various construction and oil exploration projects, some of which caused contamination of surrounding areas.[28] Because radioactive elements often emit radiation for hundreds of years, the effects that nuclear power and weapons developments have already had upon the environment will continue well beyond the next century. Radiation carried by the wind also falls on adjacent countries and circles the globe.

As nuclear power plants proliferate around the world, these reports from the Soviet Union have heightened awareness of risks from generating station accidents that have occurred in England, Japan and the United States, as well as from earlier nuclear weapons testing by all the major powers.[29] Although Soviet excesses probably were on a scale unmatched elsewhere in the world, they were not alone in using questionable judgment about nuclear development. Even after the U.S.S.R., the U.S. and Great Britain stopped testing nuclear bombs above ground in 1963, France continued to do so until 1974, and China until 1980. France resumed nuclear weapons testing, despite international objection, in 1995. Within the U.S., over 100 nuclear bomb tests were conducted in Nevada above the ground until 1963, with others continuing below ground thereafter. Later a nuclear power generating plant was constructed over a known earthquake fault in California. More recently, a defective American nuclear reactor slowly released its radioactive water into Lake Erie. With the exception of Three Mile Island, nuclear power generating mishaps in the U.S. rarely receive wide publicity.[30]

The ending of the Cold War and the collapse of the Soviet Union have diminished the likelihood of a globally devastating nuclear exchange between the world's two major military powers. However the continuing sale of nuclear materials (as well as the sale of sophisticated military technology and equipment) to the ambitious heads of several less powerful states simply shifts the locus of nuclear problems geographically, making them more difficult to control through central decision-making. In addition to international proliferation of nuclear arms, production accidents and the problems implicit in storing atomic fuels and wastes pose still unsolved dilemmas for all countries that use atomic power.

During the period of increasing nuclear activity since World War II cancer rates have risen constantly, including the rates of cancer in children.[31] A correlation does not prove cause and effect, of course; however these developments are consistent with current understandings of how exposure to radioactivity affects mutation within the human body. Physicians have responded to increased cancer rates by trying to lessen the amount of radioactivity to which patients are exposed in the course of medical treatment, ordering fewer x-rays, for example. Some physicians, banding together as Physicians for Social Responsibility, have publicized health dangers from the nuclear weapons race and urge international nuclear disarmament.[32] Meanwhile engineers continue to search for ways to dispose of nuclear power wastes that will not endanger health, a problem yet to be satisfactorily solved as the amount of nuclear waste continues to grow.[33] The impact of nuclear activity is sure to increase with time because proliferation of nuclear weapons has spread to new countries and the search for cheap sources of power continues unabated all over the world.

Substituting non-nuclear technologies provides no simple solution to the deteriorating health environment of the planet, however. Available substitutes, both for sources of energy and for alternative kinds of military activity, are posing their own risks. International transportation of oil is producing a series of oil spills; and oil well fires that have been part of limited warfare add to global environmental problems. In the northern hemisphere, an increased use of coal to replace oil and atomic energy has produced more "acid rain."

"Acid rain" is an old problem, involving many atmospheric pollutants, but its impact is growing. Scientists have been aware since 1852 of the effects of acid rain—of industrial pollutants carried by clouds and deposited by rain on forests, crops, and streams. This was first discovered in Manchester, England; by 1881 Norwegian scientists were noting the effects of pollutants from British industry on the Norwegian countryside. By the 1930s international courts were assessing fines which recompensed nations for damage inflicted by a neighboring state's industrial pollution.[34] In early efforts to preserve areas immediately adjacent to various industrial facilities, tall smokestacks were built, but this simply pushed the problem higher into the atmosphere, spreading the damage more widely. Norway's Forest Research Institute estimated in 1989 that half of the nation's forests had been damaged by airborne industrial emissions coming from Great Britain, and probably from Canada and the U.S., with over a fifth of these forests suffering moderate to severe deterioration. Sweden now has 4,500 lakes in which no fish can live. In North America researchers have been monitoring contamination of the Great Lakes, as well.[35]

For many who use an ecological frame of reference, evidence of deteriorating health for the planet as a whole is sufficient reason to search for alternatives to *all* non-renewable power sources. More skeptical observers, however, ask what difference oil spills and acid rain now make in the actual health of the human population. After all, we have been living with the effects of the industrial revolution for more than two centuries, now, and despite some variation the overall health of the population of the world has improved. Moreover, many industrial production processes now are less polluting than they were a few decades ago. Has the health of the population actually worsened in ways that can be directly related to industrial pollution of the environment?

Yes, evidence indicates that it has. Air pollution from power sources combines with air pollution from transportation and from industrial emissions. Carbon dioxide, methane gas, carbon monoxide, hydrocarbons, and other emissions that are part of late twentieth-century economic activity affect health in basic and fundamental ways. Air pollution damages lungs and eyes, heightens susceptibility to cancer and emphysema, and increases cardiovascular stress due to lower oxygen levels in the lungs. There has been an increase in respiratory problems, including asthma, serious enough that smog and ozone alerts now are issued routinely in many metropolitan areas. Moreover, some would argue that an increase in allergy problems and more serious auto-immune diseases shows that many human immune systems have become hyperactive in response to environmental pollutants of many kinds.[36]

The health problems just listed may be simply the tip of the iceberg, however. If present trends grow stronger, as seems likely, humans in the 21st century will face even more profound changes in circumstances affecting individual health processes. For example, scientific concern has been growing about depletion of the ozone layer in the stratosphere, approximately 15 miles above the earth, which filters ultraviolet rays from the sun. The ozone layer is affected by a variety of gases rising from the earth into the upper atmosphere, and perhaps also by sunspot activity. Although scientists did not at first agree about the implications of their measurements, by 1974 sufficient evidence of depletion was available to cause concern.[37] Within four years the United Nations began sponsoring international conferences on the problem; and by 1980 there was growing evidence that the ozone layer was thinning dangerously. Between 1975 and 1984 the ozone layer over Antarctica reduced in thickness by half.[38] By September, 1992, the hole had increased another 14 percent in size, now measuring 23 million square kilometers—an area considerably larger than the continental United States.[39] Between 1980 and 1990 the concentration of chlorine atoms that affect ozone dissolution increased in the *northern* hemisphere by more than 50 percent.[40] By the winter of 1992 the ozone destroying area of chlorine monoxide in the Arctic ozone layer extended as far south as New England and there was evidence that the ozone layer is thinning over temperate zones as well.[41] These developments alarmed both scientists and health planners, since it would increase exposure to the spectrum of sunlight that produces highly malignant melanoma cancers. The germination of plants also is affected and crop yields decrease. In addition, evidence indicates that human immune systems function less effectively.[42]

For some time, scientists debated whether the change in atmospheric ozone was being produced by activity of the solar system or by industrial pollutants. That debate ended in 1984, when 150 international scientists, based at the southern tip of Chile, collected ice particles from clouds formed in the stratosphere and also from lower-lying clouds. The concentrations of chlorine monoxide in the higher clouds near the South Pole was 100 to 500 times greater than that found in clouds that had formed in the same altitudes at mid-latitudes.[43] This is happening at the North Pole as well. The implications are serious: a single chlorine atom can break up 100,000 ozone molecules before it fades away. A family of industrial products, chlorofluorocarbons (CFCs) and halons, seemed to be critically involved. The most widely used CFC (CFC-12) remains in the atmosphere for 130 years after it is released, and the shortest lived chemical of this family, halon 1211, remains active for seven years.[44] CFCs came into widespread use in industrialized nations after 1930, for refrigerants, fire extinguishers, and aerosol sprays. They also are used in the production of nylon, an ingredient in tires as well as clothing.[45]

The thinning of the ozone layer already is affecting health. Skin cancer rates in southern Chile have tripled; sheep that graze at high altitudes have developed cataracts, the reproductive rhythms of several species have been altered, and land that once produced two crops a year now produces only one.[46] Scientists predict that in the U.S. alone by 2050 there will be an additional 200,000 deaths from cancer produced by changes in the ozone. Recently the U.S. Meteorological Service added ultra-violet exposure ratings as part of its weather reports.[47]

Many people find accounts of the deterioration in global health conditions since World War II, and of their continuing impact on all of us, emotionally difficult to comprehend. It is easier to ignore the facts and trends that exist, especially since scientific evidence always is somewhat incomplete. Taking them seriously, moreover, would bring into question public and private policies affecting many areas of economic and military activity in several countries. Evidence concerning atmospheric deterioration is awkward to contemplate in the U.S.: With less than five percent of the world's population but about a quarter of the world's industrial production, U.S. industrial activity now accounts for 20-25 percent of the dangerous atmospheric emissions.[48] Perhaps understandably, U.S. policy makers have been slower than those in other highly industrialized nations to accept current scientific estimates of the extent of environmental deterioration that has occurred. In that regard, U.S. responses are closer to those found in rapidly industrializing, poorer nations like China, whose industrial emissions will soon surpass those of Japan.

Those who resisted doomsday predictions about the thinning of the ozone layer noted that differences in cloud cover, and in the height of cloud formations above the earth, affected how much ultraviolet radiation actually got through to affect life processes at the surface of the globe. Clouds at lower levels above the earth provide the greatest protection from ultraviolet rays.[49] Unfortunately, however, they also help trap heat from industrial processes, increasing the "greenhouse effect" which provides a different kind of health threat from industrial and others kinds of economic development.

In addition to the health problems that are caused by smog and other forms of air pollution in more limited geographical areas, and the broader threat posed by deterioration of the ozone layer, many scientists now believe that the collective impact of atmospheric pollution produced by human activity is intensifying a "greenhouse effect," i.e., that it is reducing the earth's ability to release solar radiation. This problem is exacerbated by the cutting of tropical rainforests, especially in the Amazon basin, and by the clearing of Siberian forests which are disappearing at the rate of 5 million acres a year. This lessens the earth's ability to absorb the carbon dioxide produced by an increasing human population, by industrial activity, and by the slash and burn preparation of agricultural fields that often follows the clearing of forests.[50] These practices are not that different from American economic practices a century ago, but the consequences now are far more serious. A warming of the earth's temperature increases malnutrition throughout the world by increasing the size of the deserts, and affecting agricultural yields. Changes in carbon dioxide and ultra-violet rays affect crops, wildlife and even fish populations, thus affecting human health both directly and indirectly.[51] Agricultural yields have been declining dramatically in the former Soviet Union and in parts of sub-Saharan Africa. These problems are expected to deepen if global warming continues.[52] Cyclical variations in average temperature let skeptics argue that these problems will be self-correcting. Available scientific evidence, however, suggests that self-correction is unlikely if present economic practices continue unabated.[53]

Already policy planners are dealing with second- and third-order international consequences of "the greenhouse effect." Malnutrition and starvation motivate people to emigrate to areas less affected by climate changes; these economic refugees, unprotected by international law or other legal agreements, often are turned away, or else must work at low wages and subsist under poor living conditions when they migrate, which in turn affects their health and the health of those with whom they come in contact. Their competition for work and the resulting low wage rates also threaten the bargaining power, living standards, and well-being of the indigenous population. Climate-induced population movement affects international relations at many levels. The contribution to air pollution, acid rain, the greenhouse effect, and thinning of the ozone layer that went unattended in the Soviet Union and its satellite states is problematic in other developing areas of the world as well.

Much of what happens elsewhere now has implications for us all. By the 1990s, a number of policy planners throughout the world were taking seriously warnings about the greenhouse effect which had been dismissed as imaginative speculation only a quarter century ago. The chemical processes involved are complex and still not completely understood. However, after describing the level of scientific certainty that now exists, a UN-sponsored Intergovernmental Panel on Climate Change concluded:

> Long-lived gases require reductions in emissions from human activities of over 60 percent to stabilize their concentrations at today's levels; methane would require a 15 to 20 percent reduction.[54]

Environmental discussion now proceeds with the realization that all these processes, which are increasing more rapidly than once thought, sometimes reinforce each other. The thinning ozone layer results not only in lower crop yields on land but in a declining phylloplankton population in the oceans. In addition to its effect on the food chain, thus, the thinning of the ozone layer lowers the oceans' ability to absorb carbon dioxide from the atmosphere. If the oceans' ability to absorb carbon dioxide declines by 10 percent, it will have an impact on the earth's atmosphere equivalent to doubling the amount of fossil fuels now being burned, thus increasing the health risks already described.[55] No one knows how long it will take for this to occur, if present atmospheric pollution practices continue. Consequently environmentalists' warnings are ignored by many policy makers in highly industrialized countries: they are accustomed to planning with three to five year goals in mind.

Unfortunately, growing environmental threats to health are not limited to the air and atmosphere. Problems with toxic wastes and with water pollution, though more localized, pose additional environmental health threats. There is mounting evidence that the incidence of cancer and other diseases varies in relation to one's distance from toxic sites.[56] Pollution also can damage links in the food chain. Fish from some waterways, for example, are not safe to eat. Moreover the consumption of food prepared from crops sprayed with pesticides, as well as the consumption of processed foods containing chemical additives and preservatives, may eventually damage at least some people's health, as current research about the effects of "adducts" on health processes makes clear.[57] Yet during our lifetime applied science has paid relatively little attention to the effects its innovations would have on larger patterns of human health.

In short, biological, social, and physical developments during the past four decades pose new global health threats, and our current health-care systems are ill equipped to deal with these new problems. We can be sure that these trends will have substantial impact on demand for disease care services over time, but we have difficulty assessing just how great an impact they will have.

Understanding the ecological context in which health problems occur adds salience to some of the concerns now addressed by advocates of holistic approaches and of prevention. The multiple effects that pharmaceutical interventions have within the body, for example, and the external environmental changes that also are affecting internal biochemistry give holistic interest in low-tech, non-pharmaceutical health interventions clearer relevance. New discoveries about how the interaction of mind and body affect basic biochemical processes that are central to health also reinforces themes this movement has explored. And discoveries of how radiation and various kinds of pollutants affect biochemical processes within the body deepens the importance of lifestyle choices that lessen susceptibility to external health threats. It is clear that prevention is the most sensible strategy to use when dealing with each of the new environmental health problems just described; but it is equally clear that prevention focused only on lifestyle choices will not be adequate for meeting environmental challenges. Prevention has to involve more than individual behavior choices. Given these new global conditions, health policy must minimize public exposure to environmental health threats, not simply provide access to disease care after-the-fact.

The Emergence of International Environmental Health Approaches

Just as it took time for epidemiologists to recognize that the various health problems facing AIDS patients all stemmed from one condition, deterioration of the immune system, so it took time for policy makers in various nations to recognize that various global crises now confronting the international community are interconnected. By the mid-1980s, however, a new global agenda for debate and action was gradually taking shape. Health issues could no longer be approached primarily in terms of care for individual diseases. Consequently the health implications of a variety of other policies had to be given higher priority than has been true heretofore.

With the passage in 1969 of the Environmental Policy Act and the establishment of the Environmental Protection Agency, it looked as though Americans might have the honor of leading the world into ecologically-guided, broader policy-making.[58] But the larger understanding of world climate changes, the thinning of the ozone layer, and the interrelatedness of survival, health, and economic development issues that emerged 15 years later was not yet available to shape the content of the American plan. After the election of a conservative American president in 1980, and 12 years of executive administrative policy favoring deregulation of industry and encouraging entrepreneurial expansion of economic activity—consequently de-emphasizing environmental protection—the U.S. lost its political leadership in this area.

By that time, however, environmental leadership was passing to the U.N., a more fitting locale to formulate global solutions to problems confronting many nations. The United Nations in fact, began monitoring worldwide environmental health problems in 1955 with the establishment of the UN Scientific Committee on the Effect of Atomic Radiation (UNSCEAR). By 1963 its documentation of world-wide health consequences from radiation had helped produce a Partial Test Ban Treaty, halting atmospheric testing by the U.S., the Soviet Union, and Great Britain. France and China, the other powers with nuclear weapons which did not sign the treaty, however, continued nuclear testing in the atmosphere until 1974 and 1980, respectively.[59] The difficulties of establishing workable agreements which protect the global environment when national political interests or transnational economic interests are at stake became clearly visible during the struggles over nuclear activity. These dynamics work on a still larger scale in current efforts to protect the biosphere.

In 1972, when the UN sponsored a Conference on the Human Environment in Stockholm, Sweden, 114 countries sent delegates.[60] The Conference's focus cut across the usual functional areas for UN activity (health, transport, agriculture, money, military security, and so forth). A new awareness of pollution as a global problem had been established; fallout from nuclear testing was producing significantly higher levels of strontium-90 in milk and vegetables in areas of the world remote from the scene of such tests.[61] The UN adopted a Declaration on the Human Environment, 109 Recommendations for Action, and established a new agency, the UN Environment Programme (UNEP), located in Nairobi, Kenya. UNEP set up an extensive Earthwatch network to monitor the quality of the environment and direct the attention of member states to emerging environmental issues.[62]

Maurice Strong, a Canadian heading the UN's new environmental program, suggested in 1972 that the new environmental situation demanded new concepts of sovereignty, new codes of international law, and new international means of managing the oceans.[63] The 20 years since the Stockholm conference have seen small moves toward a new global order in regard to the environment, but no major change in the power arrangements or in the political and economic objectives that create the global environmental crisis. The Stockholm Recommendations largely remained unimplemented.

In the meantime, the entry of the Green parties into the parliaments of several European countries kept environmental issues part of national political debates. The non-governmental social networks of environmentalists, mentioned already in Chapter 6, helped define issues that need national as well as international attention, and lobbied for the passage of ecologically relevant legislation. As those efforts went forward, the United Nations Environment Programme (UNEP) monitored the environment, documenting its rapid deterioration. It sponsored follow-up conferences and international treaty meetings, attempting to implement recommendations concerning national policies that could affect the production of acid rain, the warming of the climate, and preservation of the oceans. Public forums and negotiating sessions often failed to create joint action throughout the world, but they helped deepen awareness that serious environmental problems confront the international community. The momentum of these international meetings picked up during the late 1980s, as scientific evidence, activist lobbying, and political pressures in Europe kept national leaders aware of the salience of this agenda.

In 1985, an international conference in Ottawa, Canada, created a "30 percent club" of nations targeting themselves to cut sulfur dioxide emissions by that amount by 1993. The technique currently available for doing this is costly, and involves outfitting smokestacks with flue gas desulfurization (FGD) equipment. West Germany, one of the signatories, accomplished this task at great expense. France, another signatory, was able to do so more cheaply, since it was moving toward reliance on nuclear power. Canada, seriously affected by emissions from the U.S., also signed the treaty, but the U.S., Britain, and Poland, all major polluters, refused. Several of the other nations who signed the agreement, however, thus far have made no effort to comply with it.[64]

That same year, most nations in Western Europe and North America signed the Vienna Convention for the Protection of the Ozone Layer, limiting consumption and production of chlorofluorocarbons (CFCs) and halons. By 1989, 28 countries and the European Community had ratified the agreement. Brazil, China, South Korea, and India had not signed, partly because it would affect their ability to produce refrigerators. (The substitutes for prohibited CFCs are expensive, and are due to be phased out over time because they, too, threaten the ozone layer, though less vigorously.) The U.S., pursuing a general policy favoring deregulation of industry, initially resisted the target dates set by other nations.[65] The political jockeyings of the late 1980s and early 1990s produced considerable agreement among nation states, however, about policies that needed to be implemented worldwide. Protocols developed in meetings in Montreal, Helsinki, and London between 1987 and 1990 set targets for reduction of CFCs by specific dates.[66]

The difficulties of getting national policy to work consistently on global environmental problems came vividly in view in June of 1995, when Japanese citizens sponsored a full page ad in the New York *Times*. The ad asked Americans to write the Japanese ambassador to the United States, requesting him to urge Japan to comply more fully with the international ozone emission treaty it had signed. While Japan has reduced its production of ozone-damaging chemicals, as promised in the treaty, they reported, Japanese citizens' efforts to get Japan to stop releasing already-manufactured chlorofluorocarbons and halons into the environment were being ignored. Japanese environmentalists, consequently, urged Americans to petition the Japanese government to use the same standards for disposal of chlorofluorocarbons and halons that were being used in the United States.[67]

In 1988 Friends of the Earth, Greenpeace, and the World Wildlife Fund for Nature jointly challenged the British government to turn propaganda about the environment into action, presenting a list of 30 measures ranging from recycling resources to doubling overseas aid. They received little support in Parliament for these bills, but they began to get a more serious hearing when they joined with the Association for the Conservation of Energy (a lobby and think tank financed by manufacturers of equipment for conserving heat and energy) to discuss the greenhouse effect's implications for energy policy with the House of Common's Energy Committee.[68]

Environmentalists have had their greatest success at a national level, however, in the Netherlands. In 1988 Queen Beatrix's Christmas message to her subjects struck a strong theme of environmental crisis: "The earth is slowly dying. We human beings ourselves have become a threat to the planet. Those who no longer wish to disregard the insidious pollution and degradation of the environment are driven to despair."[69]

In 1989, the Dutch electorate strongly supported candidates advocating implementation of a Netherlands' National Environmental Policy Plan, as presented in a study entitled "To Choose or to Lose."[70] The plan directed about 3 percent of national income for environmental policies through 1994, gradually reducing environmental expenditures to 2 percent of total expenditures by 2010. Its goals included cutting energy consumption by 30 percent, reducing the acidification of Dutch soil, and disposing of wastes. The government would pay half the cost of these projects, with industry and agriculture picking up the rest. The number of cars on the road in the Netherlands has doubled in the last 15 years, and some of the earliest policies now put into law involve tax incentives to install catalytic converters on vehicle engines. Responding to inquiries from business groups, the Central Planning Bureau carried out studies assessing the financial impact of implementing these environmental policies if the Netherlands proceeds unilaterally, and also the smaller financial impact for Holland that will occur if the rest of the European Community follows suit.[71] The Dutch, in short, have now set the pace for national political action on the global environment.

They also have taken bold steps attempting to lessen the problems of AIDS and addicting drugs in the Netherlands. The pragmatic Dutch have accepted the failure of efforts to stop prostitution and the smuggling of drugs into their country. Instead, both the "sex trade" and "soft" drug sales are now legal in the Netherlands. Hard drug users are given methadone. Over a 17-year period, the percentage of Dutch youth under 22 who use heroin or cocaine has fallen from 15 percent to less than 3 percent. The government educates prostitutes as well as the general public on health issues, including protection against AIDS, and tests sex workers regularly. By legalizing and supervising drug sales, and by providing strong welfare assistance to the unemployed, the government hopes to lessen the vulnerability of poorer citizens to being recruited into the international underworld's distribution network for drugs, an arrangement that has encouraged the spread of addiction in other industrialized countries.[72] Dutch initiatives in both these areas are highly controversial and may not be acceptable elsewhere in the world, but it is clear that the Netherlands has begun to understand the nature of new global crises and to innovate on all fronts in an effort to improve the health of the environment.

Just as American health-care outcomes increasingly fell behind those being achieved in other nations,[73] so too U.S. government officials showed a much less sophisticated understanding of the nature of the problems and decisions now facing the global community.[74] Instead of undertaking new, precedent-setting actions, the U.S. government spent over a billion dollars on research to assess claims being made about the reality and severity of the crisis.[75] In April of 1992, a panel of the National Academy of Science issued a report on global warming. It concluded that there is a reasonable chance that by the middle of the 21st century global temperatures will rise from 2 to 9 degrees Fahrenheit. That threat, they concluded, is "sufficient to justify action now." The panel urged the president to develop a stronger energy plan. They called for tax incentives to help achieve a 30 percent increase in automobile fuel efficiency, and to raise automobile mileage standards immediately by 5 miles per gallon. The panel estimated that 10 to 40 percent of U.S. greenhouse emissions could be eliminated fairly cheaply, by doing such things as making buildings and power plants more energy efficient. It recommended planting millions of trees that can become collectors of carbon dioxide, a policy the U.S. administration already had endorsed.[76]

A series of international conferences during the early 1990s culminated in a UN Summit Conference on the Environment, in Rio de Janeiro, Brazil, in June of 1992. Attended by representatives from 178 nations, including more than 100 heads of state, it directed the attention of the international community to issues of global climate change, biological diversity, deforestation, and pollution of the oceans. Negotiations preceding the conference were intense. Scientists, environmental lobbies, politicians from many countries (including heads of states), and UN staff argued that the conference must include specific goals and target dates for international action to reduce the environmental threat posed by current activities. Many delegates to these planning meetings, including those from the European Community and from Japan, recommended freezing production of dangerous emissions at their 1990 levels and providing economic help to poorer nations so that they could meet these goals. Poorer nations, including Brazil, argued that debt forgiveness by international banks would be necessary for them to redirect resources toward saving the environment. They insisted that national sovereignty be respected, warning that industrialized nations must not use the current crisis to limit economic development by potential rivals elsewhere.[77]

Despite considerable international pressure, U.S. negotiators continued to resist pressure to set goals and target dates for emission controls, or to underwrite the costs of poorer nations' environmental actions; they refused to take on any commitments that might cost American jobs. President Bush, facing a tough reelection campaign with the American economy in recession, at first refused to attend the Rio Conference, then used his threatened boycott as leverage to veto or water down proposals placed before the conference. (Given the huge U.S. role in the crisis, its boycott would make UN decisions largely moot.)[78]

As U.S. delegates to the preparatory meetings for the Rio Conference tried to negotiate less stringent UN agreements, two U.S. agencies, EPA and the National Aeronautics and Space Administration (NASA), issued reports documenting the thinning of the Arctic ozone layer and reporting that the areas of depletion extended as far south as New England and France, and that emissions from the manufacture of nylon, used in everything from stockings to tires, were releasing nitrous oxide into the atmosphere with a half-life of 150 years; these emissions, combined with nitrous oxide produced by algae and bacteria, were increasing the concentration of nitrous oxide in the atmosphere by 0.2 percent a year, further eating away the ozone layer.[79] Then E.I. DuPont, the American-based corporation that is the world's largest producer of chlorofluorocarbons (CFCs) announced plans to alter production to involve less fast-acting CFCs. (DuPont hoped the Rio Summit would help it corner the market for its CFC substitutes.) President Bush thereafter made a conciliatory gesture toward other nations, announcing earlier U.S. target dates for controlling CFC emissions. He continued to veto other proposals.[80]

In Rio, delegates ratified 27 principles that should provide environmental rules for "global partnership." An abbreviated summary of their key points follows. (1) All nations have a sovereign right to exploit their own resources and to engage in economic development, but these rights should be exercised in a way that meets developmental and environmental needs of present and future generations equitably. (2) Only "sustainable development"—which does not damage the environment—is appropriate. (3) All states shall cooperate to eradicate poverty, which undermines the ability of nations to undertake sustainable development policies, and the special needs of the least developed countries shall be given special consideration. (4) States should reduce and eliminate unsustainable patterns of production and consumption and should enact effective environmental legislation, with standards set in a manner appropriate to the context of each situation. (5) States shall develop national law regarding liability and compensation for victims of pollution and other environmental damage, and shall cooperate to prevent the relocation from one state to another, in an effort to avoid such regulations, of activities that damage the environment. (6) Where there are threats of serious or irreversible damage to the environment, lack of full scientific certainty shall not be used as a reason for postponing cost-effective measures to prevent environmental degradation.

(7) National authorities should promote internationalization of the costs of environmental protection; and cost-bearing should be developed on the principle that the polluter should bear the cost of pollution, within the limits of public interest and the needs of international trade and investment. (8) States shall inform one another in timely manner of natural disasters, production accidents, emergencies, or other activities that will have transboundary implications for the environment and the health and safety of populations. (9) States shall respect international law regarding protection for the environment in times of armed conflict and shall cooperate in its further development, as necessary. (10) Peace, development, and environmental protection are interdependent and indivisible. States shall resolve all their environmental disputes peacefully and by appropriate means, in accordance with the Charter of the UN.[81]

These principles, in sum, reflect a compromise between environmental needs and the political realities of international diplomacy. Beyond these statements of principle, the Rio Conference introduced a treaty that was expected to be ratified by nearly all nations attending the summit. In it, industrialized nations agreed to try to bring emissions of carbon dioxide, methane, and nitrous oxide back to 1990 levels by the year 2000; but at the insistence of the U.S., it did not require stabilization at this level into the next century. This treaty, which will go into effect as soon as it is ratified by 50 countries, also calls for monitoring scientific advances so that further modifications can be made as needed.[82]

Another treaty, to become effective when ratified by 30 nations, commits signatories to slow the loss of plant and animal species by setting up protected areas and rehabilitating degraded habitats. It also calls on developed and developing countries to cooperate on research projects, such as the discovery of new drugs from rainforest sources. (The U.S. refused to sign this treaty, claiming that it does not provide adequate copyright and patent protection for U.S. biotechnology firms.)[83]

Other proposals regarding forestry protection provided a compromise between the U.S., which demanded a full-fledged forest treaty, and several developing countries who demanded the right to develop their own resources. India and Malaysia accused the UN of trying to internationalize a natural resource, and Brazil sought to use northern hemisphere concerns about rainforest preservation to build support for international debt forgiveness.[84]

The final document before the Rio Conference was Agenda 21, a 900-page blueprint for environmentally friendly development, prescribing action on issues ranging from ocean pollution, hazardous waste, and renewable energy to human health, poverty, and advancement for women. Staff reporters for the *Wall Street Journal* wrote that "because it had to accommodate the views of 178 nations on such a huge range of topics, Agenda 21 is a flabby and unfocused document that depends largely on political will and large-scale development aid to be carried out." Nonetheless, the creation of such an international agenda in itself marked a major change. Unfortunately, the time limit for avoiding global disaster may be shorter than that required for international political processes to unfold. By September of 1992, the hole in the ozone layer above Antarctica had grown to a size considerably larger than that occupied by the continental United States.[85]

The U.S. official stance on environmental issues changed with the election of President Bill Clinton and Vice President Albert Gore, Jr. Gore, who attended the Rio summit, has been a leading advocate for a stronger environmental protection policy in the United States for some time. Clinton appointed a strong environmentalist to his cabinet, as secretary of the interior, a position which would be key to policy regarding U.S. forests and wilderness areas. After the passage of NAFTA, however, it was not clear whether agreements regulating international trade would undercut U.S. environmental protection laws or whether U.S. policies would be extended into Mexico, where serious pollution problems went unattended.

Meanwhile, evidence of environmental change affecting global warming continued to accumulate. Between 1800 and 1994 carbon dioxide in the atmosphere increased from 280 parts per million to 358. Most significantly, worldwide carbon emissions increased 386 percent between 1950 and 1997. Four of the five hottest years on record occurred since 1990. Glaciers almost everywhere were in retreat. Oceans, which expand when warmed, had risen by 4 to 10 inches. Rising sea levels flooded crop lands in Micronesia in the Pacific and threatened to force abandonment of the island of Nokuoro, consistent with global warming predictions though not absolute confirmation that global warming is responsible. In 1995 a UN report produced by a panel of 2,000 specialists led by Bert Bolin, a Swedish climatologist, predicted that if emissions continue at current rates, global temperatures will rise an additional 2 to 6 degrees Fahrenheit by 2100 and sea levels will rise 6 inches to 3 feet, inundating islands and shorelines.[86]

The 165-nation treaty on climate change, signed in 1992, calling for voluntary emissions cutbacks, had failed. By 1995 governments agreed to negotiate mandatory emissions reductions by industrial nations. Island states proposed that by 2005 emission be cut 20 percent below 1990 levels. The European Union favored a 15 percent reduction by 2010. Japan, Australia and the United States were more reluctant. In the U.S., the leadership of the Republican caucus which swept the 1994 mid-term elections was committed to undoing environmental protection laws, which they saw as a threat to entrepreneurial freedom and consequently to economic growth. In 1997, a week before a U.N. "Earth Summit" meeting, under mounting pressure from 130 industrialists including the chief executives of Exxon, General Motors and General Electric, the Clinton administration shied away from backing specific cutbacks in carbon dioxide and other gases to combat global warming. The U.S. Senate urged the White House to make no commitments to reduce U.S. emissions unless countries with rapidly developing economies do the same, arguing that otherwise the new treaty would simply speed the shift of industrial production out of the United States and into areas not affected by the treaty. It was clear that environmental policy would remain a contested domain in American politics and administrative policy.[87]

The attention now being given to the effects of industrial activity on the global environment is realigning concerns within traditional interest groups, and even within transnational corporations. As risks from atomic energy production became visible in the 1980s, for example, investors backed away from nuclear development stocks.[88] And as problems of toxic waste disposal came to the attention of the public, pressures began to mount on firms to modify their industrial processes in the interests of health.[89] With the current understanding of how toxic the by-products of many economic activities are, major corporations face even more difficult decisions.

The new watchword within planning circles has become "sustainable economic development," meaning a growth of productivity that does not endanger the environment. Whether it will become economically feasible to stop all environmental damage remains to be seen. The refrigeration industry and the aerosol spray industries, for example, have moved quickly to substitute less dangerous chlorofluorocarbons for those previously used in refrigeration equipment, fire extinguishers, and spray cans, but the substitutes simply slow the pace of ozone depletion; they do not eliminate the danger.[90] Some major corporations, including E.I. DuPont, have begun to acknowledge the crisis. But it is clear that the large transnational corporations, including auto manufacturers and oil refineries, must soon be drawn into efforts to preserve the earth's environment. British Petroleum has taken the lead, investing heavily in solar energy. "Health policy" no longer can limit its attention to the management of disease states after they occur. Transportation, energy development, manufacturing, lumbering and forestry policies—all must now be part of health policy planning, for decisions made in these areas will have direct effects on the health of the world's populations. There is no longer an indefinite period of time to work out cooperative relationships between political and economic interests in areas that affect health.

How Do These Developments Relate to Broader Health Care Reform?

A century and a half ago the international Sanitation Society, organized by civil engineers, decided that dirt and filth were related to the international cholera epidemic of the time, after researchers traced the spread of cholera in a poor neighborhood of London to use of a pump accessing a water source that had become contaminated by feces from a nearby privy. The Sanitation Society educated the public in many industrializing countries about the importance of sanitary sources of drinking water and the disposal of human wastes, and helped create modern urban water distribution and sewage disposal systems. Twenty years later medical science discovered the germ theory of disease and began to reorient its practices around these understandings. In the meantime, operating at first independently of medical professionals, sanitary engineers created an urban physical infrastructure that may have been more important for lessening the incidence of infectious disease than medical science's eventual attack on microbes.[91]

Now the emergence of a broader ecological perspective alerts us to sources of health problems that once again go beyond the current focus of medical science. This new orientation cuts through earlier compartmentalization of the world into self-limiting categories such as health care, military policy, economic development, and technological advancement, showing how interrelated these categories have become, and how relevant they are for health and survival. Many areas of public policy and private investment decisions now have potentially important consequences for the environment and thus for health. In a period of deficit spending in the public arena and a net outflow of resources that destablizes America's position in the international economy, however, the costs of new ecological health initiatives will compete with other areas for health-care spending and public subsidy.

Identifying technological sources of current threats to health expands the arena for social conflict. It also provides a new kind of ethical base for decision-making. A scientific frame of reference now provides a grounding for moral and political judgments: Actions which disrupt the ecological balance of nature are ultimately self-destructive to humans as a whole, and consequently from a scientific perspective become both morally and pragmatically unacceptable. Since World War I the social sciences have been wrestling with the impossibility of moral neutrality in the framing of questions for inquiry, however objective one might be later when gathering data relevant to those questions.[92] The same issue now confronts the natural sciences as well.

Criticisms of an Ecological Approach to Health Care

Not all observers accept the relevance of an ecological perspective when considering health-care policy. Many are not yet convinced that there is a real environmental crisis that will seriously affect health, arguing that there is insufficient scientific evidence to justify making economic sacrifices for an unproven hypothesis.[93] Other skeptics raise three additional objections to reorienting health concerns in this way.

The first of these argues from a traditional pragmatism: Environmental concerns, while important, are fundamentally irrelevant for health-care policy because health care deals with the actual diseases that people get. In this view, measures to prevent ecological disaster may be necessary, but we must not divert resources from our present disease-care emphasis in order to work on environmental health problems; we have our hands full trying to provide all our citizens with access to basic health services.[94]

The second objection arises from a radical left political orientation: Popularizing ecological concerns is seen as simply another way to divert attention from the real problems of the masses. In the U.S., environmental concerns attract middle-class support for expenditures that leave even less money available for health care of the poor, and it can also be used as a weapon by the northern industrialized countries to prevent potentially competitive economic development in the poorest countries of the southern hemisphere.[95]

The third objection, advanced by some who take the environmental crisis seriously and see its relevance for health, is that the environmental movement has not demonstrated how to solve the problems it identifies: despite support from many levels of government and the populace, it has had little effect on those decisions about use of technology that lie at the root of the planetary crisis. Everyone is for environmentalism, much as everyone is for motherhood; but economic motivations always predominate when decisions have to be made. Consequently, in this view, the growing environmental crisis simply deepens the need for sophisticated, high-tech medical interventions to correct the damage the environment is doing to individuals.[96]

Advocates of an environmental, ecological focus for health care, in contrast, are convinced that the evidence of a mounting environmental crisis is overwhelming. They insist that it misreads scientific rigor to use debates within science as an excuse to forestall preventive actions. The scientific method, they point out, encourages doubt until doubt no longer is possible, but by that time the crisis will be beyond repair. The advice of a panel from the U.S. National Academy of Science speaks to this point: Although not all scientists are convinced that the predictions of major planetary changes being set in motion by current technological practices will actually occur, they acknowledge, there is nonetheless sufficient consensus among scientific experts about these dangers to warrant "cost-effective" preventive measures.[97]

In answer to the first objection—that pragmatically, we cannot afford to change our present approach—environmentalists join preventive health advocates in arguing that it is short-sighted and economically self-destructive to develop health-care policy that does not deal with *sources* of disease, along with the diseases themselves. Health-related *environmental* issues, they argue, are having an accelerating impact on the creation of disease problems in humans.[98]

In response to the second objection—that funding environmental health measures diverts resources away from the needs of the poor—environmental advocates answer that since low-income neighborhoods in the U.S. suffer a disproportionate exposure to environmental hazards, we cannot address their health needs without focusing on environmental risks.[99] They argue, further, that debt forgiveness to nations in the southern hemisphere in exchange for environmentally protective actions that also allow "sustained economic development" can be a practical strategy for dealing with the real needs of population groups around the world.[100] More help with population planning and AIDS prevention education, along with greater access to sterile hypodermic needles and a safe blood supply, is needed if poor nations are to have a realistic chance of improving their economic situation. What is needed most, however, is for the richest nations to decrease their consumption of the world's resources and their emission of industrial pollutants. We are poisoning ourselves and the rest of the earth's inhabitants, they argue, and must readjust our economic system so that it meets health and survival needs everywhere. The environmental crisis brings the self-interests of the rich and the poor together. A general increase in cancer rates and lower agricultural yields because of the thinning of the ozone layer is too high a price to pay, they argue, for uncontrolled industrial emissions or uncontrolled destruction of tropical rainforests; similarly, the costs of fortifying coastlines against rising ocean levels if global warming continues will greatly exceed any economic gains from ignoring current evidence of global warming. If these trends continue, they argue, the rich as well as the poor will lose.

In addressing the final objection—that because environmental problems have not been solved we should invest more heavily in high-tech medicine to deal with our new health problems rather than tackle hopeless global prevention goals—supporters of an environmental agenda admit that no foolproof formula yet exists for saving the environment; but they see evidence that a combination of current strategies—including "moral initiative" campaigns, political lobbying and organizing, and UN diplomacy—is making headway. Japan and the member states of the European Community (all major industrial powers) have supported international treaties to limit industrial emissions; 178 nations, and more than 100 heads of state, participated in the 1992 environmental summit conference in Rio. Enlightened self-interest, environmental advocates insist, now includes protecting the planet.[101]

Furthermore, some political analysts argue, cynics who insist that narrow economic self-interest will continue to prevail have failed to learn the lesson of the changing world order. The collapse of the Soviet system demonstrates the fragility of any social order too rigid to adapt to changing external circumstances. A system can collapse quite quickly, from a combination of internal and external pressures, when leaders or a coalition of interests reorient their own policy objectives and make sure that information about current problems is freely and widely disseminated. Each of the four major nations now resisting the growing environmental consensus— Brazil, China, India, and the U.S.—has a considerable block of disaffected citizens, and each (though in quite different ways) could become vulnerable to international economic pressures.

Both the liberal and conservative agendas that have guided American public policy over the last 60 years may have become outmoded in the new world context; many would argue that they are now demonstrating their limits for solving either the fiscal or the environmental problems that confront us. Perhaps new coalitions will form that address these problems more creatively. A widespread public disenchantment with established interests, combined with a growing worldwide recognition of imminent global crisis, could provide the impetus for a new international regrouping of interests and resources.

Once again, having met critiques and defenses of a new approach to health and disease, readers may draw their own conclusions. Meanwhile, there are useful lessons for current health planning.

Ecological Lessons for Current Health Planning

From an ecological approach to health, these three lessons for disease care stand out:

1. An ecological perspective—on what happens inside humans as well as on how humans fit into a larger ecosystem—fundamentally reorganizes our approaches to medicine and disease care, and points to ways that scientific medicine can begin to escape over-reliance on high-tech interventions that disrupt internal ecological rhythms. Attention to the self's own healing processes and to rhythms of neuropeptide regulation within the body will help counter the present overuse of drugs, surgery, and mechanical substitutes for human processes. Greater attention to sources of disease in the social and physical environment will lessen the need for intrusive interventions which disrupt the internal ecology of the body.

2. There is much to be gained from paying more attention to the second-, third-, and fourth-order consequences of scientific interventions. Greater reliance on less invasive, low-tech interventions can promote more effective disease management as well as protect the global environment.

3. In funding research, higher priority must be given to discovering the total environmental consequences of new technologies, whether they affect the global environment or the individual. This emphasis could lead to changes in preferred production technologies and in preferred medical treatment strategies. It could lead, for example, to greater emphasis on treatments that strengthen the body's own defense systems and less reliance on pharmaceutical interventions that target a specific problem and produce unintended side effects.

In addition, an ecological approach to health makes four other contributions to a more basic reorientation of approaches to health and disease:

1. It demonstrates that we cannot prevent serious deterioration in the health status of whole populations, nationally and worldwide, unless we deal with environmental sources of disease. These sources include toxic wastes, air pollutants, oil spills, radiation hazards, and various heat producers whose impact on global warming and on the thinning of the ozone layer affect the habitability of the planet.

2. It shows that the crisis we now face in finding resources for health care is mild compared to what probably lies ahead. Certainly the experience of other industrialized nations proves that our present resources could be reorganized to provide more effective services. But those resources will be increasingly taxed by the need to deal with environmental deterioration, a growing AIDS pandemic, problems of drug addiction, and an aging population. In this situation, setting clear priorities for research and for health expenditures becomes critical.

3. The emerging role of science in assessing what is happening to the environment offers a new basis for decision-making—and for many, a compelling new ethic: Actions which disrupt the ecological balance of nature are ultimately self-destructive to humans as a whole as well as to the larger ecosystem, and consequently are both morally and pragmatically unacceptable.

4. Ecological concerns bridge older social cleavages. An ecological approach introduces new kinds of action networks, ones that cut across economic positions and relationships to political power. It helps create networks that work globally rather than simply at the national level. These could provide the basis for a new international coalition of interests.

Solving problems that are transnational in scope will require international cooperation. Once again, as was true a century and a half ago, it seems to be time to tackle the new environmental threats to health at their source.

10

Reapproaching Health: Next Steps

Effective health-care reform has to start where we are now, but it must offer a clear vision of where we want to go; and any changes in government programs or legislation must be compatible with the political sentiments of the time. Where *do* we want to go? And how might we begin to get there?

We have twin tasks to accomplish. First, we must shift the emphasis of health care toward *health*. It must focus much more on prevention, on primary care (i.e., on early disease identification and treatment) and must use a more ecological approach to health-building (as described in Chapters 7 and 9). Only as that occurs can we begin to accomplish the second task of making health care affordable and accessible to all. Previous reform efforts tried to improve access to services and cut costs for conventional disease care, but found these problems intractable. While some currently recommended reforms are potentially useful, they have lacked a key ingredient that could affect how the present dynamic works. By shifting our emphasis toward *health*, rather than focusing primarily on the management of disease, we can begin to reduce the need for expensive disease services. We then can begin to gain the leverage needed to make reform of the disease care system more effective.

How might we begin to move in these directions? We must start where we are now, taking into account the larger changes that are occurring globally in the environment, and nationally and internationally in the social fabric of the economy. Reforms must be relevant not only to immediate issues of health-care delivery and financing but also to broader developments which shape the health issues that will have to be dealt with in the future.

Three global developments, which emerged since American health care evolved into its present organization as a health-care industry, must affect our planning. One global development changes the sources and availability of funding for health services. Another affects the nature of problems that must be addressed. The third creates a moment of opportunity for more fundamental initiatives affecting health.

First, the globalization of manufacturing and the new balance of trade have eroded American businesses' ability to fund the exponentially-increasing costs of disease care for their employees. It also has lessened the size of the tax base available to provide a public safety net as private commitment to funding disease care erodes. The down-sizing of major sectors of the economy, coupled with tax reforms that further limit government income, require new solutions to the problem of providing basic health-care services for all Americans.

Second, the nature of currently unsolved health problems is changing. On a global level the AIDS pandemic and the international distribution of illicit drugs present new kinds of health challenges; and both developments increase the number of health emergencies that require costly interventions. Increasingly, organisms that produce disease are becoming resistant to antibiotics. In addition, the deteriorating global environment is producing increases in cancer rates at all age levels. Nationally the aging of the population, as the baby boom generation enters middle age and the demographic profile of the nation changes, will increase the need for chronic disease management and long term care of the progressively disabled. All of these changing health problems increase the cost of disease care currently, and further underscore the need for a greater accent on *prevention*—to minimize the volume of future disease care expenditure by dealing now with sources of disease—at a personal, social, and environmental level. (They also guarantee that even if a shift of emphasis toward prevention occurs, disease care will remain an important part of the American economy.)

Third, on a more positive note, the ending of the Cold War has led to a changed world order, one that provides an opportunity to approach the larger ecology of health. With proper meshing of health and economic policies, the new international scene could allow redeployment of public resources. We could make American businesses more competitive by helping them develop environmentally-safe manufacturing processes that also help them compete for world markets. This would have long-term advantages for health care. It would begin to lower the volume of need for expensive disease care in the future. In addition to improving the health of Americans, a healthier environment and a stronger emphasis on health promotion should also produce lower health benefits costs for all third-party payers, public or private. This would make the cost of doing business in America lower, helping American products compete with those made elsewhere.

Each of these global developments underscores the importance of shifting our priorities toward preserving and promoting health, rather than simply managing disease. It *is* possible to begin to move in this direction, using current policy proposals for which there is strong bi-partisan support in Congress. Private innovation already underway would reinforce these directions of change. Together, these developments could provide a lever that changes how other currently proposed reforms of the health-care system would work. Although changes which are currently feasible would not solve all our problems, they would set in motion a new dynamic within health care. That could make possible still more fundamental reforms, once Congress and the public begin to understand the implications of shifting the emphasis in health care toward *health*.

This chapter recommends some first steps toward reform. A number of suggestions here build on experiments already undertaken, or on political proposals demonstrated to have fairly strong support. Thus most are both politically imaginable and economically viable, not simply visionary. Each has a chance of surviving the give-and-take of public and private policy making and implementation. Together they could begin to produce a shift of emphasis in health care. If only some of them get used, the dynamic for change will be less strong; nonetheless each would have a positive impact. As currently achievable proposals fall into place, the probability will grow that more deeply innovative reforms of the total health-care system can emerge.

This chapter identifies five overall goals involved in rethinking health: (1) shifting the emphasis toward health, (2) getting health care where it is most needed, (3) reducing wasteful use of high technology by demedicalizing life experiences, (4) shifting to lower cost, more ecologically sophisticated care, and (5) improving the health of the planet. The chapter includes examples of existing or recommended programs which further each goal. Table 10.1 outlines these five overall goals and programs relevant to them.

The next chapters will discuss ways that disease care could build on the dynamic that would be set in motion by these currently achievable reforms. Let us begin, however, with immediately possible ways to move toward the following goals: shifting the emphasis of health care toward prevention, primary care and a more ecological approach to health.

Table 10.1 Five Goals for Refocusing *Health* Care

What?	*How?*
1. Shift the Emphasis for Health Care	A. Worksite health promotion emphasis B. Defense Department prevention initiatives C. H.E.R.O. Trade Association for Health Enhancement
2. Get Care Where It is Most Needed	A. Reinsurance reform surcharge incentives B. Independent, health-oriented managed care services C. "Barefoot Doctors" training changes
3. Lower Use of High Technology	A. Demedicalizing birth B. Demedicalizing aging and dying
4. Move Toward More Ecologically-Sophisticated Care	A. Mixed-model health care B. New evaluative roles for the NIH C. A new role for the FDA
5. Deal with Environmental Sources of Disease	A. Environmentally-oriented federal research grants B. Tax incentives and technical assistance to help American-based manufacturing meet international environmental safety standards

Shifting the Emphasis to *Health* Care

Worksite Health Promotion— Prevention for the General Public

If we intervene earlier in the health-disease process, taking services to people while they are still healthy, identifying those at risk, helping them prevent the development of disease and improve their general level of health, considerable reduction in the need for more expensive disease care will occur over time. As Chapter 8 makes clear, technologies to do this effectively have now been developed, and businesses that sponsor the more successful worksite wellness programs have kept health-care benefits in line with inflation when other companies were finding health benefits costs escalating rapidly. In the spring and summer of 1994, three of the four congressional health insurance reform bills that came out of committee deliberations included provisions to reimburse employers and their employees for some of the costs of worksite prevention services through discounts on insurance premiums. The 1996 Health Insurance Reform Act made sure such arrangements, though voluntary, would not be precluded by funding arrangements for other insurance reforms.

To qualify for reimbursements, programs under the 1994 proposals would have had to engage a sufficient number of employees, and provide education, screening, counseling, follow-up, and treatment or referral programs. They would help employees reduce lifestyle and other risk factors that can be modified (such as cholesterol, inactivity, nutrition and weight management problems, smoking, or practices that increase risk of cancer, HIV or other sexually transmitted diseases). They also would help with chronic health risks or problems such as high blood pressure or diabetes. These worksite programs would promote exercise and fitness through education or actual programs at work, and include counseling and employee assistance programs that deal with areas of personal concern that adversely affect job performance, such as substance abuse, stress, or parenting. Workplace prevention programs could be reimbursed for the cost of health and safety education and prevention programs that go beyond those now required by law. They could provide prenatal counseling and education, as well as consumer education regarding health services, including programs on the development of living wills.

The 1994 Congressional bills would have made it illegal for worksite health promotion programs to share information about health risks of employees with personnel departments, other than as statistical profiles of the employee population as a whole, thus guarding against any possible punitive uses of prevention programs by employers.[1] These proposals had wide bi-partisan support, as well as endorsement from occupational physicians and nurses associations, other medical groups, employers, and vendors of such services.

Similar proposals are likely to be introduced in future legislation. It is important that this happen. Such legislation will provide an institutional base of support for moving preventive care to worksites, a move which should lower the demand for expensive health-care services. Several bills introduced into the 1995 session of Congress picked up on these themes. It seems only a matter of time until an institutionalized basis of funding for worksite prevention programs will be enacted. Hopefully such legislation will include standards for content, performance, and *outcomes* that qualify for such funding. This would introduce a new level of accountability into health-care financing.

Additional discounted rates could be given when the utilization of health-care benefits at a worksite which has a qualified wellness program falls below those of the community at large, after first taking into account any cost savings that might occur because of differences in age, sex, or occupational hazards for that group of employees.

Effective prevention programs require personalized interaction with recipients of the care. Health professionals motivate them to care about their health and help them find strategies for health improvement that respect their own lifestyle preferences. The 1995 cost for such services varied from $25 to $175 per person, annually, depending upon the needs of different employee populations and the difficulty of contacting them. Institutionalizing payment for such services will be an important step. It redirects health care toward health improvements which lower the need for evermore expensive disease care.

Effective prevention or health promotion programs do more than admonish people to change individual behaviors that put their health at risk. They help individuals discover personally enjoyable, stress-reducing ways to improve both their personal health and the social environment in which they live and work. That is why worksites are such a strategic location for health promotion programs. The culture of work, and organizational policies that affect health, all become accessible as individuals in key locations within a worksite experience health improvements and begin to understand how the health of the worksite is relevant to its overall productivity.

Extending health promotion services to public schools, as well, would be an effective way to guarantee long-term savings in the cost of medical care. This would require redirecting how some public health budgets are allocated.

Health promotion involves much more than clinically focused "prevention" efforts centering around inoculations, well-baby services and early cancer detection. Members of Congress and their staffs learned this lesson during the 1994 debates about health-care reform. So did the Department of Defense.

Department of Defense Initiatives in Prevention and Wellness

Since the end of the Cold War, the Department of Defense has been forced by Congress and military strategic planners to develop plans for operating with reduced annual budgets. This includes revamping the provision of health-care services to its personnel and their dependents. A major initiative (TRICARE) places significant emphasis on early detection and treatment, and increasingly on *prevention* of disease. Health services contracts for military beneficiaries are being offered to managed care organizations, with explicit requirements both for providing prevention-oriented services routinely and for reporting outcomes of such services. In addition, the Army is using Health Risk Assessments questionnaires, similar to those developed by the Centers for Disease Control (CDC). These are now being used with active duty personnel to identify personnel potentially at risk for disease and to track changes in their health status over time.

The Air Force now has taken a leadership role in defining optimal strategies for prevention services. Its Office for Prevention and Health Services Assessment (OPHSA) has conducted a major study to identify the "best (prevention program) practices" for use in military, community and work settings, seeking the most cost-effective strategies for *improving* the health status of populations by evaluating the corporate world's and the military's own experience with comprehensive prevention programs. The Air Force also is developing Health and Wellness Centers (HAWCs) at each military base. The Office for Prevention and Health Services Assessment is creating clinical, prevention-oriented, intake assessment tools to be used by all military-sponsored health care providers worldwide, including managed care contracts for military beneficiaries. The defense department expects health care providers to use these assessment tools to trigger appropriate preventive clinical practices, as defined by the U.S. Preventive Services Task Force and other nationally promoted, evidence-based guidelines. Because the information reporting system will include both prevention intake assessments and outcome data about health risk status, and will be available to the military, effectiveness in reducing health risks can now become part of the criteria used by the Department of Defense when awarding or renewing contracts with health care providers.[2]

These efforts are reinforced by a major Department of Defense planning effort to reposition military health-care services for the next 25 years, Military Health Service System (MHSS) 2020. The project involves collaboration between sponsored participants from military and civilian health agencies, including practitioners, researchers and academics. Although it involves planning for "downsizing," the project is in some ways reminiscent of the planning that went into Vannevar Bush's Office of Scientific Development (OSD) as part of war mobilization in World War II. (Chapter 1 describes how that operation permanently changed the relation of the federal government to health research.) The MHSS 2020 project has delineated 20 areas for attention. Twelve involve clinical issues, including a focus on wellness and preventive medicine. Three working groups deal with information monitoring, and five with administrative issues.

Documents circulated to these Defense Department working groups give a sense of the planning orientation that guides this enterprise. One scenario presented to help orient their thinking included the following predictions of how military health care might reorient itself in the near future:

> The military establishment is shrinking because of the loss of a superpower adversary and a growing national debt at home. The nature of armed conflict is changing....American medicine is going through major turmoil in an effort to compete while ruthlessly controlling costs. The shift is toward managed care with a primary care focus and ambulatory treatment. Physician extenders and alternative forms of therapy are on the rise. The information age is... causing power and responsibility to shift from the medical establishment to payers and individuals. A global concept of health is emerging. We will soon have the tools to predict an individual's risk for future illness and take measures to prevent it. The emphasis will be on a holistic view of health which also focuses on achiev-

ing human potential, healthy communities and protection of the environment for a meaningful and sustaining society. Military medicine will shrink in size and focus attention on a broad definition of readiness. Efforts will be toward responsive active duty care. The Department of Defense will accept full accountability for care of family members and retirees. It will invest heavily in ways to keep beneficiaries healthy and to enable them to manage their own well-being. At most locations the responsibility for delivery of that care will be privatized. Even where there is a major military medical presence, integrated delivery systems will rely on contracts and purchased services to fill in the gaps in the most cost-effective manner.[3]

Another planning document comments: "The biggest change will be in our whole approach to health. Today we have a medical system narrowly focused on sickness. What is health?"

The discussion that followed this question defines health in terms reminiscent of the World Health Organization's definition of health as "a state of complete physical, mental, and social well-being and not simply the absence of disease or infirmity." The Defense Department planning document discusses personal, community, and ecological health. Personal health, in addition to "being fit and healthy," includes belonging to a community of people, having control over one's life, and access to education, rewarding work, a decent place to live, and safety. The planning document addressed the importance of fairness, equity, and cooperation for a healthy community. "Ecological health requires using nature's productivity without damaging it. ... Individuals must start taking responsibility for their own health and we must all work toward achieving sustainability for our society." [4]

This is not the place to describe the MHSS 2020 project's discussion of broader changes in medical treatment and the organization of health care that may lie on the horizon. Nor is this the place to assess the likelihood that this planning exercise will actually translate into fundamental changes in all Defense Department health-care practices and contracting. That assessment lies beyond the scope of this study. It *is* clear, however, that a much greater emphasis on *health*, in the senses described in this book, now informs the thinking and planning of health officers in the Defense Department. The Department of Defense initiative seems likely to shift the focus of care, redirecting health-care providers across the nation who provide services for military beneficiaries. Providers will have to pay much more attention to the maintenance and enhancement of health, rather than simply respond to health's breakdown.

A major regrouping of health-care resources seems to be on the horizon. Congressional action may create an institutionalized basis for funding prevention for the general population, with services based at worksites. That, however, is likely to remain a voluntary choice for individual businesses. The defense department initiative could refocus clinical service delivery toward health promotion in the capitated payment plans that service military beneficiaries. Business analysts note that where a new approach captures 15 percent of a local market, the entire market begins to adapt.[5] In communities with a large military presence, defense department managed care contracts could have that kind of market impact. Because military contracts for managed care are made predominantly with the larger managed care plans that operate nationally, the new requirements for managed care contracts with the military provide an institutional lever that could shift the emphasis of capitated payment plans much more toward maintenance and improvement of *health*.

Health Enhancement Research Organization (HERO)

As the institutional pressures and incentives just described were developing, Bill Whitmer, organizer of the Worksite Health Promotion Alliance (that had sponsored the legislative proposals to fund worksite health promotion) and Mark Dundon, the chief executive officer of a chain of Catholic hospitals, jointly sponsored meetings that brought together doctors and administrators from several hospital chains, insurance company executives, leaders in the health promotion field, innovative program vendors and some academic researchers. Their conversations led, in November of 1995, to the establishment of the Health Enhancement Research Organization (HERO), a consortium to provide better research on cost-effective ways to encourage health promotion. In addition, HERO provides a network of resources and expertise to help capitated payment plans move into cost-effective care that promotes health enhancement. Participating insurance companies announced plans to offer differential insurance rates to encourage cardiovascular and cancer risk reduction behaviors. Vendors of health promotion program and benefits services agreed to merge their current data sets in order to discover how costs are affected when persons with identified health risks improve their health status. HERO, itself, now sponsors on-going research on the relative cost-effectiveness of various kinds of health enhancing programs, and makes expert consultation available to its membership. The formation of HERO provides a new kind of trade network to help shift the health-care paradigm from a system based on diagnosiis and treatment toward one centering on prevention. Hospitals and other service providers expressed interest in shifting the focus of their services forward on the health-disease continuum, which they saw as the best way to survive in an era of capitated payments.[6]

These three developments—the institutionalizing of funding for prevention and health promotion programs at worksites, Defense Department health services reorganization to place more emphasis on health promotion, and the establishment of a networking organization to document cost-benefits of health promotion programs and services and to provide expertise to capitated payment plans that want to move in this direction—will help bring an emphasis on *health* into the mainstream of American medical services. This shift of emphasis seems to be increasing in momentum. Its pace could increase still more, if additional providers of managed care services can be encouraged to enter the market, who have a mission to get health-oriented services to populations that now lack basic health care.

Getting Health Care Where It Is Most Needed

Reinsurance Reform

The Pepper Commission and the Clinton Health Insurance Reform Task Force struggled with fair ways to share the increased costs of including previously-excluded populations in insurance coverage. The option they recommended—single community-wide rates for health insurance premiums—spreads the burden of these increased costs evenly among all insurance purchasers of an area. However, community rating does little to motivate health-care providers— especially those receiving capitated payments—to welcome enrollees for whom it might be harder or more expensive to provide services. Community rated premiums, moreover, would put businesses which paid for worksite health promotion services at a competitive disadvantage with those which did not: This added business expense could no longer be recouped through lower insurance premiums, which now result from employees' decreased use of disease-care services. The community-rating solution to fair distribution of insurance costs, on closer analysis, was severely flawed.

Hoping to preserve prevention incentives and also to motivate more health-care providers to reach out actively to now-avoided populations, a group of policy planners turned away from community-rated premium prices as the device for sharing these increased costs. Instead, they looked to simple reforms of *reinsurance* practice.

Every health-care provider or insurer runs the risk of cost over-runs that could bankrupt them—either because of a run of too many high-cost patients being served under pre-set, capitated payments or DRG formulas, because of services given to individuals who cannot or do not pay their bills, or the like. Almost all health-care providers and insurers, consequently, protect themselves through reinsurance. The purchaser of reinsurance determines the level of risk that can be absorbed, and purchases a reinsurance policy that will reimburse for losses beyond the deductible level chosen. At present reinsurance is purchased from companies all over the world, with rates based on the purchaser's previous history of reinsurance claims.

Why not create a single national reinsurance pool, which would spread the risk of loss among a larger set of providers and primary insurers? This could lower basic reinsurance premium rates, much as the creation of common purchasing pools lowers the cost of health insurance premiums for small businesses.

Then a surcharge could be added to the reinsurance premium to cover the costs of reimbursing providers who take responsibility for more than their share of now-avoided populations (i.e., those with pre-existing health problems, residents of inner city neighborhoods, people outside the metropolitan areas, persons of limited income without health insurance, or the like). This surcharge could be redistributed periodically among providers of health care who actually provide health services to these now-avoided populations.

A reinsurance surcharge would share the *risks* inherent in serving now-avoided population groups evenly among all providers. The surcharge would make serving these populations a *protected* risk for those who actually assume the responsibility. In fact, health-care providers who discover cost-effective, consumer-oriented ways to take care of these enrollees would make a greater profit by serving those others avoid.

The reduced basic reinsurance premium charges created by the national risk pool would lessen the financial burden of this surcharge for health providers. The surcharge is a fair burden for health providers and insurers to assume, since they are the ones with most to gain financially from covering an increased proportion of the population. Most providers, no doubt, will increase their fees enough to cover any difference in reinsurance costs, if the surcharge exceeded premium savings. Thus the cost would be spread evenly across the population, without destroying market incentives for more cost-effective care.

This proposal has circulated informally among insurance companies, regulatory agencies, and others with direct expertise in the area. After finding general enthusiasm for reinsurance reform, Senator James M. Jeffords, Republican from Vermont, agreed to sponsor such a bill. As this book goes to press he has been waiting for a propitious moment to introduce the proposal, either as a bill of its own or as an attachment to other legislation. Little opposition is expected once providers as well as insurers understand the benefits it will produce for all parties.[7]

Can such positive incentives really shift health-care providers' decisions about whom to enroll or their choice of location in which to provide disease-care services? For some, probably. Can it provide a shift of practice on a sufficient scale to make basic health and disease care services available to everyone? It could help, by providing incentives for new providers, for specialists retooling in response to the growth of managed care, and health-care professionals already oriented toward serving neglected publics to enroll more of these people under their care. It might be especially attractive to professional groups that currently are looking for new markets for their services. Nurse associations, and nurse practitioners in particular, might be especially attracted to opportunities to serve now-neglected populations if they could be reimbursed through reinsurance surcharges. They might be especially interested in introducing prevention-oriented variations of managed care, once the risks involved become more protected.

Prevention-Oriented Managed Care

Most current "managed care," with primary care physicians deciding what services are needed, operates within the organizational constraints of a large disease-care delivery service which needs to keep its full complement of staff efficiently occupied. Managed care organizations often are quite effective at allocating time uses of their staff and at rationing care—discouraging some clearly inappropriate referrals and treatments. Most have been less effective at encouraging prevention, health promotion, and guided self-care—major potential cost savers.

Making prevention-oriented "managed care" more independent of control by larger provider organizations could help change the demand pattern for disease care. Health insurance reform could allow nurse-run prevention services (such as the Visiting Home Nurse Association, public health agencies, or other nursing services) or other appropriately staffed preventive health services to enter into flexible "managed care" contracts. They would sell their services to consumers and take responsibility for providing all health needs, negotiating appropriate supplementary primary and secondary disease care services, and hospital care. They would have to provide a full range of prevention services, plus oversight, referral, and follow-up for disease care, as needed. They should be empowered to use both nurses and paraprofessionals, under appropriate supervision, for such services as monitoring prenatal health and nutrition, or providing simple primary care services, with appropriate referrals. This could help bring services to residents of communities where there is a shortage of physicians.

Nursing education develops a more holistic sense of the patient than does current medical school training. Nurse-run, prevention-oriented managed care, consequently, may be more effective. Quality checks by public health officials, or licensing groups should be a condition for continued licensing to provide services.

Legislation will be needed to protect the ability of nurse-run prevention services to contract for disease services, by giving them the legal right to broker contracts for primary care, catastrophic and Long Term Care services and requiring other service providers to bid for their services, when requested. If this were done, physicians and HMOs no longer would have a monopoly in determining effective demand for health-care services.

Reinsurance reform could provide a source of funding needed to make outreach services to now underserved populations economically viable. Once a reinsurance surcharge to all providers and insurers is in place, any provider who makes competent services available to now-avoided populations should be eligible for reimbursement from that pool. Nurse-run services would have to compete with other care-providers. This competition would help guarantee that a high quality of service is available to these populations.

Nurse-run outreach services could also provide health-oriented managed care for acute and chronic high-cost illness. Each year about 20 percent of the population accounts for about 80 percent of health-care costs. While much of this spending is for hospital services, some non-hospitalized, chronic conditions also are quite expensive.[8] "Managed care," i.e., cost-effective oversight of the use of health-care services, has been used to control access to specialists, to hospital admittance, and to emergency services. Once one is diagnosed as needing such care, however, and especially as having a chronic health problem, less attention is paid to its cost-effective management. Referrals for more expensive treatment no longer is what needs monitoring. Instead, other help may be needed.

Some managed care plans are now assigning "case managers" to enrollees with chronic health problems. Such services need to be consumer-oriented and to address health improvement, not simply cost control.

Chapter 8 described Federal Express' strategy for targeting and working with employees who are the highest-cost users of health-care benefits. Their "pareto group" consists of 19 percent of the employees each year whose care accounted for 80 percent of health-care benefits spending in the past year. They are given personalized services, aimed at helping them find cost-effective services and developing an appropriate program of health improvement, not simply of disease management. This strategy helped Federal Express hold health benefits spending flat—even with the general inflation—over an eight year period when other company's health benefits costs were skyrocketing. Legislation could encourage wider use of such services by making these costs deductible from insurance premiums for catastrophic care. Targeting the high-cost users of disease care services for consumer-oriented services that strengthen their own health-building capacity would be an excellent use of resources. Nurse-run, *health*-oriented managed care services could do this well.

American "Barefoot Doctors"—Lessening the Need for Emergency Room and Intensive Care

The neglect of primary services to the poor and residents of inner city and rural neighborhoods leads to inappropriate use of Emergency Room services and to strikingly higher fatalities when these people become hospitalized.[9] Particularly tragic are the low birth-weight babies who end up in neonatal intensive care units, treated at great expense and often suffering permanent disability, many of whom would have grown to normal birth-weight if their mothers had proper nutrition and prenatal health supervision during pregnancy.

Some nations have made impressive strides in improving the health of their poorest citizens, by rethinking how health services are delivered to them. The U.S. could learn from their example. In China, Cuba, and Tanzania, for example, where funds for health care are limited, training paraprofessionals to help with the day-to-day health problems of the general population has given the poor access to basic health services. "Barefoot doctors" (to use the expression coined in China) have been sent out pro-actively to worksites and to underserved neighborhoods, providing simple primary care and prevention services. They have been backed up by nurses, who were responsible for supervising the quality of care these paraprofessionals gave, and who could help with more complicated problems. The nurses, in turn, had a chain of command above them, so that problems not appropriate for their level of training were referred to physicians.

Using health-care providers of lower skill levels, tiered levels of supervision, and the triaging of care so that patients received the level of skill that was needed for their situation, these countries produced striking improvements in mother, infant, and child mortality and in the basic health of their poorer populations.[10] American worksites are beginning to discover the value of on-site health promotion. Primary care clinics also have begun to take a leaf from this international record: More primary care now is given by nurse-practitioners and physicians' assistants. We could extend that lesson further, using nurse-run health maintenance services to reach out actively to inner city and underserved populations, with nurses supervising other paraprofessionals.

New health-care legislation should include reform of Licensed Practical Nurse, Nurses Aide, or other certified paraprofessional training programs so that graduates can assist in providing appropriate basic services for prenatal care, including health and nutrition education, and very simple primary care services in underserved communities or neighborhoods, under clear guidelines about when to refer to health professionals with more training. Such legislation should include incentives to recruit residents in housing projects and other underserved neighborhoods for this paraprofessional training, and allow nurse-run preventive services to contract for the paraprofessionals' services and supervise their performance. If this happened, we could begin to get basic health services to population groups that now most lack them. Some might object that this creates a two-tiered level of care, with the poor receiving lower quality care. However, if training and supervision is appropriate, this need not occur. We could, instead, create more humane communities of nurturant care. To make sure they work well, the design and implementation of such programs would need careful attention.

Demedicalizing Life Experiences

Demedicalizing Birth

There is widespread agreement that Cesarean delivery and the use of Neonatal Intensive Care occurs much more often in the United States than should happen if adequate and appropriate health care were available to all. Chapter 3 discussed some of the reasons why each occurs with the frequency that it does and the often unnecessary costs both in terms of money and of human suffering that this use of health resources incurs. As noted earlier, the growing movement toward midwife-assisted births, toward natural child birth, and also toward home birth where conditions warrant it and emergency back-up services are easily available, demedicalize the experience of the beginning of life. Research has shown that all of these practices are appropriate for large segments of the population, but that pregnancies need careful monitoring if a less medicalized approach to birth is followed.[11] If American Cesarean delivery rates approximated those found elsewhere in the world where high standards of modern medicine are practiced, there would be considerable cost-savings for the health-care system as a whole.

Another change also would help. The rate of premature births among U.S. working women is three times as high as that in most European countries. This increases use of neonatal intensive care. Between 1961 and 1985, the proportion of women working within one month of delivery doubled. Women with jobs that are physically demanding or keep them on their feet all day, who work during the last two months of gestation, have higher rates of premature delivery. Three quarters of U.S. working women now work outside the home during the last trimester of pregnancy.[12] The U.S. currently allows *unpaid* maternity leave, but this is not sufficient. If insurance companies offered rate discounts to employers who provide paid maternity leave, we might begin to change the need to over-use neonatal intensive care units.

Demedicalizing the Experience of Aging and Dying

About $50 billion of Medicare spending in 1995 went for the medical care of the roughly 2 million Medicare enrollees in their final year of life. At least a quarter of this paid for services that clearly assist aging and dying patients—home health services, skilled nursing, some doctor's services, hospice care, and the like. About $35 billion went for hospital costs for these dying persons, not quite half of it spent during their last *month* of life. Although Medicare enrollees in their last year of life comprise only 5 to 6 percent of the total Medicare population, they account for half of the Medicare enrollees whose care is in the top one percent of costs.[13] Too much of this spending goes for heroic interventions that retard the speed of dying while disrupting the personal processes that allow one to leave life with grace, dignity, and a sense of completion. Only 3 percent of the Medicare recipients who die each year were able to take advantage of hospice services, a much more humane as well as less expensive way to meet the end of life. There often are waiting lists for hospice care.

Greater development not only of hospice care for the dying but also of consumer-oriented case management services for the progressively disabled are becoming higher priorities as the numbers of older Americans and persons with AIDS increase. We could shift the spending for services to the progressively disabled in directions that improve quality of life while reducing costs. Patient-oriented managed care could provide services for the aging and for persons with chronic conditions who are becoming progressively disabled, assisting with the practical details of maintaining quality of life as their ability to be personally independent declines. Some need oversight of prescriptions—double-checking to make sure that medications prescribed by various physicians do not create joint side-effects that are deleterious to health, or help in knowing when to take which medications, when many are prescribed together.

Many would benefit from purchasing services for home health-care equipment and pharmaceuticals. While much attention has been given to high prices charged by pharmaceutical companies for new drugs used with catastrophic illnesses, few have noted the high mark-ups that many *distributors* of drugs and home health-care equipment and services regularly add to their wholesale costs. Some pharmaceutical distributors now acquire the life insurance policies of AIDS patients, giving them credit for home health drugs, equipment, and services, sometimes at 100% mark-up over already high wholesale prices. This practice exhausts credit rapidly and sometimes leaves patients destitute in the last stages of their illness.[14] Many of the same drugs, home infusion equipment, and services needed by AIDS patients are used with other expensive chronic health problems as well, at similar prices. An Internet program could be developed to make price comparisons available for major drugs, home care supplies and equipment used by AIDS patients. This could be expanded to cover the drugs and equipment needed for most expensive chronic disease conditions.[15] Once this is available, persons who know these markets can offer to manage purchasing services for insurance companies, Medicare and Medicaid, the major third-party payers for catastrophic illness care, as well as individuals themselves.

This chapter includes purchasing services for chronic disease-care as part of new initiatives that emphasize health, because health-oriented managed care for those who have become incapacitated must include attention to all of their needs, including their use of more conventional medical treatments. These services would logically fall together, rather than be parceled out to different kinds of "managers" of the person who needed assistance.

Patient-oriented managed care for the aging, the progressively disabled, and the dying also would involve assistance, when requested, in developing living wills—clear indications to medical professionals of the circumstances in which one does or does not want heroic interventions to be made to try to extend one's life. It would make available hospice services (at home or in a hospice center) where one can die free of pain but without further efforts to sustain life. For some, it would also involve counseling, support groups or buddy-systems to help people who are dying. A number of the AIDS programs, which work with persons dying much earlier than they had expected, recruit volunteers, train them and support them emotionally as the volunteers provide both practical daily assistance and personal support as AIDS patients do their own dying work. One highly successful AIDS support program in San Francisco (Shanti) describes its mission in these terms:

> Dying is about transformation. [Our organization] attracts people who are concerned with transformation in their own lives. Our volunteers like to hang out with people who are busy with the transformation process. It helps them with their own.[16]

If dying well were approached as a part of health, not simply as disease or the breakdown of the body, and if appropriate support services were made available to those going through this transformation, demand for heroic, high-tech life-extenders would decline. Too much of health-care spending currently goes for persons in the last year of their life. Many could receive services more relevant to their own life situations, at considerably less cost, if we re-orient the kinds of services that routinely are available. The popular culture is moving in this direction. It is time to develop the support services that make this a practical choice for individuals and families.

Prevention-oriented services will help shift the focus toward health. In addition, we need to begin to shift the focus of all health care in more ecologically-sophisticated directions.

Shifting the Emphasis of Health Care Toward Lower Technology and More Ecologically-Sophisticated Care

Mixed Medical Models (Providing More Ecologically-Sophisticated Care)

Insurance companies and some forward-looking HMOs already are beginning to fund alternative and complementary treatment strategies that go beyond the assumptions of medical science. A number of the more popular alternative treatment approaches, including acupuncture, biofeedback, yoga, and the chiropractic, utilize discoveries of older, non-scientific medical traditions. They often are more nearly in tune with recent research discoveries about health-building processes of the body and the larger ecology of health and disease than are the more invasive, high-tech practices of the health-care industry. Clinical studies have documented better health outcomes, at lower cost, for patients using alternative medicine for *certain* health problems, including especially cardiovascular disease.[17] These have encouraged some of the more progressive health insurance companies to reimburse the costs of such treatments.[18] A small but growing number of managed care organizations offer their clients a mixed medical model that includes conventional medicine, alternative medical clinics, and prevention programs. They hope to attract an important market segment that already uses all these health strategies. National surveys show that a third of the American public, including many of the better educated and more affluent members of the public, now is using alternative health practitioners.[19] These health-care providers hope to lower costs by keeping their clientele healthier and by using lower-cost treatment strategies as a first line of defense, with modern, high tech medicine as a back-up when needed.[20] Meanwhile, King County (greater Seattle), in Washington state, has established a publicly funded alternative medical clinic to make such services available to the less affluent public.[21]

These mixed-model reforms of HMO and insurance reimbursement practice are at an early stage as this is written. They will require little legislative encouragement, though some states may need to loosen their current restrictions on who may perform some health-care services. It is significant that this mixed medical model is being introduced within managed care organizations with per capita funding limits that require clear outcome accountability. If the mixed model can thrive within the organizational constraints of an HMO, it has the potential to transform 21st century medicine. If it cannot, the mixed medical model will have to develop its own funding solutions.

One serious problem that limits movement in this direction is the shortage of well-documented evaluative data to help clinicians choose among alternative approaches. That could change, however, with a change in directives given to the National Institutes of Health, which already has in place the organizational capacity to undertake such evaluation.

New Roles for the National Institutes of Health

Congress could direct NIH to increase its budget for the Office of Alternative Medicine, directing it to increase its evaluation of traditional herbal remedies used in various parts of the world, of acupuncture, and other unconventional treatments that claim to strengthen the body's own health processes, looking especially at their use with AIDS and cancer patients. NIH also could require more thorough investigation of *all* drugs and treatment strategies in terms of their second- and third-order consequences— their short and longer term side effects—and in terms of the relative cost-effectiveness of various strategies for treatment that are currently available. NIH would not have to increase its budget in order to do this; instead it could redirect how current research allocations are used. NIH's findings could then be made part of required Continuing Medical Education for physicians.

What would it take to provide a realistic basis for evaluating the relative effectiveness of currently conventional medical practices and alternative health-care strategies? Clear criteria regarding demonstrated efficacy (with more federal study of alternative treatments)? A ranking of various methods for treating a disease condition—in terms of regularly occurring short and long-term side effects and the frequency with which people who use a method then come in for treatment of another condition resulting from the original intervention in their own body's functioning? A ranking in terms of a treatment modality's ability to strengthen the body's own health processes as well as its ability to counter an immediate problem? Cost-benefit comparisons of different modes of treatment? All would be useful.

With this information available, insurance companies could be encouraged to modify their reimbursement formulas to pay for less expensive treatments that have a documented effectiveness, letting more people use them. Present insurance reimbursement formulas—which are natural extensions of Blue Cross-Blue Shield's origins as an effort to keep hospitals in business—discourage consumers from using treatments that do not involve pharmaceuticals, physicians services, or hospitalization. Consequently these formulas help maintain the constant cost acceleration in medical care. With better information, that could change.

Such studies could move disease treatment in more sophisticated, ecologically cognizant directions while at the same time encouraging the use of lower tech interventions, thus saving costs. Without such a knowledge base, insurance carriers are unlikely to expand the range of treatments they will cover to include lower cost options, because they currently do not have well-documented evaluations of their efficacy. (As funds were redirected in those ways their redeployment also would slow the pace of development of ever more expensive high-tech diagnosis and treatment strategies.) A change in NIH's mandate and role, thus, could be an important part of cost containment, and could help move health care in more efficacious, cost-effective directions.

Who could be most effective in helping Congress and NIH leaders see the possibilities inherent in such a change of emphasis? The role of citizens' lobbies and informal friendship networks in Congress in establishing NIH's Office of Alternative Medicine in the early 1990s provides one scenario for how such changes might occur. Conferences of researchers, examining the joint implications of various thrust areas of medical research (discussed in Chapter 9) for new approaches to treatment and healing, also could help create such a climate. Private foundations, centers for the study of alternative medicine at some of the major universities, and the new Office of Alternative Medicine in NIH might cooperate in such a project. These efforts could encourage more effective cost containment for present disease care while also helping move care in a more ecologically sophisticated direction.

New Roles for the Food and Drug Administration, the States, and Congress

State and federal authorities have begun to develop a new public strategy for dealing with *sources* of disease. It is now well established that use of nicotine is an important factor leading to cancer and heart attacks, the major causes of death in the U.S., and that the breakdown in health caused by its use is a major source of health-care costs now charged to Medicare, Medicaid, and private insurers. Establishing the culpability of tobacco companies, rather than blaming individual smokers for their addictions, marks a new strategy for dealing with the problem.

Both the White House and members of a commission established by Congress to advise it in regard to tobacco urged Congress to give the Food and Drug Administration unrestricted authority to regulate nicotine as a drug. We finally seem to be understanding the importance of dealing with disease at its *source.* A new public policy seems to be emerging, one that could hold considerable promise for the future.[22]

The public and private reforms described in this chapter will help shift the focus from disease management toward prevention of disease and toward more ecologically-sophisticated health-building. Yet the ongoing deterioration of the global environment threatens to overwhelm the ability of individuals to maintain their own health processes. How can these problems be addressed? Tackling the problems would involve integrating health and economic planning. We may be at a juncture in time where this is possible.

Improving the Health of the Planet: Environmental Health Policies

How can we affect environmental sources of disease, including pollution of the American environment and health risks created by such global phenomena as the thinning of the ozone layer and global warming? Can Americans participate in the world political economy in ways that protect their economic interests while also lessening the current U.S. threat to global health and survival because of the disproportionate contribution to global warming and to the thinning of the ozone layer that comes from American economic activity?

The end of the Cold War and the emergence of a new global order may open up possibilities for moving in new directions on these fronts as well. Parts of the American economy that fall into the military-industrial complex of interests have depended heavily on government contracts for their prosperity. Would it be possible to redirect some of the government grants and contracts long given to these interests, so that they simultaneously help America's balance of trade and protect the global environment?

For example, the federal government could help industrial firms develop alternatives to present manufacturing techniques that endanger the atmosphere. Defense spending now involves important funding for manufacturing industries. Why not redirect some of this spending more effectively? We might, for example, set the following priorities for government business subsidies: (1) helping defense industries diversify so that they are not primarily dependent upon military policy for their prosperity; (2) providing technical assistance and tax incentives to American-based industry to make manufacturing processes conform to current international proposals for environmentally-safe, sustainable economic development; (3) directing federal research grants toward the development of products and processes that have a high priority for ensuring the safety of the planet: substitutes for CFCs and other chemicals which threaten the ozone layer or which contribute to global warming; the development of more effective, renewable energy sources, so that the global economy relies less on atomic fuels and coal and oil-based sources of energy; development of an effective substitute for the internal combustion engine. This book has documented the remarkable impact on disease care development that has come from federal medical research grants. Public encouragement of product development and of manufacturing processes that help restore the health of the environment and that are also cost-effective could change the dynamic of environmental destruction that now threatens us all.

What do we need? A replacement for the internal combustion engine; a way to make nylon that does not damage the environment, or environmentally-friendly products that could substitute for nylon; renewable, environmentally friendly alternatives to atomic fuel, oil, gas and coal as sources of energy; safer ways to dispose of toxic substances. Once such products are available, at a reasonable cost, they will be more attractive than current products and manufacturing and waste disposal processes that are destroying the health of the planet. Market forces will then lead to a rapid reallocation of business investment capital, to take advantage of new opportunities for gain.

Large transnational corporations, including auto, oil, and chemical companies, must be drawn into efforts to preserve the earth's environment. Transportation, energy development, manufacturing and forestry policies now need to be part of health policy planning.

If current Department of Defense health initiatives produce agreement that reducing environmental health threats should be part of military health planning, an incentive system could be developed to encourage this kind of activity. When awarding defense department—or other governmental— contracts, after taking into account price competition among bidders, preference could be given to companies whose entire product lines conform to current international standards for environmentally-sustainable production.

During the Carter administration, from 1976 to 1980, the U.S. government began to create incentives for environmentally responsible innovation. The time was too short to accomplish these goals and the priorities of the succeeding administrations were quite different. It is time for us to rediscover this kind of agenda, and to make health-implications a heavier factor in setting priorities for public use of economic development funds. If U.S. businesses became pace-setters in environmentally relevant innovation, it would have a major impact on business practices throughout the world. But even if they only changed the American contribution to global environmental problems it would benefit the entire planet.

Government programs are not enough, though they could play a critical role in helping create a momentum for change. Foundations and business groups also could play a role, creating forums in which these concerns and possibilities are addressed. Universities could become an active part of the solution, helping direct attention to problems demanding attention which also open new business possibilities, and they could actively encourage their faculty to undertake types of research that help spur these kinds of changes. Networking could create new creative coalitions of business and development partners.

These areas of policy innovation would enhance American-based industry's ability to compete in the new world market while also helping change the patterns of environmental pollution which now threaten the health of the planet and its residents. Given the interlocking of investment patterns across industries, such a shift in use of government resources need not threaten present private investors. If new jobs are created, current defense workers can be retrained to take advantage of new opportunities.

Innovations identified in this chapter shift the emphasis in health-care delivery toward prevention, health promotion, and greater availability of basic disease care services. Some innovations direct services to where they are most needed, or lessen dependency on high technology. Others begin to move toward more ecologically-sophisticated care or provide strategies for dealing with environmental sources of disease. These innovations reinforce one another's impact. Broad-based current support for many of these ideas and the institutional sources now sponsoring them creates a momentum which could set a new dynamic in motion. Can this provide the leverage needed to make reform of disease care more effective? If so, how?

Chapter 11 returns to the current mainstream debate about reforming the American health-care system, suggesting how steps recommended here could provide a lever that changes how other reform proposals would work. It may yet be possible to get appropriate levels of care to all the population, at a cost Americans can afford.

11

Reapproaching Problems of Cost

It is time to start again, rethinking what it will take to get adequate health care to all Americans at a price we can afford. Any new proposals must take into account the very real constraints on problem solving that became visible during health insurance reform efforts of the 1990s, but we must not remain stymied by these limits. Instead we must look for ways to reframe the problem to be addressed that can let these circumstances work for us rather than against us. Is it possible to take advantage of the core visions that have guided previously contending strategies for reform but move beyond them? Would it be possible to combine the strengths of single payer, market force, and managed competition plans, doing so in ways that overcome the various fatal flows (discussed in Chapter 5) which prevent any one of these current health policy strategy contenders from providing a usable solution to our dilemma? How can the movements toward a re-emphasis on *health* (discussed in Chapter 10) affect our choices?

These are the questions this chapter will address. Taking advantage of what has been learned in earlier parts of this book, this chapter will reframe the problem to be addressed and will propose a way to recombine elements from previous proposals to create a different route through our present impasse.

Constraints

There are several very real constraints on policy choices that must be taken into account when making new policy proposals. Six constraints severely limit what can be done. However, there are also potential strategies for dealing with each of them.

(1) The American legislative process is not well designed to accomplish a total overhaul of anything as complex as the American health-care system. Key decision-makers can change every two years. Many legislators do not understand how market dynamics affect health care. Moreover, the legislative process is vulnerable to special-interest politics. That often

gives current funders and providers of services veto power over proposals that would directly affect them. Consequently, legislative proposals need to be relative simple and to provide win/win solutions to potential conflicts of interest that affect various stake-holders and the public.

(2) Both state and federal tax bases are shrinking and there is little public support for general tax increases, considerable competition for use of public revenues, and pressures to reduce government deficit spending. Consequently, unless or until public sentiment shifts to favor more public funding of health care, any expansion of coverage for lower income people and the growing number of elderly will require a *redirection* of public revenues. It will also require development of new kinds of revenue sources. However, in the present political climate, these cannot be imposed on employers or the general public. They will have to involve win/win trades for those most affected.

(3) Not only state and federal third-party payers but also the businesses which finance a major portion of current health benefits spending have become unwilling to remain captive to constant escalations in the costs of health care. Few private households can absorb the difference. Consequently we no longer can deal with cost increase by shifting the burden from one payer group to another. Instead we will have to address sources of cost increase more directly, and the incentives toward cost increase that affect different areas of health provision. Rather different strategies for cost containment may be needed for various parts of the health-care market. We may need a set of incentives that influence behavior choices of health-care providers, health-care consumers, and third-party payers. Past experience suggests that positive incentives are more effective than regulatory control in changing the day-to-day dynamics of health-care consumption.

(4) Leaders of the health-care industry, which has replaced manufacturing as the largest employer of American workers and which is a vital part of current American economic prosperity, will not sit idly by while would-be reformers attempt to regulate it, to nationalize it, or to eliminate some of its key players. Moreover, the economic health of the nation needs this sector of the economy to remain strong—but to do so in ways that strengthen rather than deplete other sectors of the economy. Past strategies for cost containment and health-care reform have pitted one interest group against another. New approaches to cost containment will be needed that provide more nearly win/win solutions for all the key parties, including the public.

(5) Over the past 25 years health-care providers, from hospitals and managed care plans to individual physicians, have shown remarkable ability to subvert efforts at cost containment, turning them into practices that further their own goals of providing high quality (often meaning expensive, high-tech) care while increasing their income. Price controls have not

worked. Neither have "supply-side" economic strategies limiting the amount paid per illness or limiting the amount of money paid annually per person.

Some would argue that the fatal flaw in past cost containment efforts was the lack of a single payer that could enforce cost containment policies consistently and prevent health-care providers from playing one funding source off against another. Given the first two constraints listed above, however, that kind of solution is not currently feasible politically—and the Canadian single-payer system, whose costs are second only to those in the United States, is having its own severe cost containment problems. Consequently approaches to cost containment cannot rely primarily on regulation or restraint. They must provide positive incentives to providers, to consumers of their services, and to third-party funders which will enlist their active cooperation. Also needed are strategies for reducing demand for particularly costly services that are not used cost-effectively. New approaches must identify acceptable, less expensive ways to deal with the health problems involved and be able to help third-party payers encourage the most cost-effective care.

(6) Finally, the market system, if left entirely to its own devices, will continue to weaken what remains of the current health-care safety net— because broader economic dynamics will pull both business and government even farther back from captive commitment to health-care funding. The challenge, consequently, becomes that of finding ways to restructure present market dynamics so that all the public gets access to basic health care and so that any resulting growth in health-care funding *strengthens* rather than depletes the economic health of other sectors, public and private.

None of the organizing principles previously proposed for health-care reform can achieve its goals within this set of constraints. However some *elements* from each strategic approach operate reasonably well within these limiting conditions. The planning task, thus, involves crafting new *sets* of strategies that jointly remain viable within these constraints. They should address the "bottom-line" concerns of advocates of currently contending strategies for reform, so as to produce solutions that can get wide support. Ideally, these solutions should mutually reinforce one another's impact.

If neither single payer, nor market force nor managed competition offer a workable larger strategy, what might work better? Is there another organizing principle that could incorporate the strengths of each of these earlier approaches, while still operating within the limits of the very real social, economic and political constraints we face? Can we reframe the problem to be addressed in a way that takes advantage of all that we now know?

The rest of this book proposes one way to reframe problems of cost and access to health care so that they can be addressed within present social, political and economic constraints. It suggests ways that "bottom line" concerns of the three currently contending policy perspectives could be addressed jointly. (A central goal for single-payer advocates is guaranteeing access to care for everyone; free market advocates seem most concerned to minimize government regulation and coercion and to avoid disruption of present market dynamics; while managed competition advocates seem most concerned about achieving universal access in a way that lets the health-care industry thrive while also keeping costs within acceptable limits.) If these concerns are respected and addressed together, considerable support for new proposals should result. The discussion which follows uses 10 proposals for cost containment now recommended by one or another of the contending policy camps, but reorganizes some details of each proposal to take advantage of the health-oriented developments recommended in Chapter 10. Although few of the details are original, a new framing of the problem(s) to be addressed lets earlier proposals work together in new ways.

Some readers will like the proposals spelled out here. Others will not, or may prefer to combine these ingredients in different ways to set a different organizing principle in motion. That is all to the good. What is needed is a new level of dialogue that lets us step outside the frames of reference that have limited our ability to think in new ways about the problems that must be addressed.

I invite readers to lay aside their earlier reactions to specific proposals that were previously developed as part of now-contending policy positions. Some of these proposals will have quite different implications when used within a new reframing of the problem, in combination with other ingredients of a solution.

Reframing the Problem

The proposals which follow reframe the problem to be addressed, in the following ways:

(1) They ask whether different dynamics affect prices and overconsumption of disease-care services in various sectors of the health-care market. This analysis identifies currently costly but wasteful uses of disease-care services that might be approached in new ways, and recommends positive incentives that could influence consumption choices. Some incentives affect providers of disease-care services, others affect immediate consumers of these services, while still others are relevant for third-party payer decisions. The analysis argues for funding major sectors of the health-care

market differently, so that cost-containment incentives most appropriate for that sector can be used.

(2) This discussion proposes four different strategies for funding particular health and disease care services, rather than assuming that each requires the same kind of "protected risk" solution involving prepaid insurance (our current general funding strategy).

(3) It redivides the public/private health-care market, doing so in ways that anticipate future demands for care and that free up more public funds to subsidize health costs of the non-elderly poor. It also identifies additional potential sources of funds to help subsidize health-care costs for low-income populations.

(4) It reduces legislation to the minimum required to set private initiatives properly in motion, proposing win/win trades where conflicts of interest might intervene.

(5) It reduces regulation to a necessary minimum, relying, wherever possible, on positive incentives rather than coercion to produce needed changes in behavior.

(6) It makes use of *health*-oriented strategies described in Chapter 10 (a) to reduce need for more expensive health care and (b) to create a safety net that allows low-risk experimentation with more innovative cost-containment strategies.

(7) Whenever possible, these recommendations use proposals that can be initiated through private initiative and thus are not captive to the legislative process. Preference is given to proposals that can reinforce movements now underway toward health promotion and toward addressing personal, social and environmental sources of disease. Preference is given, as well, to cost-containment incentives that address *sources* of cost increase, not simply the consequences of cost dynamics.

Only a few of the proposals that follow are original to this book. What is new is the combination of strategies used, and the reframing of the problems to be addressed, which lets this combination of strategies set a new dynamic in motion.

A New Organizing Principle: Flexible Collaboration in a Redivided Health-Care Market

The set of proposals which follows creates a new kind of public/private collaboration in a redivided health-care market. This redivision of the market allows use of different funding strategies for each, and reliance upon positive incentives rather than regulatory control to redirect public and private spending for health care. At its heart lie flexible partnerships for different health-service needs, and new strategies for funding low-income populations.

Central Problems We Must Solve

We must identify sources of excessive spending for disease diagnosis and care that do not enhance the quality of life for those who receive these services. Then we can introduce more cost-effective substitutes for procedures that waste public and private resources, freeing up funds to provide better access to basic health-care services for people now neglected.

Are there areas of health care that now consume inappropriately large proportions of total health-care spending? A look at current spending patterns identifies some clear candidates.

The high cost of dying is one obvious candidate. Increased use of living wills, and wider development of hospice services could reduce inappropriate uses of high technology with the elderly, often improving the quality of their remaining life while also reducing health expenditures on the last year of life, perhaps by half. In 1988, only three percent of Medicare patients who died used hospice services. That proportion could increase if more attention were directed to making this option more widely available. Since payment for most medical costs of the dying elderly come from public sources (through Medicare and Medicaid), living wills which decline heroic intervention in the last stages of life and increased use of hospice services would release a major block of funds that could be used to subsidize health costs of the younger poor. Proposals that help demedicalize the end of life should receive high priority.

Similarly, greater investment in prenatal care would sharply reduce Medicaid spending for neonatal intensive care of low-birthweight infants. Small changes in maternity leave policies could do the same for the private insurance market. (As noted earlier, the U.S. has three times the rate of premature births as is found in Europe.[2] Enough is known about causes of premature birth to prevent or greatly reduce their frequency.)

We might also learn from the example of Federal Express, discussed in Chapter 8. Federal Express kept its own health benefits spending even with inflation (when other health costs were doubling) by identifying each year those employees who had been the highest cost users of health services. Reaching out actively to them, nurse health counselors helped these people discover cost-effective ways to manage their ongoing disease problems, and encouraged them to improve their general state of health. Considerable public funds could be redirected toward people now left out of health-care coverage if Medicare and Medicaid had similar programs for their highest cost users of health care.

In 1990, $425 billion of direct health-care spending was for the treatment of chronic health problems, three fourths of all health expenditures. About 39 million Americans have more than one chronic health problem.[3] If even 20 to 30 percent of the cost for the more catastrophically expensive chronic disease care could be saved through equally helpful but more cost-effective management of these conditions, another major block of money would be available to be redistributed for other uses.

Chapter 10 has identified current strategies and proposals that could help reach each of these cost-reduction goals while *improving* personal services to the individuals affected. These sources of potential cost savings involve better management of current health-care practices. In addition, unnecessary waste of health-care resources occurs because of the overuse of health insurance.

Finding Additional Solutions to the Problems of Cost

The discussion which follows assumes that the following basic reforms of health insurance already are in place: the establishment of voluntary purchasing pools that enlarge the risk pool and thus lower the cost of health insurance premiums for small businesses and the self-employed; a backup system utilizing access to the Federal Employees Health Benefits Plan's risk pools to guarantee access to health insurance for anyone lacking access to another voluntary purchasing pool;[4] no insurance discrimination against people with pre-existing health problems; and a reinsurance pool surcharge to be redistributed among health-care service providers who enroll now-neglected populations. These proposals either are already law or seem to have strong legislative support. Such reforms provide a start, but more changes are needed. The cost of insurance is now too high for *everyone*, not simply for small employers, the self-employed, and those with known medical problems. More basic changes will be needed.

Managed care does not solve these problems. Although it limits access to more expensive services, this does little to lower health insurance costs. The savings that come through gatekeeper rationing of access to more expensive care are turned into profit rather than into lower premium rates. Moreover, other than by avoiding hospital use altogether when it can, managed care does little to produce cost-effective use of services once one is past the gatekeeper; there unnecessarily high costs too often continue.

A shift in strategies for funding different *kinds* of health-care services could result in further lowered costs and more effective care. As cost containment problems get tackled more effectively, current health-care spending can be redirected in ways that guarantee access to basic health-care services for all Americans.

Earlier market-oriented proposals for lowering the cost of health insurance more basically were discussed in Chapter 5. As now proposed, these involve fairly high risks, either to individuals, employers, or the insurance pool itself, and thus come into conflict with the need for protection that underlies our present practices. However, if there were safety nets that guaranteed protection, several of the proposals would become much more interesting. Let us retrace the arguments of Chapter 5, noting how the consequences change when using different incentives and different kinds of shared and protected risk, once health-oriented innovations, discussed in Chapter 10, are in place to provide a safety net.

Chapter 5 noted that our present approach to all health-care financing puts more resources into health insurance premiums than is necessary. This happens because insurance is now used to protect against most health expenditures, rather than only the more expensive ones. High-deductible insurance policies are one way to change that. They separate the source of payment for catastrophic and non-catastrophic health-care costs. These do not need to shift the burden of non-catastrophic health-care costs to private households, as previous discussions of catastrophic insurance policies have assumed. If each area is approached separately, rather than combined together, a more flexible set of strategies becomes possible. Several recommended health steps from Chapter 10 would let us lower costs for both kinds of care.

The highest health-care costs have been hospital services, long-term care, and non-hospital care of catastrophically expensive chronic health problems. For decades, these costs have risen much faster than the general rate of inflation. The cost of catastrophic care could be addressed more effectively, once the health innovations discussed in Chapter 10 are in place. Moreover, this could be done without endangering the vitality of hospitals as one of the important growth sectors of the economy.

Lowering the Cost of Catastrophic Care

Previous efforts to control the growth of hospital and other catastrophically expensive costs have largely failed. Ironically, the latest effort to contain health-care costs by reducing utilization of hospital services has boomeranged. The reduced hospital census has increased per-person daily hospital rates. Fixed operating expenses now have to be divided among a smaller hospital population base. Thus per-person costs have continued to rise. Meanwhile, outpatient costs have risen as well.

The Canadian solution, in which provincial health departments give hospitals fixed annual operating budgets and require hospitals to serve all who come, without further charge, probably would not work in the U.S., for reasons discussed in Chapter 5. However, a variation on that strategy might work quite well.

Hospitals with their specialists and their high technology, although an expensive part of the American health-care system, are not, in themselves, undesirable. Rather, it is the overuse of high technology and specialized services which is the problem. Similarly, there is nothing wrong with hospitals continuing to be a high growth sector of the American economy—so long as public and private third-party payers and private households do not become captive payers for the constant cost increases. That happens now because of the arrangements used to pay for hospital services. Thanks to economies that prevention and mixed model strategies for care make possible, it would be possible to reapproach hospital financing in ways that more effectively limit the obligations of most third-party payers and most private households, while still letting hospitals increase their income and upgrade their technology.

Hospital Capitation

The government, large employers, large purchasing pools, managed care plans, and other groups that have a sufficient pool of potential hospital users to make this strategy practical, could stop paying for the treatment of individual illnesses. Instead they could offer capitation plans that provide hospitals with a fixed income based on the number of persons for whom they would assume responsibility if hospitalization is needed. Various payers might negotiate different capitation rates, based on the frequency with which their enrollees need hospital care, and the severity of the problems they tend to have that require hospitalization. Since hospitals are already at a highly sophisticated level of technology, capitation contracts could specify that all enrollees under a capitation plan are entitled to use the services and technologies that are *currently* "state of the art," at the discretion of attending physicians. Supplementary insurance would be available to private households that wished to have immediate access to all the technology that will be developed in the future, just as soon as it is available within a particular hospital. Continued technological advancement could occur, consequently, but it would be paid for out of discretionary income by those who want the latest "state of the art" high technology treatment to be available to them.

Although limiting access to the newest technology for persons in hospital capitation plans would produce two tiers of treatment, this would not result in poor services for the general public. U.S. treatment levels already are more advanced than is available in most other countries. It would, however, limit captive costs that third-party payers now must pay. Anyone who wanted "the latest" would be free to use their discretionary income to help pay for it. Moreover, contracts could stipulate that once the acquisition costs of new equipment have been paid off their contract's capitated patients will have access to that equipment, as well. Thus technological progress in medicine could continue, but be financed out of the discretionary income of wealthier segments of the population, rather than as a captive cost to third-party payers.[5]

If this strategy were pursued for limiting the costs of hospital care without stopping hospital growth, health-oriented strategies discussed in Chapter 10 would be useful for both hospitals and the groups contracting for their capitated services. Hospitals would have a new incentive to explore less costly routes to care, and mixed medical models for the treatment of chronic disease might be used much more frequently. (For example hospitals across the country already are beginning to use the Ornish plan for cardiovascular recovery and improvement. It uses stress reduction, low-fat nutrition, social support groups, relaxation and Yoga stretches as components for its holistically integrated therapy. If hospitals were receiving capitated payments for all services to patients, these lower-cost treatment strategies would become all the more attractive.) The *payers* of the capitated rates also would have strong incentives to include their enrollees in proactive health promotion programs that can lessen the need for hospitalization. As payers' needs for services lessen overall, they will be in position to bargain for better capitation rates for the hospital services. Other proposals of Chapter 10 also would be relevant. Managed care purchasing services to assist with cost containment for the care of persons with severe chronic diseases, targeted health improvement services for individuals whose health has broken down, and care strategies that lessen the need for heroic interventions at the beginning or end of life, all would help reduce immediate costs and position a third-party payer to bargain for lower capitation rates for hospital care.

In short, the addition of *health*-oriented innovations of the kind already recommended would make it possible to reapproach hospital funding, lowering overall costs and discouraging overutilization of the more expensive services. As we shall see, complementary strategies for lowering costs of other kinds of health care would make it practical to add additional services to basic health insurance plans. These could meet emerging needs for elder care while also freeing public funds to help subsidize health-care costs of the younger poor—who all too often now are left out of health-care coverage because of public commitments to care for the elderly. This could help lessen competition for care between the generations.

Funding Long-Term Care and Other Catastrophic Costs

By using the principles of shared and protected risk more creatively, separating catastrophic and non-catastrophic care needs and financing them in different ways, the real costs of "insurance" for both kinds of care can come down. This proposal provides three different strategies for funding health needs. First, capitation rates handle hospital costs. Second, non-catastrophic health expense are handled through employer/employee "self-insurance," which will be described shortly. "Insurance," in its more classic sense, is reserved for high-cost expenses that do not involve hospital use. This would make it possible to include Long-Term Care insurance as part of catastrophic coverage for the entire population.

Care for the partially or completely disabled, either at home, in the community, or in nursing homes, currently is the monster in the closet for American health care. The size of the elderly population will increase rapidly in the coming decades, as will the number of AIDS patients. Many young people also need such services because of accidents or exposure to violence. Few Americans have private long-term care insurance at present, so premium costs are quite high. (Only those who expect to need the care in the near future tend to buy this kind of insurance; thus a narrow risk pool raises the cost of long-term care insurance.) However, if *everyone* had long-term care insurance, risks would be shared across the entire population and rates would drop.[6] It would be a fair addition to basic insurance, since all age groups now face some risk of needing this protection.

If this were done, managed care and purchasing services for persons with costly chronic illness and for the progressively disabled, discussed in Chapter 10, would be critical for keeping these costs within manageable range. Mixed medical care models also would be relevant for the management of some of these patients, as would development of services that help demedicalize the process of aging and death. Health-oriented innovations, in short, could make universal long-term care insurance affordable in the long run. They also would add an important humanizing impetus to services directed toward the end of the life span.

Moving long-term care expenses into the private market would let us absorb the growth in the number of elderly needing care and growth in the size of the population dealing with AIDS. This could be done without exhausting public funds or preventing payment for the care of the able-bodied poor. It would, in fact, free up a sizable portion of public funds now committed to care for the elderly, making them available to redeploy for other needs that now have to be ignored.

Funding Care Given Outside of Hospitals

Reducing the Cost of Insurance Premiums. To lower health insurance costs, some have suggested limiting insurance coverage to catastrophically high medical claims—a proposal that would drastically lower third-party obligations, but would transfer many health-care costs to private households. Instead, third-party payers could continue to take responsibility for the total health needs of those whose health care they fund, but finance each category of health care differently. For example, employers or other third-party payers could "self-insure" for non-catastrophic health-care costs but buy high deductible health insurance to protect themselves (and their employees) from devastatingly expensive health costs. As Chapter 5 has noted, a number of small businesses in Michigan use this principle of shared risk, with employers being responsible for the first $2,000 of an employee's family medical expenses before the insurance policy reimburses for health-care costs. They save $600 per family per year in premium costs. Employers gamble that only a few families will have high expenses and thus that the employer will pay out less in the long run than if full coverage insurance had been chosen. That gamble has paid off. Some small employers who participate in this kind of shared-risk plan have reported a 44 percent reduction in health benefits spending. Yet they remain fully protected against the occasional, catastrophically costly medical emergency that could overwhelm their resources if they were fully self-insured. Meanwhile employees remain fully protected.

Increasing Savings from Shared Risk. When employers share this kind of risk with an insurance company, it makes good financial sense for them to sponsor worksite health promotion programs that reach out to employees, helping them improve their health and avoid illness. It also makes sense for insurers to offer premium discounts as incentives for companies to offer high quality worksite health promotion programs. This lessens the risk employers take on when self-insuring for some health-care costs and also lessens the risks to insurers. Moreover, proactive prevention services provide a safety net that could allow employers to gradually share risks and potential health-care savings with employees, giving them an incentive to use disease-care resources wisely. Here's how this could work.

When employers take out high-deductible health insurance policies for their workforce, but pay the other costs themselves, they usually ask employees to share part of these costs. In the Michigan example, families paid the first $200 to $300 of their own health-care costs, before being reimbursed by the employer or the insurance company. Thus what looks like a $2,000 per family potential liability for the employer is cut almost in half. (Add together the employee's deductible expense and the $600 the employer saves in premium costs for each family every year. This leaves the employer facing at most a cost of $1,100 to $1,200 for some families, while saving up to $600 in insurance costs for every family that spends less than their share of the deductible.) Proactive worksite health promotion programs help minimize the risk of costly illnesses for employees, making this a safer risk.

In addition to encouraging health improvement, worksite health promotion programs can provide protective monitoring of employees' health. (Present experience with proactive worksite programs of this type provides reassurance that most employees welcome this kind of health monitoring, and do not find it intrusive.) This health monitoring can make it safely possible to extend the principle of shared risk and shared savings to employees as well as the employer, increasing their own motivation to spend health resources wisely.

In years that the total savings from lower health insurance premiums is greater than the employer's deductible health expenses, these savings could be shared between the employer and the employees. Health savings accounts could be set up for each employee, and made accessible to that employee when the savings account has accumulated a balance of $1,000 (half the size of the deductible required before insurance reimburses). Thereafter the employee could assume responsibility for the first $1,000 of expenses, the employer for the other half of the deductible. Over the years, cost savings could continue to be split between employer and employees. As the savings accounts grew larger, any surplus above $1,000 could be available as an Individual Retirement Account, providing future security, or for discretionary use by the employee. If Health Savings Accounts were used in this way the risk to the employer would gradually go down, and the employee would have a positive financial incentive to make wise health-care purchases.

Without the safety net of preventive health services, this proposal could be dangerous—and costly in the long run. In order to acquire savings funds, some employees would neglect their health at times when problems could be corrected inexpensively. However, if participation in a prevention program that monitors health status were required in order to be eligible to get an employer-paid health savings account, the risk of health neglect would be negligible. In short, when the safety net of preventive services is in place, it becomes practical to separate catastrophic and non-catastrophic health costs, and to use high deductible insurance policies. Employers can use the principle of shared risk to lower their health benefits obligations. They also can extend the principle of shared risk and shared potential gain to their employees, establishing health savings accounts which then lessen the employer's obligations under the shared risk deductibles.

Would all employees want the responsibility of choice that goes with the concept of Health Savings Accounts? Probably not. Some might opt for the peace of mind that comes from putting themselves in a managed care plan that made wise choices *for* them about what kinds of services are needed. It would be quite possible to pay for such services out of a health savings account; managed care plans almost surely would adapt their financial arrangements to deal with two-part payments, for catastrophic and non-catastrophic health care, if these kinds of arrangements became popular. Health-oriented innovations once again would make a difference in how managed care would work. H.E.R.O. and other competing trade groups that might emerge could help capitated payment plans learn how to do *health enhancement* cost-effectively. In addition to the large managed-care plans now available, independent, health-oriented managed care services would offer individualized attention. Some, such as those that might be run by Planned Parenthood, religious organizations, or public health agencies, might focus care toward the special concerns of particular groups of users. Health savings accounts and managed care could take us in different directions; but they could also work together, if the health-oriented innovations discussed already were part of the picture.

Health Savings Accounts, Chapter 5 cautioned, could destroy the health insurance market. If currently standard low-deductible health insurance policies are available along with high-deductible policies and a health savings account, the healthy will choose health savings accounts. Most people with more expensive health problems will continue their conventional, low-deductible health insurance. This raises the cost of health benefits rapidly: The healthy take out in savings what previously was used to subsidize the higher costs of the unhealthy. Meanwhile the cost of insurance premiums skyrockets, since only the higher cost patients remain in the insurance pool. This proposal, however, is quite different. By extending the health savings accounts to all employees in a contract, the insurance pool is protected. If participation in a health promotion program that monitors individual health status is an eligibility requirement for the health savings accounts, the health of the individual participants also is protected. Substantial savings for both employers and employees could result. Equally important, the costs of health insurance would be low enough to let a number of smaller, marginally profitable businesses offer this health benefit to their employees. This would lower the number of Americans who require public subsidies in order to have health insurance.

Some risk remains, of course. A few people will ignore their health counselor's advice, just as they now ignore that of their doctor. Most will not, however. Effective health counselors seek out their clients and motivate them to care about their health.

Handling catastrophic and non-catastrophic health-care costs separately, through high-deductible health insurance, opens up possibilities for real savings for non-catastrophic care, thanks to the safety net that prevention programs puts in place. These programs provide more than a safety net, however. By directing health-care interventions to an earlier point on the health-disease continuum, proactive health promotion programs can reduce the level of *necessary* spending, as well as make it possible for people to safely reduce their consumption of more expensive and optional health-care services.

Changing Provider Incentive to Overutilize Services

The discussion thus far has focused on employers, their employees and families, and hospitals, suggesting ways that basic costs for health care could come down by extending the principles of incentives, and of shared and protected risk into new areas, once a basic safety net of health-oriented services were available. There has been little discussion thus far of physicians, the key gate-keepers whose individual decisions *in fact* are the primary determinant of which services get used. Professional values of physicians emphasize giving the highest standard of care to every patient. At present, the "highest standard" usually means "state of the art" —i.e., high tech— care. Sometimes this results in better patient outcomes; at other times it simply increases the cost of care. The real battle is not between high-tech and low-tech care. Sometimes one, sometimes the other, sometimes something in between is most appropriate. The real issue involves making sure that resources are not wasted and that ecologically sophisticated care, which strengthens the health-building potential of each individual, is available.

Education. New roles for the National Institutes of Health, proposed in Chapter 10, if coupled properly with continuing medical education courses for physicians, could help shift physician's sense of options when caring for patients. It will be important to make sure that both cost and *effectiveness* become major criteria used to choose treatment plans. Medical science research has opened up a much more sophisticated understanding of the health-disease process, and of the internal and external ecology of health and disease, as Chapter 9 describes. Medical practices, however, still remain too focused around earlier, single-cause understandings of the origins of disease. They often use biochemical or mechanical interventions that ignore the body's own health-regulating processes. Changing those approaches could lead to more cost-effective care. NIH could play a critical role in helping this occur.

More will be needed, however. We will also need to address the overuse of medical specialists, as well as sources of overconsumption of health-care resources by physicians. Some of the overuse of resources by physicians stems from self-protection, and some from self-interest.

Reducing Over-Specialization. So long as the majority of American physicians remain specialists with little responsibility for the ongoing care of patients, costs for care will be high. A start has been made on correcting that problem, through pressures on medical schools to change the ratio of general care physicians to specialists among those currently being trained. In addition, the move toward managed care, the creation of mammoth, quasi-monopoly networks of provider organizations, and the buying up of physicians' practices by capitated payment plans will force a number of specialists to do primary care medicine. Gatekeepers in managed care plans will direct too few patients to medical specialists to let the current number of specialists thrive in the new market. These market pressures to retool professionally create a moment of opportunity to help physicians develop a more ecologically sophisticated understanding of how to organize medical interventions. We should not let the opportunity slip by.

Malpractice Reform. One of the reasons medical specialists get overused in American medicine is for referrals made by other physicians, not because they believe it will benefit a patient, but in order to protect themselves in case they are sued, a practice which adds greatly to the cost of day-to-day health care. In addition, malpractice insurance has become so expensive that general practitioners now abandon some areas of practice. Few primary care doctors still deliver babies, for example, because of the cost of malpractice insurance. There is considerable sentiment now in favor of malpractice tort reform. If done well, it could lessen the use of specialists.

We could take a lesson from Sweden and institutionalize the settling of claims by establishing No Fault Malpractice Awards.[7] A certain number of medical mistakes will occur in any system of medical care. Highly invasive medical procedures will have a predictable volume of mistakes, and the consequences are grave for the patient. Currently damages are collected only through suit. Lawyers get no compensation if they lose the case, but usually collect one third of the damage award in cases that they win. Not surprisingly, they often urge their clients to ask for very large awards. If medical injuries were treated like workman's compensation claims, however, that dynamic would change. If someone is injured on the job there are pre-established compensations to which one is entitled. Few cases go to court; instead the injured person files a claim, with supporting evidence, and compensation is automatic unless the claim of damage on the job is disputed.[8] Malpractice compensation could work in the same way. It need not preclude law suits for punitive damages in cases where gross incompetence has resulted in serious injury or death, but the number of suits would be far fewer than at present and less money would be spent paying for damage claims or lawyers fees. If procedures were institutionalized for dealing with problems of malpractice, more than money would be saved.

Semi-adversarial relations now characterize many doctor-patient interactions. Without worry about law suits, much more cooperative interactions could return. A different kind of calculus could inform decisions about which tests, procedures, and referrals are appropriate.

The steps recommended in Chapter 10 as ways to demedicalize the experience of birth, aging, and death might have even greater impact on the current overconsumption of physician services. Malpractice reform could help encourage this trend. Physicians are freer to "work with nature" when they have clear directives from patients and when a disappointing outcome will not lead to lengthy legal involvement or financial loss. Each of these areas of reform—the demedicalizing of life events and the reform of malpractice compensation—would strengthen the impact of the other. They are a natural combination.

Positive Incentives. These two areas of reform do nothing, however, to change the positive financial incentives that encourage physicians to use resources in questionable ways. Chapter 5 discussed one strategy that some capitated payment plans use to change physicians' interest in providing the most expensive care for each patient. About 15 percent of the physician's compensation is withheld until year's end, and distributed differentially among the physicians as reward for "cost-effective care". Physicians whose patients cost more than average receive a less than average "merit" payment at year's end; those whose patients cost little, get more than their expectable share. This strategy pits self-interest against professional norms to provide the "best possible" standard of care. It may save money, but does not protect interests of the patient. There must be better ways to be cost-effective.

There are. A mixed medical model that encourages more ecologically-relevant strategies for health improvement saves money while improving health. More investment in prevention and general health promotion for patients keeps people healthier and reduces the need for disease care services. H.E.R.O.'s analysis of cost-effective strategies for health enhancement, described in Chapter 10, offers a preferable route to the same end. In capitated payment plans physicians benefit from less expensive use of services. Substituting cost-effective improvements rather than withholding services should work better for everyone.

Reapproaching Health Benefits Packages.

The problem of unintended incentives to overconsume health-care resources is more complex for health care providers who work on a fee-for-service basis. When they are paid for each service delivered, there is a natural tendency to provide the maximum possible service, so long as payment for it is guaranteed. As Chapter 5 noted, benefit packages can work as a "pork barrel" for health-care providers who work on an indemnity plan. Each guaranteed benefit can be prescribed with full confidence that it will be reimbursed by the third-party payer, with little need to justify its choice for use with a particular patient. Because patients do not pay for these services directly, or pay only a portion of their costs, they rarely question the judgment of the physician who recommends particular kinds of care. Under these circumstances the professional ethic of providing the "best possible care" provides a comfortable rationalization for ordering expensive services that may be of only marginal benefit to the patient, and ignoring less expensive alternatives. This is why struggles between labor and management about which health services to include in benefits contracts have been so intense. Specifying benefits helps create a demand for them, either on the part of the doctor or the patient. Any service that is specified for reimbursement gets used more frequently, independent of changes in demonstrated *need* for that service.[9]

Historically, U.S. third-party payers have approached the problem of incentives to overconsume health services in a variety of ways. Many have ignored the problem, paying for "all necessary services," with no cap on the amount of benefits to be paid. Other third-party payers modify "all necessary services" to exclude some costly ones that are used by only a minority of their enrollees, or place an upper limit on reimbursement for certain specified services. This shifts these costs onto private households, yet does nothing to lower the "pork barrel" impact of unlimited payment for all other services. Increasingly, therefore, third-party payers are moving to capitated payment plans which limit their annual liability. Managed care plans specify how much can be spent overall, and use physician gatekeepers to decide what services are needed by whom. This rations care, trading "pork barrel" incentives for other incentives to maximize income by providing fewer services for the same amount of money. There are better ways to approach overconsumption of health services.

Ideally, any real need of a patient for services should be met, and no services should be given that are not clearly useful for that patient, so long as a third party is obligated to pay for the services. Patients as well as physicians should have some say about what is needed or useful. Moreover, everyone should have the same access to needed services, independent of their personal wealth. Managed care gives everyone the same "right" to care, but largely ignores patient choice. (Point-of-service managed care offers a compromise, letting patients choose additional services or use providers who are "outside the network" but pay more when they do so.) If we use some of the strategies already proposed for lowering the basic costs of care while shifting the emphasis toward *health*, it might be possible to change the dynamic of self-interest that leads physicians to over-prescribe or under-prescribe services and patients to accept this or to ask for services of questionable value.

Each person or family has different needs for health services. Not everyone benefits from physician-controlled "managed care" or prefers it. Managed care also adds administrative costs that are not needed for other systems, and at times, cumbersome decision rules. Additional routes to economy are needed.

A "capitated payment" approach to benefit packages might innovate in ways that both save money and create flexibility to fit each household's needs. The federal government could allow, as tax-free benefits, a specific dollar amount. That amount would equal the current "best price" for funding hospital capitation payments, catastrophic insurance for long-term care and other non-hospital costs that exceed a high-deductible threshold, plus the cost of funding "self-insurance" arrangements for non-catastrophic care. This tax-free level would leave households free to use indemnity insurance, managed care or health savings accounts to pay for basic health services, with the backup of hospital coverage and catastrophic insurance for other needs. Anyone could use more costly personal or bargained "benefits" options, but these would be counted as discretionary spending and would be taxable. For their basic health needs, many households might choose to use independent, health-oriented managed care services described in Chapter 10. Professionals would direct them to choices that improve health, rather than simply use disease services "efficiently." This kind of managed care could benefit households financially, as well as lower overall costs for services.

A "capitated" approach to benefits has several advantages. It preserves access to all needed services, while ending "pork barrel" pressures to over-consume; it lets each household choose the form of service that works best for it; and it generates additional public revenue out of discretionary health-care spending. This could help generate additional tax revenue to subsidize health costs for low income households, and would do so in a way that treated all Americans equally. All would have tax-free access to funding for basic health services, regardless of the level of their personal income.

With these proposals, we are beginning to see a domino effect. It is set in motion by health-oriented innovations that provide a safety net making it possible to experiment more basically with approaches to shared and protected risk in the funding of health-care services. Each innovation in the funding of care, in turn, is augmented by *health*-oriented innovations that increase its impact. As the momentum builds, it becomes possible to innovate still more basically in the way that funding arrangements themselves work. Third-party payers, the recipients and also the providers of health-care services all gain positive incentives to make more cost-effective use of disease-care services, and to do so in concert rather than in opposition to each other. The reorientation toward *health*, thus, gives a focus that allows both long-term and short-term economies. Without the shift of emphasis toward health, seen in the rather concrete steps discussed in Chapter 10, these approaches to cost containment would not work. They provide both the direct and indirect impetus that might change the cost dynamic that now makes health care constantly more expensive. Moreover they do so while still protecting the vitality of this sector of the economy.

Thus far most of the proposals have been congruent with a market-focus for reform. Some of the cost-containment steps, however, require additional national legislation—establishing a common national pool for reinsurance (and imposing a surcharge on all health-care providers) in order to share their costs more equitably, and requiring everyone to have catastrophic and long-term care insurance. In addition, tax law changes would establish an annual limit on tax-free health benefits, in order to generate additional income to subsidize health costs of persons who have either low or no income. They would also establish protection against cost-shifting to employees, and rules for appropriate uses of health savings accounts. Health savings accounts would only work if the strategy is used universally within an insurance risk pool, but this strategy could be optional from risk pool to risk pool, and thus would not have to be universal. Legislation that made it easier to set up voluntary purchasing pools for insurance, and that protected those who used them, would help, as would directives to the Federal Employees Health Benefits Plan to provide a backup purchasing pool for non-federal employees who chose to use it.

All of these legislative packages seem politically possible and economically sound. In addition, four of the 10 steps to reorient the system toward health would benefit from national legislation: setting up discounts on insurance policies or providing other incentives to help fund worksite health promotion programs; legislation to aid the establishment of independent, health-oriented managed care services; changes in the training requirements for licensed practical nurses and authorization for various combinations of health-care professionals to offer basic services; and directives to the National Institutes of Health to make comparative assessments of treatment strategies. These also seem politically possible. Together these proposals could change the present dynamic toward constant cost escalation at the same time that they move us closer to a real *health*-care system.

A Summary of the Larger Strategy Proposed for Cost Control

Reframing the problem to be addressed has made it possible to combine proposals from all of the currently contending strategies for health-care reform, creating new possibilities for cost containment. Redividing the health-care market's funding in ways that encourage additional public/private partnerships opens quite different avenues for problem-solving. It is time to summarize the argument of this chapter, showing which proposals address issues of cost containment, the provision of more cost-effective care, and the generation of new funding sources that can subsidize health needs of the poor. (Table 11.1 provides a graphic overview, suggesting how each proposal would affect the larger dynamic at work.)

Cost Containment. Six proposals from this chapter change the nature of the dynamic which now holds third-party payers, private households and health-care providers captive to pressures toward more cost increase than is needed for good care:

1. Hospital capitation rates guarantee a basic annual income to hospitals, bargained-for in terms of actual health services provided to an enrollee group through hospitals. Meanwhile, optional, supplemental hospital insurance allows for continued technological development for hospitals, now financed out of discretionary income use, rather than through captive payments.

2. Universal catastrophic insurance, which covers the cost of all health services that are not hospital-based, above a specified deductible amount, provides "protected risk" against high cost illness. (So does guaranteed access to hospital care at a capitated rate.) Long-term care would be included in all catastrophic insurance policies, which would be universal, so that all Americans were covered.

3. Insurance discounts to employers who provide qualified worksite health promotion services to their employees spread shared and protected risks more evenly between the "self-insured" and insurance companies, while encouraging lower utilization over time of expensive disease care services.

4. "Non-catastrophic care" (i.e., all other health services including part of the cost for preventive and health promotion services) would be funded through employer or other third-party payer self-insurance and employer-generated health savings accounts. This change takes the bulk of health-care transactions out of the insurance market and makes possible a different kind of calculus for use of optional services.

5. Universal access to insurance purchasing pools, which would also bargain for hospital capitation rates, guarantee all Americans insurance at comparable, reasonable rates.

6. A "capitated" health benefits structure sets tax-free benefits at the most cost-effective rate needed for hospital capitation payment, "self-insurance" for the first $2,000 of costs, and high deductible, catastrophic insurance for all other health costs, including long-term care. (This covers all

health needs, allows flexible choice of services, but ends "pork barrel" incentives to overconsume. The health-oriented initiatives described in Chapter 10 provide a safety net protection for this combination of share and protected risk.)

More Cost-Effective Care

Six additional proposals could help moderate the health-care system's current preference for high-tech solutions, independent of their relative utility for particular problems.

1. Health savings accounts give users an incentive to make cost-effective optional choices (while preventive services provide a safety net discouraging unwise economies).

2. "No fault" malpractice insurance reform lessens pressure on physicians to prescribe services of questionable health value which now are recommended to protect physicians from law suits.

3. These two reforms should reinforce other organizational dynamics that will encourage more specialists to offer primary care services.

4. Education proposals of Chapter 10 could help physicians more generally move toward more cost-effective, ecologically-relevant choices for disease care.

5. Capitation agreements for hospital rates; and

6. Capitation rates for tax-free health benefits both would reinforce the shift of emphasis toward the most cost-effective care, by damping the "pork barrel" incentive of current benefit structure formulas.

Needs of the Poor

Finally, proposals discussed in Chapters 10 and 11 identify three possible sources of funds needed to subsidize those now left out of health care.

1. A reinsurance surcharge would let costs of serving now-avoided populations be partially subsidized by the entire pool of health-care providers who purchase reinsurance.

2. A new form of health-oriented managed care and purchasing services for persons with costly chronic health problems could lower present public outlays for their care, freeing some of this budget for redeployment to other poor persons.

3. Shifting long-term care to the private insurance market and including it as part of universal catastrophic health-care insurance frees considerable Medicare and Medicaid money for redeployment to other needs of the poor.

(Additional possibilities for subsidizing health-care costs of those now left out of health insurance will be discussed in Chapter 12.)

New approaches to cost containment, made practical by a shift of emphasis toward *health,* can begin to make American health care more affordable. Could these approaches to cost containment also affect problems of access to basic health-care services? If so, how? Chapter 12 addresses this question, suggesting how reforms discussed in Chapters 10 and 11 could help move us toward universal access to basic health-care services.

TABLE 11.1 Lowering Costs in Order to Improve Access to Health Care

Proposed Reform Strategy	*Implications of Reform Strategies for Cost Containment*	
	a. Changes dynamic keeping payers/users captive to cost increases	*b. Affects incentives toward expensive care*
1. Hospital capitation rates	•	•
2. Universal catastrophic health insurance (including long-term care)	•	•
3. Employer-generated health savings accounts plus employer-self-insurance to pay for other health costs)	•	•
4. Purchasing pools	•	
5. "Capitated" benefits formula	•	•
6. No-fault malpractice insurance reform	•	•
7. Incentives for specialists to provide primary care	•	•
8. Physician education re: cost-effective, ecologically-relevant care		•
9. Reinsurance surcharge		•
10. Health-oriented managed care and purchasing services for persons with costly chronic health problems		•

12

Reapproaching Problems of Access

As Chapter 11 has demonstrated, a shift in emphasis toward *health* makes it possible to approach issues of cost containment for disease care in new ways. This chapter takes advantage of the reframing of the problem presented in Chapters 10 and 11 to suggest ways to open greater access to basic health services for those now left out. It closes with a summary of how the full set of proposals sketched out in these three chapters could work together.

Improving Access to Care

Table 12.1 identifies eight groups within the population that have had difficulty getting the health-care services they need.

TABLE 12.1   Americans with Problematic Access to Health-Care
Insurance or Services

1. People with Pre-existing Medical Conditions
2. People Who Change Jobs
3. Small Businesses and the Self-Employed
4. The Working Poor who lack Health Insurance
5. The Unemployed who are not on Medicaid
6. Many Medicaid and Low-Income Medicare Enrollees (because primary care physicians often will not accept government discounted payment rates)
7. Inner City Residents Who Lack Access to Primary Care Physicians
8. Citizens Who Live Outside the Standard Metropolitan Areas

Legislators have been most concerned with access problems of middle-class constituents—those with pre-existing medical problems, small businesses and the self-employed who face excessive premium rates, and persons who lose their insurance coverage if they go from job to job. They have paid less attention to the unemployed who lack Medicaid, the working poor who have no health insurance, low income Medicare and Medicaid enrollees who have health insurance but have difficulty finding primary care providers willing to accept their discounted payment schedule, or persons who lack geographic access to health-care services. The innovations discussed in Chapters 10 and 11 would make it possible to approach the access problems of these groups as well. Here is one way this could work.

Three issues must be addressed in order to increase access to care. The first involves getting basic services to people in geographic locations where few physicians now offer basic primary care. The second involves finding funds to subsidize the working poor and those without employment who now lack health insurance. The third concerns ways to absorb low-income Medicare and Medicaid populations into general health care so that they are not discriminated against because public funds offer discounted payments far below the income health-care providers can make in the private market. Each of these problems can be approached through a series of steps that build on the momentum of reforms discussed in Chapters 10 and 11.

Getting Services to People in Underserved Areas

Current health policy proposals gamble that government offers of capitated Medicare and Medicaid payments for residents living in underserved areas will motivate managed care plans to extend their services. Many hospital systems are reorganizing to provide primary and secondary health services for capitated payment, as a survival strategy in the new health-care market. Some hospitals are likely to bid for contracts to cover enrollees who live in under-served areas. This offers no guarantee, however, that services will be made easily accessible or that basic health services will be delivered regularly to these people.

Another approach to this problem has been sketched out in three proposals of Chapter 10, which could supplement or replace the current thrust of reform. Allowing independent, health-oriented managed care plans to compete for these contracts, plans run by nurses or other health professionals who contract for other services, as needed, can help extend geographic coverage for the population. Nurses are much more widely distributed throughout the population and could be recruited and trained to provide a range of basic services, with access to physician backup as needed. Allowing nurse-run managed care plans to also supervise services of licensed practical nurses, whose training has been upgraded so that they can do simple monitoring of basic health conditions and provide some proactive prenatal care to the rural and inner city poor will help still more. Together they would provide an American equivalent of the Barefoot Doctor approach that has improved basic health status for under-served populations in several parts of the world. All this becomes more feasible financially if Reinsurance Reform provides a surcharge pool that is redistributed among all health-care providers in proportion to their enrollment of now neglected segments of the population who might need more expensive service delivery.

Current capitated payment proposals and this alternative could work together. Basic health-oriented services will receive more emphasis, however, if community-oriented, prevention-focused agencies hold the basic contracts for enrollees in now under-served areas and negotiate for other services, as needed. They could partner with larger managed-care services, so long as the larger provider systems give supplementary services rather than determine how basic care will be organized for enrollees in these areas.

As funds become available, health professionals with vision respond to new opportunities. In addition, as specialists in over-supply find fewer opportunities to practice in metropolitan suburbs—because of the spread of capitation plans for health-care delivery which need fewer specialists, and because malpractice reform leaves physicians making less "defensive medicine" referrals—more physicians will offer primary care, and some will go to now-avoided communities that need their services. The combination of opportunity and changing circumstances for nurses and physicians should lessen the geographic maldistribution of health-care services.

Health Insurance for the Working Poor

The safety net that proactive prevention services provides can make it possible to lower the cost of health-care benefits. If this happens, more businesses will be able to provide all or at least part of the cost of health insurance for their employees. The Clinton health insurance reform task force recommended an employer mandate, legally obligating businesses to provide health insurance to their employees, along with federal subsidies to reduce the liability of marginally profitable businesses for health insurance costs. Chapter 4 discussed the financial and political objections that eliminated an employer mandate when Congress began rewriting the legislation. Some businessmen argued that it could cost the economy a million jobs. Whether or not that forecast is accurate, political opposition from small businesses effectively killed legislative requirements that businesses *must* finance health insurance for their employees. It seems clear that we cannot force all employers to pay for health insurance for their employees.

That, however, does not mean that it is politically impossible to mandate employers to make *access* to health protection available to all employees, at group rates. Here is one way that could work.

Creating a Health Protection Mandate

An employer mandate could be modified to become a Health Protection Mandate, guaranteeing all Americans access to hospital coverage, as well as to catastrophic and long term care insurance. It could require employers to assist in making such coverage available to their employees by providing access to group-rate contracts unless employees use another route for health cost protection. Health benefits costs could be paid by employers, by other sponsoring groups that act as a third party payer, by employees, or through government subsidies for some low-income Americans who do not have other routes to health protection, or through any combination of these funding routes. Whoever pays these costs would get the tax credit that is available. If costs are jointly paid by employer and employee (or by any other entity that pays taxes) the tax credits would be shared. The payer could count as a deductible business expense each year the cost of the least expensive basic package of catastrophic and non-catastrophic health protection that is available. Any employee who paid all or part of that cost could deduct it from his or her taxable income.

It would be important to discourage shifting onto workers, the government, or other third party payers the cost of health benefits employers *now* pay. To protect wages, there could be a heavy tax penalty for any employer who stops claiming business expenses for the amount paid—unless the employer can show an equivalent increase in wages to employees, spread evenly across the employee population. Because health benefits are, in fact, a part of wages, any future insurance discounts given because of lowered use of health benefits should be shared between the employer and the employees and so reported on the employer's IRS form.[1]

Chapter 11 discussed ways to lower the cost of basic health protection. Some employers who cannot now provide health insurance for their employees might be able to afford the lower cost proposals spelled out there. Others might be able to pay for part of it. The federal government, for example, now assumes that Americans will spend about 7.5% of their adjusted gross income for health care, and subtracts that amount before allowing itemized deductions for health-care expenses. Some employers might offer to pay for catastrophic and long-term care insurance and to subsidize the *difference* between 7.5% of an employees adjusted gross income and the $2,000 needed for a health savings account. Some of the employers who currently offer no health benefits almost surely will refuse to pay any employee health costs. Rather than remain stymied by present political constraints, we could reach a compromise requiring employers to provide the centralized accounting that would make it practical for their employees to get health protection at group rates. There should be less resistance to a mandate for employers to make services accessible, so long as there is flexibility about how these services will be financed. In some cases, employees with higher incomes might contribute this amount themselves, and claim it as a deduction from their taxable income. The working poor whose employers provide no payment for health insurance and the unemployed will need other funding routes, which will be discussed shortly. The self-employed who lack access to private health cost protection purchasing pools, but who are not the working poor, could buy into the Federal Employees Health Benefits Program. They could use the IRS tax payment mechanism to reimburse the government through their quarterly payments, subtracting their tax-deductible health benefits allowance from what they otherwise owe.

This solution to the Employer Mandate ignores questions of "fairness", of who *should* pay for health costs. Many would prefer employers to provide health-care coverage as part of wages, or else to have free, i.e., publicly supported, health care. Neither of these options seems politically possible at this point in time. Consequently one must rely on proposals that could get services to all who need them, with federal subsidies for those who lack some other means to pay for them.

Subsidizing Low-income Populations

Even if all employers provided health insurance for their own employees, the current down-sizing of American businesses means that considerable subsidy will be needed for those left out of paid employment. Medicaid has not been absorbing these people. In addition, if employer-paid health insurance remains optional, many of the working poor also will need help. Additional sources of funds must be found to meet the survival problems of the economically disadvantaged, including the need for access to health care. What can be done, in a practical way, to fund health needs of the poor?

Redirecting Tax Revenues

This discussion already has identified two sources of new funding that could help subsidize the younger poor, which become possible as health-oriented innovations allow more flexibility in allocating resources. First, transferring long-term care to the private market, as a universal insurance requirement, frees up considerable state and federal funds that now go for long-term care. Second, a cap on tax-exempt health benefits spending, made possible by new ways to finance basic health protection, would raise additional revenue. More expensive health service choices would be counted as discretionary spending, and taxed, once a less expensive way to cover *needs* replaces "pork barrel" incentives of specified benefits packages. In addition, Congress is exploring proposals to sharply increase the tax on tobacco, earmarking a portion of this revenue for health services to some of the currently uninsured.[2] Other "sin taxes" might be acceptable to the public and generate revenue, as well.

Additional funds will be needed. They are not likely to come from traditional sources. Each year fewer businesses provide health benefits for all their employees and the larger companies, which have traditionally provided employee health benefits, are drastically reducing the size of their work force. Laid-off workers often are going into jobs with lower wages and no health benefits. Because of tax reforms of the 1980s and past sluggish growth of the economy as a whole,[3] public revenues have not kept up with increased needs to subsidize health costs of the poor. Additional sources of revenue are likely to be needed. Where might they be found?

The problem is not that insufficient funds are flowing through the economy. Rather, funds are now flowing in directions that do not solve such public problems as access of the poor to health services. Some additional sources of funding might be tapped, either through legislation or private initiative.

New Funding Sources to Explore

Can sources of funds be found in the private (and therefore voluntary) economy that could begin to meet health needs of the poor? Simply asking this question may be morally offensive to some. Many would argue that the state *should* take responsibility for the well-being of all its citizens, and that it is a mistake to look in other directions for a solution. Others may object that private solutions mean voluntary solutions, which can be quite unstable as economic circumstances change. For almost fifty years now, however, private interests have provided funding for the health needs of most Americans. American third-party payer private health insurance is a voluntary system (albeit often and originally with the pressure of union contracts behind it). We have found few moral problems in using these private sources of funding for the bulk of health care in America. Employers have an institutional interest in maintaining a healthy workforce and thus for the most part have been a reliable private and voluntary source of funding for health care. What is needed is private income that gets regularly generated through normal market dynamics, and which could remain consistently available to subsidize health costs.

Are there other institutional interests besides employers or the government that have a stake in the successful resolution of problems in getting access to health-care services for those now left out? And could there be ways to tap voluntary flows of funds in the private economy so that more of them become relevant to the health-care needs of people with low income who now have no health insurance? What kinds of public/private partnerships could be established to guarantee that basic health-care services get to people who now are left out of health-care funding?

We already have a demonstration of how alternative institutional sponsorship might work. Some African-American religious denominations, as well as individual congregations, have begun to explore ways to play a different role in meeting the practical health and welfare needs of impoverished neighborhoods. Facing the fact that the neighborhoods for which they feel special responsibility are currently a low priority politically, and that people are hungry, sick, and dying prematurely, churches and other neighborhood institutions have begun to play new economic roles in their communities, creating and sponsoring economic "enterprises for service" that can redirect how money flows into and out of low income communities. Their goal is to tap into money that is already circulating in the private economy, finding ways to redirect some of it to fund basic needs of low-income neighborhood residents, including their need for health care. A particularly innovative approach currently is being demonstrated by the Institutional Leadership Conference, a coalition of African-American leaders from twenty-two urban communities, and its Detroit affiliate, People Aspiring to Create Hope (P.A.T.C.H.).[4]

Sometimes African-American churches and their broader coalitions generate income by endorsing business enterprises that sell products or services to members of the local community. In exchange they receive sales commissions, which can be ongoing, and sizable. Sometimes they introduce insurance companies, health-care service providers or business services to local small businesses or to benefits departments of large corporations, to school districts, hospital systems, or the like. Through endorsement by "faith communities" and the coalitions they organize, new competitors gain entry to these markets. In return, the endorsers receive sales commissions for each employee who designates this competitor as part of their annual benefits selection. Because the "faith communities" accept a moral responsibility to investigate the quality of services given before endorsing a particular competitor in the market, public and private benefits departments and small businesses often welcome the recommendations churches provide, while also welcoming the opportunity to aid lower income populations. (For some corporate officers and public servants this provides an opportunity to express a moral commitment to the broader community and also represents a valuable public relations opportunity.)[5]

In addition, some "faith communities" and the coalitions of local institutions they help organize are directly sponsoring their own "enterprises for service", not-for-profit businesses whose operating surplus can be used to meet local community needs, including health care. Sometimes charitable trusts give them grants to acquire a high profit-margin business which can also employ neighborhood residents. Sometimes they become agents for an insurance company. At other times local businessmen (funeral home directors, or others with regular cash flow) loan money to start new enterprises. They take advantage of "empowerment zone" policies to generate *community* income which can be used for public need.[6]

In short, these private "moral communities" are beginning to step into the vacuum left by the collapse of New Deal programs that implemented public moral commitments. They are creating morally-focused economic enterprises that can tap into the flows of money already circulating in the private economy and redirect some of them for public needs.[6]

Because African-American religious institutions historically have served as community centers and have identified the survival and social needs of their neighborhoods as part of their spiritual ministry, they are uniquely prepared to pioneer as moral economic entrepreneurs creating "enterprises for service". However in their own response to crises of the homeless many "faith communities" outside African-American neighborhoods have also begun to express their faith through direct services to those most in need, providing food kitchens and emergency shelter. Once African-American religious institutions demonstrate how to play new moral roles in the private economy there is no reason that their example cannot become imitated more widely. When religious institutions act on behalf of those left out of the system, they often have a powerful impact on many individuals who share their moral vision and who are in a position to make economic choices that can assist their cause.

The genius of the "enterprise for service" strategy lies in its ability to tap into existing money flows in the private economy and to redirect them for public service. Unlike taxes, doing business with "enterprises for service" imposes no additional costs on those who cooperate with these efforts. Unlike philanthropy, the investor gets back an immediate, tangible gain in addition to the moral satisfaction of helping others.

Can this new strategy provide sufficient funds and institutional sponsorship to meet the needs of all who now are left out of access to health care? Probably not. Almost surely, however, it can do three things that are deeply needed at present. It can lessen the crises facing some of the most disadvantaged Americans. It can provide a moral leadership that helps mobilize business and health-care professionals to cooperate in new ways to get services to those now left out. And it can keep leaders in business, politics, and middle class America searching for solutions to problems not effectively addressed by current political formulas. If commitment to meeting the real needs of all Americans solidifies, political options will change. These new enterprises can help to create such commitments, but in a way that breaks through earlier notions of public and private charity. They begin to create partnerships rather than dependencies. They demonstrate that untapped money can become available and that important segments of the community *care* about public needs. They could begin to build a different kind of momentum for problem-solving, which could change national political priorities.

If churches and other community agencies were available to receive income and enroll those without health insurance, several private sources might generate additional income to help guarantee access to health services. Some sources of support might involve simply redirecting funds currently "lost" to those who pay them. Hospitals, businesses and individuals with a high volume of phone calls could use a carrier who is willing to donate a percent of the volume to a fund for health services for the poor. Credit card interest could be used in the same way.

It is essential, of course, that funding sources be consistently available. Thus *donations* cannot become the primary source for additional funding to meet the health needs of those now left out. There is no reason, however, that charitable contributions could not become a supplementary part of the solution. Health services to the poor already has become an attractive target for individual giving as a Designated Gift category through United Way campaigns. Agencies that supplement health insurance could be added to these lists. Other income could come through special offerings from churches.

Because many of the poor live together, in lower-income neighborhoods, local institutions, including especially churches and non-profit coalitions they could organize, could receive donations earmarked to fund health services for those now left out of the system. They then could act in lieu of an employer, enrolling people and negotiating appropriate prices and services.

In addition, such sponsors could ask health-care providers to donate a portion of their co-pay charges to help subsidize insurance costs for the poor, to offer discounted rates, or to designate other sources of contributed income, in exchange for access to a new pool of enrollees whose costs would be partially paid by the sponsoring agency, thus reducing providers' overhead from unreimbursed services to the poor.

Church coalitions or other community agencies could enter into partnerships with existing health-care providers. Some "enterprises for service" would be appropriate vendors to larger hospitals or other health-care providers, as described above. The income earned could then be used to provide needed supplementary services in a neighborhood, beyond those a managed care plan normally provides. The local sponsor, for example, might fund a nurse-run clinic to provide primary care services to the uninsured, and might offer health-oriented case-management outreach services to an entire neighborhood. It might sponsor neighborhood community gardens and other nutrition projects that improve the health of the neighborhood. This would lower costs for the managed care group, who might be asked to reciprocate by providing physician backup services for the local agency's health work. (Plans are underway in Detroit to create such a partnership.)

If community agencies demonstrated this kind of capability, some might be able to play a still larger role. It might be possible for them to get a state or federal waiver and to become the recipient for Medicare/Medicaid capitation payments. They then would be in position to sponsor all people in the neighborhood, much as a large employer sponsors its employee population—negotiating services for the entire neighborhood, providing universal access to care.

If local agencies sponsor health-care services, small businesses that cannot pay full health benefits for their employees could contribute a portion of those costs to the local sponsor, as tax-deductible contributions. Larger businesses might make charitable, tax-deductible contributions for this purpose. This would improve their potential labor pool while also affecting their own health benefits spending. Larger businesses now absorb much of the cost of services given the poor who cannot pay: Daily hospital charges include "overhead" for unreimbursed emergency room services and other expensive care for the uninsured poor.

Many *recipients* of "donated" insurance might also contribute a small percent of their income to its cost, thereby retaining their own independence and self-respect. In short, if we cannot get legislative agreement to find tax revenues for this purpose, several sources of donations might supplement other funds in order to get health services immediately accessible to all, while public demand for *guaranteed* access is building. If many groups and organizations "voluntarily taxed" themselves 1% or half of 1% of whatever income source made most sense to them, a groundswell of support for needs of the poor could begin. As that momentum builds, public demand to commit tax resources for this purpose would increase markedly. Private funding thus could be a catalyst to change public policy. Enough groups have something tangible to gain from such a voluntary commitment to make this worth pursuing now.

Encouraging Medicaid Participants to Help Control Costs.

Additional funds could come from present tax revenue if we replaced current Medicaid formulas with the same principles for cost reduction that have been recommended for the private market. Extending this principle to Medicaid enrollees might free additional funds so that more people could be covered.

Many states now pay a lower rate for Medicaid services. In many states hospitals and physicians, for example, get reimbursed at 60% of the rates they charge private insurance. A number of for-profit hospitals, consequently, refuse to take Medicaid patients and the practice of refusing Medicaid patients also is quite widespread among private physicians and dentists. It seems probable that many health-care providers who now *take* Medicaid patients use income generating strategies that were used during the Nixon and Reagan eras to evade price controls. (When prices are controlled, more diagnostic tests and services are prescribed. When prices are controlled by diagnostic category—as in DRG reimbursement procedures—diagnostic entries are chosen that anticipate higher expenses and maximize income; in addition, fewer services are given.) Since Medicaid patients do not pay for services received, they have little reason to question why services are given to them.

At present, most Medicaid reform efforts focus on shifting Medicaid recipients into managed care plans. This approach may improve access to basic health-care services for Medicaid enrollees with "normal" health-care needs who live close to service delivery sites or who have their own transportation. For those who live farther away, assignment to managed care plans may increase income for the health-care provider while providing few services to the Medicaid recipients. Medicaid enrollees with expensive health problems may find managed care gatekeeping a frustrating and at times life-threatening hindrance. Rather than self-insure, as Medicaid has done up to now, the new managed care programs for Medicaid hope that offering health providers "shared risk" access to the Medicaid population will lower total state and federal outlay.

But why not also experiment to see whether Medicaid recipients might respond to the same kind of incentives being proposed for the rest of the population? If they did, it could lower the total health bill in ways that *benefit* the poor directly and could let them help subsidize the cost of other low-income citizens, as well, through the savings for their own health-care costs that they create. Medicaid participants who now consume a high volume of services, without much personal choice about which services are used, might respond quite differently if they had opportunities for shared risk and shared gain that would become available to the rest of the population. Their greater financial vulnerability makes it necessary for them to have protected risk throughout. However, Chapter 11 has proposed ways to let employees share risk and gain with employers, while staying protected against financial loss or dangers to health. The federal and state governments could try a similar approach to Medicaid enrollees, setting up a few experiments to see whether the same principles could work with this population group, as well.

An Experiment with Low-Income Populations

This book's discussion of ways businesses can give employees a stake in cost-efficient use of health services might also apply to publicly funded health-care recipients. The federal and state governments, like private business, could approach the funding of catastrophic and non-catastrophic health needs differently. Public third party payers could calculate their current Medicaid per-capita costs for health care. Then they might experiment on a state or county basis with alternative approaches to funding catastrophic and non-catastrophic health needs of the Medicaid population. In one state, for example, hospitals might be offered a capitation rate for all federal or state employees and long-term care insurance might be purchased for them at the rate calculated for the population as a whole. Medicaid enrollees then would be folded into the federal employee health insurance pool. (Their costs could be calculated separately if this seemed wisest.) They could be given a health savings account that could be used either for membership in a capitated payment plan for managing their health needs, or they could choose the lowest cost indemnity options available to federal employees through the Federal Employees Health Benefit Plan. This would help end discrimination against recipients of public aid by service providers. The fact that one was a Medicaid enrollee would become invisible.

The rationale behind experimenting in this way is that it might improve both cost and access. The public gamble would be that many Medicaid recipients currently receive more services and diagnostic tests than they need for good health care, and that changes in funding practices could correct for this in the same ways that private businesses could give providers and their own employers different incentives for health-care spending. Medicare and Medicaid entitlements represent the same kind of "pork barrel" incentive for providers to order "the best" whether or not it is in the best interests of the patient. Because public third party payers enforce a sharp discount on price (far below the discount large private employers negotiate) one might expect a number of health-care providers to compensate for this by providing extra services which can be billed, or by accepting capitated payments but providing few services. For this experiment Medicaid recipients would pay "market rates" but the purchasing power of the federal employee pool would be used to negotiate the most favorable market rates currently achievable for the general population.

Medicaid recipients, like many employees, would be offered a choice of how to deal with the first $2,000 of their health-care expenses—the part not covered by guaranteed insurance. They could either use a managed care plan that emphasized prevention and health enhancement or could enter into a protected-risk, shared-gain contract with Medicaid. Those who chose the latter option would enroll in a proactive health promotion service, which would monitor their basic health. In either case costs of noncatastrophic care would be paid for out of a health savings account set up in the recipient's name. Medicaid recipients could use the health savings account to reimburse providers (including their prevention or managed care contractors) for health-care services. The health savings account could only be used to pay for health services; however, any interest it accumulated would stay in the account. Each year Medicaid would add sufficient funds to each savings account to reinstate its original balance.

If Medicaid found it was spending less per-person (after adjusting for inflation) than occurs under the system now in operation, it would keep half of this amount, and share the other half of the savings with the Medicaid recipients, adding it to their savings account. The health savings could be used only for health spending, so long as the balance was $2,000 or less. If savings accumulate beyond $2,000, the recipient would have the right to spend the surplus on investments that would decrease the likelihood that they will need to receive public assistance in the future. Schooling costs, down-payment or mortgage payments for a home, and similar uses that would help stabilize finances could be paid for with this money. If the health savings accounts had an account number that flagged them as publicly subsidized, it would be relatively easy for banks and other financial institutions to monitor expenditures from these accounts, to make sure they conform to legal requirements. The government's surplus, if this experiment works, could be earmarked for health-care subsidies to low-income populations. Thus economies that Medicaid recipients generated out of their own wiser use of resources would benefit both themselves and other poor people. Although they pay no taxes, they would help shoulder their portion of public responsibility for others.

This experiment would let us see what happens to availability of services for the poor, if they "disappear" into purchasing pools and into the negotiated pricing mechanisms used with the larger population. It also would demonstrate whether protected risk and shared gain can help to stabilize public health-care spending. This model, if successful, also could be used with subsidies to the working poor. The public funder simply substitutes for an employer when developing protected-risk and shared-gain strategies with the recipients of the subsidy. (The public funder also substitutes for an employer in terms of shared risk/shared gain relations with providers of care.)

Would this kind of system be applicable to Medicare as well? Perhaps. However, careful experimentation should precede trying it more widely.

Even if the system works well, however, distrust of changes not fully understood might emerge among those currently enrolled in Medicare, so that it would become politically costly to enact: The elderly may prefer to keep their present entitlements in tact, and politicians are sensitive to the backlash that developed over earlier proposals to introduce catastrophic care insurance for Medicare. If so, entry into Medicare could be frozen with its present cohorts. Current Medicare participants could continue to receive their present services, while the aging baby boom cohorts could be directed toward more cost-effective care.

Good, proactive prevention services would have to be available in all communities where the experiment was tried, to protect the poor from unwise economies in basic health care. If the experiment works, health-oriented prevention services will proliferate rapidly, once there is a clear market for them. It would be important to expand this kind of program incrementally, however, first documenting the availability of high quality prevention services in communities before shared risk plans are introduced. This should not create an insurmountable problem. Many public health agencies would quickly adapt to the new market opportunity.

Moving Toward Universal Access to Care

The proposals discussed in this chapter provide no guarantee that every American will have access to basic health-care services, although they could vastly increase the number who get the care they need. While they are no final solution, these proposals provide a new flexibility for addressing the problem of access. They could help build momentum that let a more total solution emerge, because they would help build new public-private partnerships that begin to shift public priorities. Only when that shift occurs is universal access to health services likely to become a reality. The innovations discussed in chapters 10 and 11 suggest ways to free up public funds which could be redirected to increase access to care for those now left out. This chapter has suggested ways to begin making services available to those who most need them, and to build stronger public support for a more basic shift in policy priorities.

A Summary: Strategies for Dealing with Cost and Access

Table 12.2 summarizes the proposals made thus far in Chapters 11 and 12, and suggests how each would affect the larger dynamic at work.

TABLE 12.2 Lowering Costs and Improving Access to Health Care

	1. Cost	Implications for 2. Access	
Proposed Reform Strategy	*a. Changes dynamic keeping payers/users captive to cost increases*	*b. Affects incentives toward expensive care*	*c. Provides new sources of funds to subsidize the poor*
1. Hospital capitation rates	•	•	•
2. Universal catastrophic health insurance (including long-term care)	•	•	•
3. Employer-generated health savings accounts plus employer-self-insurance to pay for other health costs)	•	•	
4. Purchasing pools	•		
5. "Capitated" benefits formula	•	•	•
6. No-fault malpractice insurance reform	•	•	
7. Incentives for specialists to provide primary care	•	•	
8. Physician education re: cost-effective, ecologically-relevant care		•	
9. Reinsurance surcharge		•	•
10. Health-oriented managed care and purchasing services for persons with costly chronic health problems		•	•
11. Funding projects which redirect money flows in the private economy for use by local churches and other agencies that will sponsor access to health services for the uninsured poor			•
12. Absorbing Medicaid population into the Federal Employee Health Benefit pool and providing protected-risk, shared benefit incentives for cost-effective use of services (with prevention safety-net)		and also lessens discrimination against them by providers	•

Equally important will be the improvement in access to care resulting from health-oriented innovations already discussed in Chapter 10. Proactive, worksite health promotion programs will bring health improvement services and basic health-risk monitoring directly to worksites, where many employees have no other regular, ongoing health care. Independent, health-oriented managed care services, particularly because of their use of non-physicians—the American equivalent of barefoot doctors—can bring care to many who now are left out of primary care. Health-oriented managed care can also provide purchasing services and other managed care functions for the chronically ill and progressively disabled so that these patients get the services they need at a reasonable cost. More ecologically-sophisticated treatment strategies, the demedicalizing of life events so that heroic interventions into birth and death requiring high technology are used only where unavoidable, and implementation of environmentally sound economic development policy that reduces exposure to life-threatening sources of disease, all reduce costs of care.

As a result, the public and private sectors will have more ability to pay for the needs for health and disease care that lie ahead. This lets services become available to many who otherwise would be ignored—because public funds have already been allocated and costs to business for health insurance became too great for many employers. In short, the movement toward *health* which the innovations noted in Chapter 10 accelerate makes it possible to approach the full set of problems in health-care reform.

All this requires relatively little legislative change or new tax revenue, compared to the single payer or managed competition proposals that were under discussion in the early 1990s. Tables 12.3 and 12.4 summarize the legislation needed to make these changes.

TABLE 12.3 Health insurance legislation that would be needed for health care to reorient itself toward lower cost and increased access to care

---

1. Health Insurance Reforms:
   A. Voluntary purchasing pools for insurance (with backup from the Federal Employees Health Benefits Plan purchasing pool)
   B. Insurance discounts for contracts that include worksite health promotion
   C. Universal requirements to have hospital coverage as well as catastrophic and long-term care insurance
   D. A Health Protection Mandate in which employers provide access to group-rated health cost protection
2. Reinsurance Reforms affecting Health-care Providers
   A. Creating a single national pool for health-care reinsurance
   B. Adding a surcharge to be redivided among insurers on the basis of their enrollment of populations known to have higher health-care costs

---

Table 12.4 Recommended Federal Actions to Encourage Better
Health for All

1. Changes in Tax Law:
    A. Setting tax-deductible health benefits annually, as best price
       available for mix of catastrophic and non-catastrophic health
       protection and hospital care
    B. Authorizing any payer of these benefits to take the tax deduction
       with protections of worker income to prevent cost-shifting
    C. Authorizing establishment of health savings accounts and setting
       conditions for use of these accounts whenever publicly funded

2. Steps to Encourage Innovation in Health-care Delivery:
    A. Enabling legislation to establish independent, health-oriented
       managed care services
    B. Directives to National Institutes of Health for new kinds of evalua-
       tion of treatment methods, with responsibility to educate physi-
       cians about comparative findings
    C. Authorize experiments in publicly funded health care:
        1. Capitated hospitalization payments for federal employees
        2. Shared-risk health savings accounts for Medicaid recipients
        3. Folding Medicaid recipients in with federal employees for
           health benefits pools and services

3. Redeploying Federal Business Subsidies to Encourage Environmental
   Health Protection
    A. Assistance from defense budget to help defense industries diversify
    B. Technical assistance and tax incentives to help American businesses
       meet current international standards for environmentally-safe
       economic production
    C. Federal research encouragement to develop products and processes
       that lower environmental exposure to health risks
        1. Replacement for the internal combustion engine
        2. Substitutes for CFCs that damage the ozone layer
        3. Environmentally friendly substitutes for gas, oil, coal, and
           atomic sources of energy
        4. Safer ways to dispose of toxic substances

Additional, though still more controversial, legislation (outlined as part
three of Table 12.4) could help integrate health policy with economic development concerns. These would take advantage of this moment in history to redirect federal business "subsidies" that have been part of the Cold
War. These can simultaneously encourage economic prosperity for Americans in a changing world market and lessen exposure to the life-threaten-

ing health risks that come from national and international military and manufacturing activity. (For example, if increasing rates of cancer could be reversed, there would be enormous savings of health-care resources as well as an inestimable improvement in the quality of human life.)

This book has presented a series of fairly daring proposals, which invite us to think in new ways about how to lower the cost of health care without putting the health of the population at risk or subjecting health-care providers to regulations many will evade. These proposals recognize the importance of health care to the economy as a whole. Thus while offering opportunities to lower *captive* costs—to public and private third party payers and to private households—they preserve the ability of health care to prosper economically. These strategies cannot work well unless they have the safety net of a relatively few, concrete innovations that shift the focus of care toward *health*. Once these are in place and begin to exert their own influence, there is something of a domino effect, as one reform strategy after another begins to work in a different way.

Some readers will like these suggestions. Others will not. Those who are loyal to a particular approach to reform may find ingredients from other approaches unpalatable. Others may be deeply skeptical about some of the assumptions that underlie this proposal. If so, I invite them to try their own hand at putting together an equally comprehensive but better set of proposals that can work within the current constraints affecting health policy choice, also noting how an emphasis on *health* can affect the whole.

Chapters 10, 11, and 12, however, reframe the nature of the problem to be addressed and demonstrate a new way to combine some of our best thinking, to date. They address sources of disease and sources of cost increase, refocusing resources to improve *health* and in the process shifting the nature of disease care in more ecologically sophisticated directions. Each part reinforces the impact that the others would make.

The package of reforms sketched out here is imaginable and would be relatively simple to introduce. Most pieces redirect present spending, rather than require major new sources of funds. A number of the proposals could be introduced without requiring new legislation. Others build on proposals that already have considerable bipartisan support. New ingredients discussed here and in Chapters 10 and 11 change the impact that some earlier proposals would have by themselves, however. I believe these new proposals would attract support from various public constituencies. Rather than pitting one interest group against another, this set of proposals moves toward win/win solutions for all. They simplify government and business spending and bureaucratic administration, minimizing regulation while helping redirect resources to places where service is most needed. The overall cost of health care can go down, if we provide better prevention services, make insurance cheaper but more comprehensive, use health savings accounts to encourage better choices of health-care services, and change the dynamic affecting growth of hospital costs. Then, by redirecting public spending, it should be possible to subsidize all of the poor, including the working poor, so that they can get health services on the same basis as other Americans. Quality and freedom of choice can be protected, while discouraging waste of resources.

Is all this too good to be true? Perhaps—and yet perhaps not. I have sketched broadly here, without doing the fine-tuned cost-accounting that will show how well all the pieces fit together in economic terms. That task needs to be done—and almost surely will be, if policy makers or the public find the suggestions attractive. Almost surely, some parts will need redesigning so that this works in practice. My intent here is not to argue for every detail of this particular plan. Rather, I want to open a new kind of dialogue about health-care reform, showing how a shift in emphasis from disease to *health* changes our options. As single payer advocates, believers in the free market, and those who opt for managed competition reassess the situation, I urge them to learn from one another, and to explore how refocusing on *health* strengthens what they are trying to accomplish.

In Conclusion

As American health care continues to change, the revolution that made modern medical science preeminent a century ago is being superseded by an equally profound reorganization. Both the underlying *ideas* on which health care is based and the *organization of care* is changing, as is the way all this relates to larger social, economic, and political forces.

This book has traced both changes in ideas about health and disease that have occurred during the past half-century and changes in the organization of health-care services during the same period of time. A series of social, economic, and political developments at a national and international level led to new ways to organize and fund health-care services. All industrialized nations were building their health-care systems on the model of applied medical science, with research-based care the ideal for service delivery. In the U.S., because of earlier political circumstances that prevented the creation of a nationally coordinated health-care system, the organization of American health care went in rather different directions than were being pursued elsewhere in the international economy. Medical service delivery gradually evolved into a health-care industry, recognizing itself as such and organizing accordingly. Health care became one of the most vibrant sectors of the American economy, frequently a leader in economic growth, and the largest employer. Its research-based medicine focused on the use of pharmaceuticals, mechanical devices, and surgery, intervention strategies that reflect an earlier view of the body as a machine, paying relatively little attention to internal processes of problem-solving that occur normally. Federal funds stimulated medical research which worked from these premises, and American medicine developed increasingly sophisticated high technology to aid in the diagnosis of medical problems and to "regulate" body processes that had gone out of control. It paid relatively little attention to the prevention of disease or to the encouragement of natural health-building processes. It ignored almost completely mental, social, or environmental factors that affect biochemical processes. The result has been a technologically sophisticated but increasingly expensive health-care delivery system that now threatens the financial stability of the third party payers—businesses and government—that pay the bulk of health-care costs. They have become captive to the constant increase in costs that are part of

American health care. Now, however, new research discoveries and renewed respect for other medical traditions around the world are beginning to change our focus for attention.

This book has traced the evolution of American health-care organization in some detail, showing how innovations arose in response to moments of crisis or opportunity that were created by changing national and international political and economic developments. It has shown how the health-care industry model for service delivery became ever more expensive, affecting the well-being of both business and governmental funders, and growing beyond the ability of most private households to finance. It has noted wide-ranging efforts that have been made to control costs, and their persistent growth, regardless of which strategies were tried. The abandonment of major health-care legislative reform in 1994 was not that different from what happened with earlier attempts to find a political solution to the emerging dynamic. As happened earlier, the organization of health-care services has continued to evolve, despite legislative stalemate. Unfortunately, it is evolving in ways that try to protect the interests of major funders rather than correct the underlying dynamic which leaves more and more Americans without access to basic health-care services. This has happened before, and it does not bode well for the future.

This book has argued that health reform will continue to falter until we shift our focus for attention more fundamentally. We need to find better ways to address *sources* of disease and health, not simply to manage disease problems after they develop. Attempts at health-care reform must address underlying sources of cost increase, rather than simply trying to limit their consequences. These sources include a preference for use of constantly evolving high technology, rather than using this as a fall-back strategy when simpler interventions do not work; a preference for highly specialized services that do not address health-building as a whole so that overall health improves; funding arrangements that encourage use of many costly services; and the organization of health-care services to maximize profit. (Even "non-profit" health-care providers like to generate an "operating surplus"—excess resources that do not have to be distributed to shareholders.)

Much of this book has explored efforts to rethink basic approaches to health care, noting lessons to be learned from previous efforts to move beyond medical science's almost total dependence on biochemistry and its preference for high technology. It has noted other innovations that refocus services to encourage health building rather than attend primarily to the management of disease. This book has noted, as well, how research understandings have grown beyond the practices that much of current health-care delivery still uses. Contemporary medical science research has replaced the germ theory of disease and the principle of a single cause (and single cure) for each disease. In their place, growing out of DNA research, comes an understanding that information transfer lies at the heart of health and disease. Genetics gives each generation a set of instructions for how to solve various survival problems. Interactions with the larger environment, including interactions with other species that enter our bodies, environmental chemicals that become part of our cells, and our own mental and emotional reactions to our larger environment, alter the information flow that affects how our biochemistry works. In place of the germ theory of disease now comes an understanding of the ecology of the self. The metaphor of the body as a machine is replaced by the mind-body as an active problem solver. In place of "blind" biochemical reactions we now explore the self's interactive dialogue with its environment. As understandings have grown about the immune system, genetic mutation and other processes of the body and the mind, a much less passive, much more ecological understanding of human health processes is emerging. Unfortunately, most medical practice has not yet adapted to the implications of these discoveries. Our high-tech interventions, in consequence, become simultaneously remarkably sophisticated and yet often quite crude, in the sense of throwing off larger sequences of internal activity and immobilizing balances that still are at work.

International developments, chronicled earlier in this account, are producing a series of emerging health problems that the health-care industry is poorly equipped to meet. Had this account stopped with a discussion of the mainstream of health-care delivery and legislative efforts to reform it, it would be a depressing story. Each of the problematic trends—in emerging needs for care, in growth in the costs for care, in inability of third party funders or private households to continue as captive payers with no end in sight—continues. For half a century we have been rethinking and reforming health-care delivery. Clearly we need a new vision. Now we are beginning to have one.

Some contemporary health delivery is developing ways to work with the natural ecology of health rather than to ignore it. This shift of attention to *health* costs less, and discourages the onset of disease. It involves attention not only to biological and biochemical processes, but also to the emotional, social, and physical environments with which we interact. This book has drawn attention to social experiments that now are pursuing these newer understandings of how health can best be encouraged, noting strengths and weaknesses of each approach, looking for lessons to be learned that might be applied more widely.

Chapters 10, 11, and 12 address health-care policy more directly. They note emerging international developments which affect the nature of health problems that must be addressed, setting limits on resources available for earlier styles of care and creating opportunities for broader integration of health and economic policy. Chapter 10 has identified steps now underway that can provide an institutional shift reorienting us toward *health*. Chapter 11 reframes the nature of the problem to be addressed, proposes some new forms of public/private collaboration within a redivided healthcare market and suggests ways the institutional shift toward *health* described in Chapter 10 could be used in combination with current proposals for health insurance reform to solve our current dilemmas of cost containment more satisfactorily. Chapter 12 suggests ways the new reframing of the problem would let us reapproach problems of access to care. If these chapters were successful they will have opened a different kind of dialogue about where we can go from here, and how. Whether or not readers endorse this particular combination of strategies, they now have an invitation to enter into a dialogue about how to move disease care into a *health*-care system.

We need to see clearly where we are now. Two images of our situation come to mind. The first image—of a growing cancer—provides an appropriate analogy for health care's cost inflation. The second image — of a crew bailing water out of a boat rather than patching the hole where the water comes in, as the boat drifts toward rapids and then a waterfall — reminds us of previous efforts at health-care reform. It is time to do something differently.

We also need a clear vision of what we could do differently. Fortunately, not all approaches to service delivery involve a cancerous growth in cost over time. Fortunately also, other approaches to health care have also been afloat. Their advocates have been learning how to steer more successfully through the current of cost inflation which threatens to drown us, while also discovering where to look for leaks and how to plug them. That is what the second half of this book has been about.

These dramatic images suggest impending crisis in the not-too-distant future. Another image, consequently, may be equally useful. The Chinese symbol for "crisis" combines two pictograms. One signals "danger"; the other, "opportunity".

We face real danger, but also a moment of unusual opportunity, thanks to the rethinking of options that has occurred already, and the changes in the national and international world order that can let us redeploy resources. By refocusing on health and understanding the ecological character of health and disease, we can begin to head in new directions. Momentum to do so already exists. This is a moment of unusual opportunity that occurs before we enter a period of danger. It is time to act. Let us make the most of it.

Appendix: Tables

TABLE 1.   National Health Expenditures in real $, constant 1982 $, and as percent of the GNP, by year (in billions)

Year	Actual Costs	Costs in 1982 $	Percent of GNP
1950	$12.1	$57.5	4.6
1955	17.9	69.2	4.7
1960	27.1	89.7	5.3
1965	41.6	125.3	5.9
1970	74.4	182.8	7.3
1971	82.3	191.0	7.5
1972	92.3	204.7	7.6
1973	102.5	216.2	7.5
1974	116.1	226.3	7.9
1975	132.9	239.0	8.3
1976	152.2	254.5	8.5
1977	172.0	265.4	8.6
1978	193.4	277.1	8.6
1979	216.6	286.5	8.6
1980	249.1	296.9	9.1
1981	288.6	311.7	9.5
1982	323.8	323.8	10.2
1983	356.1	335.3	10.5
1984	387.0	346.8	10.3
1985	420.1	359.7	10.5
1986	452.3	369.5	10.7
1987	495.5	385.0	10.9
1988	544.0	404.5	11.2
1989	604.1	428.4	11.6
1990	662.2	448.3	12.2
1995	(est.) 1007.0	(est.) 560.4	(est.) 15.0

Data sources for Table 1: Health Care Financing Administration, Office of the Actuary: Data from the Office of National Cost Estimates, 1991; U.S. Department of Health, Education, and Welfare, Social Security Administration, *Social Security Bulletin*, December, 1970. Constant 1982 dollars were computed using Table B-3, Implicit price deflators for service products, 1929-1990, 252, in U.S. Government, *Economic Report of the President. Annual Report of the Council of Economic Advisers, Appendix B: Statistical Tables Relating to Income, Employment and Production*, 1991. Sources for 1991-1995 data: Health Care Financing Administration, Office of the Actuary, and the Congressional Budget Office for projections. Population estimates and projects from the Social Security Administration.

TABLE 2. Influences on Inflation: Comparisons of changes in the
          consumer price index (CPI)

Year	Total CPI	All Health Care	Hospital Room	Energy: Fuel Oil and Coal
1967	100.0	100.0	100.0	100.0
1970	116.3	120.6	145.4	110.1
1972	125.3	132.5	173.9	118.5
1973	133.1	137.7	182.1	135.0
1975	161.2	168.6	236.1	253.8
1980	246.8	265.9	418.9	556.4
1981	272.4	294.5	481.1	675.9
1985	322.2	402.1	710.5	619.5
1988	354.5	402.1	880.6	504.5
1990	391.3	577.3	1138.9	429.0
1991	407.8	627.7	1246.1	430.7

This table compares the relative change in prices for all consumer items, with the relative increases in prices for health care as a whole, for hospitalization, and for energy (fuel). The CPI sets 1967 prices at 100.0 and then computes changes from that base-line price. CPI figures for 1988 had been calculated at 1982 prices in government tables, but were recalculated here to fit the earlier comparison point with 1967 prices.

Data sources for Table 2: Table 138, Index of Medical Care Prices, 1970, 1986, 1991, and Table 738, Consumer Price Indexes by Major Groups: 1950-1991, in U.S. Government, *Statistical Abstracts of the United States*, 108th and 112th editions, Washington, DC: U.S. Government Printing Office, 1988, 1992.

TABLE 3.   Business Health Spending as Percent of Corporate Profits

| | *Business Health Spending as a Share of:* | | | |
| | *Labor Compensation* | | *Corporate Profits* | |
Year	*Wages & Salaries*	*Fringe Benefits*	*Before Taxes*	*After Taxes*
1965	2.2%	22.4	8.4	14.0
1970	3.5%	29.2	19.8	36.1
1975	3.5%	29.2	19.8	36.1
1980	5.8%	31.7	27.3	42.6
1985	7.2%	38.9	51.3	89.9
1986	7.5%	40.5	57.5	110.4
1987	7.3%	40.8	48.5	90.1
1988	7.7%	43.2	48.3	84.8
1989	8.1%	45.1	55.1	98.3
1990	8.5%	45.5	(est) 61.1	(est) 107.9

The righthand column compares health care costs for business with after taxes profits. The 1980s figures reflect both a declining profit picture for business (see Table 4) and a constantly rising health care cost. These comparisons make business' interest in an alternate way to handle health care for employees immediately understandable.

Data source for Table 3: K.R. Levit and C.A. Cowan, "Business, Households, and Governments: Health Care Costs 1990." *Health Care Financing Review* 13(2), Winter 1991, 88.

TABLE 4.   The Changing Profit Picture for American Manufacturing
                Corporations

| Yearly Average | Corporate Mfg. Profits | | Manufacturing Profits | |
	Actual $ (billions)	(1982 $) (billions)	As % of all corporate profits	Change in profitability
1950-1964	$21.6	($66.5)	51.1%	+37%
1965-1972	37.4	(83.6)	46.2%	+26%
1973-1980	61.8	(97.1)	42.5%	+16%
1981-1983	72.2	(72.8)	38.8%	-33%
1984-1990	101.5	(90.6)	33.7%	+24%
1981-1990	82.6	(76.2)	35.4%	-21%

Changes in manufacturing profitability reflect changes in average profits for manufacturing corporations, in constant $ for the time periods specified in comparison with the preceding time period.

Data source for Table 4: Constant 1982 dollars were computed using Table B-3, Implicit price deflators for durable and non-durable goods, 1929-1990. Table B-88 and B-89, Corporate profits by industry, 1929-1988, 350-351, in U.S. Government, Economic Report of the President. Annual Report of the Council of Economic Advisers, Appendix B: Statistical Tables Relating to Income, Employment and Production, 1992.

TABLE 5. U.S. Private Corporations, Direct InvestmentAbroad (in billions)

	Actual dollars			In constant 1982 dollars		
	1970	1980	1987	1970	1980	1987
Manufacturing	32.3	89.2	126.6	76.9	104.1	107.6
Petroleum	21.7	47.6	66.4	51.7	55.5	56.4
Other	24.2	78.8	115.8	57.6	91.9	98.4
Total	78.2	215.6	308.8	186.2	251.5	262.4
Major Recipient						
Canada	22.8	45.0	56.9	54.3	52.5	48.3
United Kingdom	8.0	28.6	44.7	19.0	33.4	38.0
West Germany	4.6	15.4	24.5	10.9	18.0	20.8
Switzerland	1.8	11.3	20.0	4.3	13.2	17.0
Japan	1.5	6.2	14.3	3.6	7.2	12.1

Data source for Table 5: U.S. Department of State, Bureau of Public Affairs, "Foreign Direct Investment in a Global Economy," based on U.S. Department of Commerce data, Washington, DC, March 1989, 7. Constant 1982 dollars were computed using Table B-3, Implicit price deflators for gross national product, 1929-1990, 290-291, in U.S. Government, *Economic Report of the President. Annual Report of the Council of Economic Advisers, Appendix B: Statistical Tables Relating to Income, Employment and Production,* 1991.

TABLE 6.   Employment Status of the American Population 16 Years Old and Over: 1950 to 1991

		Labor Force				
		Employed			Unemployed	
Year	Number	Resident Armed Forces	Civilian	Number	% of labor force	Not in labor force
1950	63,377	1,169	58,918	3,288	5.2	42,787
1960	71,489	1,861	65,778	3,852	5.4	47,617
1965	76,401	1,946	71,088	3,366	4.4	52,058
1970	84,889	2,118	78,678	4,093	4.8	54,315
1975	95,453	1,678	85,846	7,929	8.3	59,377
1980	108,544	1,604	99,303	7,637	7.0	60,806
1985	117,167	1,706	107,150	8,312	7.1	62,744
1990	126,424	1,637	117,914	6,874	5.4	63,262
1991	126,867	1,564	116,877	8,426	6.6	64,462
DIST. (%)						
1950	59.7	1.1	55.5	3.1		40.3
1960	60.0	1.6	55.2	3.2		40.0
1970	61.0	1.5	56.5	2.9		39.0
1980	64.1	.9	58.6	4.5		35.9
1990	66.6	.9	62.2	3.6		33.4

(In thousands, excepts as indicated. These data exclude institutionalized populations in the U.S. Annual averages of monthly figures are based on Current Population Survey section 1 and Appendix III. See *also Historical Statistics, Colonial Times to 1970*, series D 11-10 and D 85-86.)

Data source for Table 6: U.S. Department of Labor, Bureau of Labor Statistics, Bulletin 2307 and *Employment and Earnings*, monthly.

TABLE 7. Corporate Contributions to U.S. Tax Revenue

Year	Taxes as % of GNP	% of tax revenue coming from corporations
1966	18.6	32.7
1967	18.7	30.3
1968	19.8	30.5
1969	20.7	27.6
1970	19.2	25.5
1971	18;.4	26.6
1972	19.1	24.3
1973	19.4	24.4
1974	20.0	22.7
1975	18.4	22.9
1976	19.1	22.9
1977	19.3	22.5
1978	19.6	22.5
1979	20.1	20.5
1980	20.3	19.7
1981	20.9	19.1
1982	20.1	15.3
1983	19.4	17.1
1984	19.2	18.0
1985	19.6	16.7
1986	19.6	16.2
1987	20.2	17.2
1988	20.0	17.2
1989	20.2	16.0
1990	20.3	15.5

Data sources for Table 7: Table B-8, Gross National Product by Sector, 1929-90 (in billions), 296, and Table B-81, Federal Government receipts and expenditures, national income and product accounts, 1960-90, 381, (percentages were computed for this table), in U.S. Government, *Economic Report of the President, Annual Report of the Council of Economic Advisers, Appendix B: Statistical Tables Relating to Income, Employment and Production.*

TABLE 8.   Changes in Total Federal Expenditures

Year	Actual dollars (in billions)	Constant 1982 $ (in billions)	Percent change
1960	$93.9	$380.2	15.2%
1965	125.3	445.9	17.3%
1970	207.8	564.7	26.6%
1975	364.2	637.8	12.9%
1980	616.1	729.7	14.4%
1985	1017.5	933.5	27.9%
1990	1273.0	1032.4	10.6%
1960-70	+113.9	+184.5	+48.5%
1970-80	+407.3	+165.0	+29.2%
1980-90	+255.5	+303.7	+41.5%
1960-90	+1179.1	+652.2	+171.5%

Data sources for Table 8: Table B-79, Federal and State and local government receipts and expenditures, national income and product accounts, 1929-1990, 379, with constant 1982 dollars figures using Table B-3, Implicit price deflators for federal expenditures, 1929-90, 290-291, in U.S. Government, *Economic Report of the President, Annual Report of the Council of Economic Advisers, Appendix B: Statistical Tables Relating to Income, Employment and Production.*

TABLE 9.   Changes in Federal Expenditures for Personal Health Care Costs

Year	Actual costs (billions)	Costs in 1982 $ (billions)	Medicare enrollees (millions)
1965	$3.4	($10.2)	n.a.
1970	10.4	(25.6)	20.5
1975	21.3	(38.3)	25.0
1980	42.5	(50.7)	28.5
1985	69.0	(62.2)	31.9
1990	113.9	(77.1)	34.2

Data sources for Table 9: Actual costs: Health Care Financing Administration, Office of the Actuary. Data from the Office of National Health Statistics. Reported in *Health Care Financing Review*, vol. 13, #2, 86. 1982 constant dollar equivalents figured using the Implicit price deflator for service industries, Table B-3, in U.S. Government, *Economic Report of the President*, 1992. Medicare enrollment figures from Table 575, Medicare Program—Enrollments and Payments, 1970 to 1990, U.S. Bureau of the Census, *Statistical Abstracts of the United States*, 112th edition, 1992.

TABLE 10.   Changes in Health Care Spending and Military Spending as percent of federal spending and as percent of gross national product (GNP)

Year	Federal Outlays		Gross National Product	
	Health	Military	Health	Military
1960	3.1%	52.2%	5.3%	9.5%
1965	3.8%	42.8%	5.9%	7.5%
1970	8.5%	41.8%	7.3%	8.3%
1975	10.0%	26.0%	8.3%	5.7%
1980	11.7%	22.7%	9.2%	5.0%
1985	12.5%	26.7%	10.5%	6.4%
1989	14.7%	26.2%	11.6%	5.9%

Data sources for Table 10: Health Care Financing Administration, Office of the Actuary, Office of National Cost Estimates, April, 1991, and Table 533: National Defense Outlays and Veterans Benefits, 1960 to 1989, 330, U.S. Bureau of the Census, *Statistical Abstracts of the United States*, 110th edition, 1990.

TABLE 11. Changes in the Annual Federal Deficit and the Gross
           Federal Debt ($ in billions)

Year	Federal Deficit		Gross Federal Debt	
	Actual $	1982 $	Actual $	1982$
1950	$3.1	$12.97	$256.9	$1074.9
1955	3.0	11.03	274.4	1008.8
1960	0.3	00.97	290.0	941.4
1965	1.4	4.0	323.2	956.2
1970	2.8	6.6	382.6	911.0
1975	53.2	89.7	544.1	917.5
1980	73.8	86.1	914.3	1066.9
1985	212.3	191.4	1827.5	1647.9
1990	220.4	178.8	3206.3	2600.4
1950-60	-2.8	-12.0	$34.0	$133.5
1960-70	2.5	5.6	91.7	30.4
1970-80	71.0	79.5	532.0	155.9
1980-90	146.6	92.7	2292.0	1534.0
1950-90	217.3	165.8	2949.4	1525.5

Data sources for Table 11: Table B-76, Federal receipts, outlays, surplus or deficit
and debt, selected fiscal years, 1929-1990, 375; Constant 1982 dollars were computed using Table B-3, Implicit price deflators for gross national product, 1929-
1990, 290-291, in U.S. Government, *Economic Report of the President. Annual Report of
the Council of Economic Advisers, Appendix B: Statistical Tables Relating to Income, Employment and Production.*

TABLE 12A. Costs for health services & supplies, by amount & type of payer:
Who is bearing the brunt of increasing health care costs?
—In Actual Dollars

	Health Care Costs in Actual Dollars				
Year	Total Health Care Costs (billions)	Business (billions)	Govt. (billions)	Private Households (billions)	Others (billions)
1965	$38.2	$6.5	$7.9	$23.1	$0.7
1970	69.1	15.1	18.9	33.6	1.5
1975	124.7	28.8	38.5	54.9	2.5
1980	238.9	64.8	76.7	90.9	6.7
1982	309.4	90.7	97.7	118.7	2.3
1985	407.2	115.0	128.3	152.0	11.9
1986	438.9	127.3	135.9	162.7	13.0
1987	476.8	133.6	149.6	179.8	13.8
1988	526.2	153.1	163.4	194.3	15.4
1989	582.1	169.7	184.6	210.3	17.5
1990	643.4	186.2	212.9	224.7	19.6

Data sources for Table 12A: Health Care Financing Administration, Office of the Actuary, Office of National Cost Estimates, April, 1991. Compare with tables reported in Katherine R. Levit, Mark S. Freeland and Daniel R. Waldo, "Health spending and ability to pay: Business, individual and government," *Health Care Financing Review*, Spring 1989, (10), #3, 3, which were figured before the Health Care Financing Administration recalculated health care spending. 1982 figures in tables 12 and 13 came from this issue, before the recalculation. Constant 1982 dollars were computed using Table B-3, Implicit price deflators for service products, 1929-1990, 290-291, in U.S. Government, *Economic Report of the President. Annual Report of the Council of Economic Advisers*, Appendix B: Statistical Tables Relating to Income, Employment and Production, 1991.

TABLE 12B. Costs for health services & supplies, by amount & type of payer:
Who is bearing the brunt of increasing health care costs?
—In Constant 1982 Dollars

| | Health Care Costs in 1982 Dollars | | | | |
Year	Total Health Care Costs (billions)	Business (billions)	Govt. (billions)	Private Households (billions)	Others (billions)
1965	$115.1	$19.6	$23.8	$69.6	$2.1
1970	169.8	37.1	46.4	82.6	3.7
1975	224.3	51.8	69.2	98.7	4.5
1980	284.7	77.2	91.4	108.3	8.0
1982	309.4	90.7	97.7	118.7	2.3
1985	347.7	98.2	109.6	129.8	10.2
1986	358.6	104.0	111.0	132.9	10.6
1987	370.5	103.8	116.2	139.7	10.1
1988	391.2	113.8	121.5	144.5	11.4
1989	412.8	120.4	130.9	149.1	12.4
1990	435.6	126.1	144.1	152.1	13.3

Data sources for Table 12B: Health Care Financing Administration, Office of the Actuary, Office of National Cost Estimates, April, 1991. Compare with tables reported in Katherine R. Levit, Mark S. Freeland and Daniel R. Waldo, "Health spending and ability to pay: Business, individual and government," *Health Care Financing Review,* Spring 1989, (10), #3, 3, which were figured before the Health Care Financing Administration recalculated health care spending. 1982 figures in tables 12 and 13 came from this issue, before the recalculation. Constant 1982 dollars were computed using Table B-3, Implicit price deflators for service products, 1929-1990, 290-291, in U.S. Government, *Economic Report of the President. Annual Report of the Council of Economic Advisers,* Appendix B: Statistical Tables Relating to Income, Employment and Production, 1991.

TABLE 13.   Percent of Health Care Costs Borne by Each Payer Group

Year	Total Health Care Costs	Business	Govt.	Private Households	Others
1965	100.0	17.0	20.7	60.5	1.8
1970	100.0	21.8	27.4	48.6	2.2
1975	100.0	23.1	30.9	42.4	3.6
1980	100.0	27.1	32.1	38.0	2.8
1982	100.0	29.3	31.6	38.4	0.7
1985	100.0	28.2	31.5	37.3	3.0
1986	100.0	29.3	31.0	37.1	2.6
1987	100.0	28.0	31.4	37.7	2.9
1988	100.0	29.1	31.1	36.9	2.9
1989	100.0	29.2	31.7	36.1	3.0
1990	100.0	28.9	33.1	35.0	3.0

Data sources for Table 13: Health Care Financing Administration, Office of the Actuary, Office of National Cost Estimates, April, 1991. Compare with tables reported in Katherine R. Levit, Mark S. Freeland and Daniel R. Waldo, "Health spending and ability to pay: Business, individual and government," *Health Care Financing Review,* Spring 1989, (10), #3, 3, which were figured before the Health Care Financing Administration recalculated health care spending. 1982 figures in tables 12 and 13 came from this issue, before the recalculation. Constant 1982 dollars were computed using Table B-3, Implicit price deflators for service products, 1929-1990, 290-291, in U.S. Government, *Economic Report of the President. Annual Report of the Council of Economic Advisers,* Appendix B: Statistical Tables Relating to Income, Employment and Production, 1991.

TABLE 14A. Growth in Number of HMO Plans

Year	All Plans	Group Plans[1]	IPA Plans[2]	Mixed Plans
1976	174	122	41	--
1980	235	138	97	--
1985	478	234	244	--
1987	647	238	409	--
1989	604	219	385	--
1990	572	212	360	--
1991	553	168	346	39
1992	555	166	340	49
1993	551	150	332	69
1994	540	117	319	104
1995	550	107	323	120

[1]Group plans include all staff group and network model HMOs.

[2]Individual Practice Associations HMOs operate under contracts with an association of physicians from various settings (a mixture of solo and group practices) to provide health services.

Data sources for Table 14A: The data in this table are reworked from Table 136 Health Maintenance Organizations (HMOs) and Enrollment, According to Model Type, Geographic Region, and Federal Program: United States Selected Years 1976-95, in U.S. Department of Health and Human Services, Public Health Service, *Health United States, 1995.*

TABLE 14B.   Growth in Number of HMO Enrollees[1]

Year	Total Enrollees[2] (in millions)	Medicare Enrollees[3] (in millions)	Medicaid Enrollees[4] (in millions)	Percent of total Population Enrolled in HMOs
1976	6.0	--	--	2.8%
1980	9.1	0.4	0.3	4.0%
1985	21.0	1.1	0.6	8.9%
1987	29.2	1.7	0.8	12.2%
1989	31.9	1.8	1.0	13.0%
1990	33.0	1.8	1.2	13.4%
1991	34.0	2.0	1.4	13.6%
1992	36.1	2.2	1.7	14.3%
1993	38.4	2.2	1.7	15.1%
1994	42.2	2.5	2.6	16.1%
1995	46.2	2.9	3.5	17.7%

[1]Data as of June 30 in 1976-84, December 31 in 1985-87, and January 1 in 1989-95. Medicaid enrollment in 1989-90 are as of June 30. HMOs in Guam are not included prior to 1995.

[2]Data for 1989 and later include enrollment in managed care health insuring organizations.

[3]Federal program enrollment in HMOs refers to enrollment by Medicare beneficiaries where the Medicare program contracts directly with the HMO to pay the appropriate annual premium.

[4]Federal program enrollment in HMOs refers to enrollment by Medicaid beneficiaries where the Medicaid program contracts directly with the HMO to pay the appropriate annual premium.

Data sources for Table 14B: The data in this table are reworked from Table 136 Health Maintenance Organizations (HMOs) and Enrollment, According to Model Type, Geographic Region, and Federal Program: United States Selected Years 1976-95, in U.S. Department of Health and Human Services, Public Health Service, *Health United States, 1995.*

TABLE 15.   Trends in Community Hospital Utilization Rates

	Percent of Occupancy, by Type of Hospital			
Year	*All Hospitals*	*Private Non-profits*	*Public Comm. Hospitals*	*For-Profit Hospitals*
1972	75.4	77.5	71.0	68.7
1973	75.7	77.9	71.4	68.3
1974	75.6	77.9	71.0	67.5
1975	75.0	77.5	70.4	65.9
1976	74.6	77.2	69.8	64.8
1977	73.8	76.4	68.9	64.6
1978	73.6	76.2	69.2	63.8
1979	73.9	76.5	69.5	63.9
1980	75.8	78.2	71.1	65.2
1981	70.0	78.6	71.6	66.4
1982	75.3	77.8	71.1	65.6
1983	73.5	75.8	70.4	63.1
1984	69.0	71.4	66.2	57.0
1985	64.8	67.2	62.9	52.1
1986	64.3	66.8	62.7	50.7
1987	64.9	67.6	63.1	51.1
1988	65.5	68.2	63.9	50.9
1989	66.2	68.8	64.9	51.7
1990	66.8	69.3	65.3	52.8

Diagnostically Related Groups (DRG) Reimbursement for Medicare hospital patients was introduced in 1983.

Data source for Table 15: Table 1, Trends in Utilization, Personnel, and Finances for Selected Years from 1946 through 1990, Table 2a. Utilization, Personnel and Finances in Short-Term Hospitals, in American Hospital Association, *Hospital Statistics*. Chicago: American Hospital Association, 1989-1990, 2-8.

TABLE 16.   Changes in the Number of Nonprofit and For-Profit Hospital Beds

Year	All Hospitals	Private Non-profits	Public Comm. Hospitals	For- Profit Hospitals
1946	473,000	301,000	133,000	39,000
1950	505,000	332,000	131,000	42,000
1955	568,000	389,000	142,000	37,000
1960	639,000	446,000	156,000	37,000
1965	741,000	515,000	179,000	47,000
1970	849,000	592,000	204,000	53,000
1975	947,000	659,000	215,000	73,000
1980	992,000	693,000	212,000	87,000
1981	1,006,000	706,000	213,000	88,000
1982	1,015,000	712,000	212,000	91,000
1983	1,021,000	718,000	209,000	94,000
1984	1,020,000	717,000	203,000	100,000
1985	1,003,000	708,000	191,000	104,000
1986	982,000	690,000	185,000	107,000
1987	961,000	673,000	182,000	106,000
1988	950,000	668,000	178,000	104,000
1989	935,000	661,000	172,000	102,000
1990	929,000	657,000	171,000	101,000

Diagnostically Related Groups (DRG) Reimbursement for Medicare hospital patients was introduced in 1983.

Data source for Table 16: Table 1, Trends in Utilization, Personnel, and Finances for Selected Years from 1946 through 1990, in American Hospital Association, *Hospital Statistics*. Chicago: American Hospital Association, 1989-1990, 2-7.

Chapter Notes

Introduction: The Deepening Crisis

[1]V.R. Fuchs, "The best health care system in the world?"

[2]U.S. Dept. of Health and Human Services, *Health Status of the Disadvantaged Chartbook.*

[3]E. Friedman, "The uninsured: From dilemma to crisis" (hereafter called "The uninsured"); P.F. Short, *National Medical Expenditure Survey: Estimates of the Uninsured Population, Calendar Year 1987: Data Summary 2*; D. Chollet and F.J. Mages, *Uninsured in the United States: The Nonelderly Population Without Health Insurance, 1988.*

[4]Robin Toner, "Lobbyists scurry for a place on the health-reform train," New York *Times*, March 20, 1993, 142, 1; Christi Harlan, John Connor, and Thomas T. Vogel, Jr., "Securities firms set ban on political gifts," The *Wall Street Journal*, Oct. 19, 1993, C1.

[5]Clyde H. Farnsworth, "Soaring costs for health care touch off service cuts and fees," New York *Times*, Nov. 14, 1993, A4.

[6]E. Friedman, "The uninsured".

[7]A.C. Enthoven, *Theory and Practice of Managed Competition in Health Care Finance.*

[8]Participants in the Airlie House and first Waldorf-Astoria conferences heard presentations by Herbert Benson, Harvard Medical School, on the role of stress in creating susceptibility to illness; Ken Pelletier, the Department of Behavioral Medicine at the University of California Medical School in San Francisco, a pioneer in biofeedback (mind-body) control of physical states; Gay Luce, writer and innovator who was working with new approaches to the problems of aging; Tom McEwen from the Mellon Foundation; and Archie Cochran, a policy analyst from the United Kingdom.

[9]NBC, "What price health?" NBC Special Report, 1992.

[10]See Table 1 in Appendix.

[11]See Table 3 in Appendix.

[12]E. Friedman, "The uninsured".

[13]*Ibid.*

[14]E.P. Steinberg, J. Feder, and J. Hadley, "Comparison of uninsured and privately insured hospital patients: Condition on admission, resource use, and outcome."

[15]A.R. Hinman, "what will it take to fully protect all american children with vaccines?"

[16]E. Friedman, "The uninsured."

[17]S.A. Schroeder and L.G. Sandy, "Specialty distribution of u.s. physicians—the invisible driver of health care costs."

[18]V.R. Fuchs, "The best health care system in the world?"

[19]M.I. Taragin, et al., "Physician demographics and risk of medical malpractice."

[20]A. Cranston, "AIDS update."

[21]See Alvin R. Tarlov, Barbara H. Kehrer, Donna P. Hall, Sarah E. Samuels, Gwendolyn S. Grown, Michael R.J. Felix, and Jane A. Ross, "Foundation Work: The Health Promotion Program of the Henry J. Kaiser Foundation," the Henry J. Kaiser Family Foundation Annual Reports, and interview with Lawrence W. Green, May 28, 1989.

[22]R.R. Clayton and C. Ritter, "The epidemiology of alcohol and drug abuse among adolescents"; P.M. O'Malley, et al., *Quantitative and Qualitative Changes in Cocaine Use Among High School Seniors, College Students, and Young Adults.*

[23]Marlise Simons, "Massive ozone and smog defile Atlantic skies," New York *Times*, October 12, 1992, A1.

[24]Alicia Hills Moore, "The other worry: Atomic wastes," *Fortune* 118: 114, August 1, 1988; "Further study needed," *Bul. Atomic Scientists*, 46:4, July-Aug., 1990; "Catch-22", *Bul. Atomic Scientists*, 46:6, Sept.,1990; "Toxic wasteland," 40–43; J. Griffith, et al., "Cancer mortality in U.S. counties with hazardous waste sites and ground water pollution," 69-74; K. Baverstock, et al., "Thyroid cancer after Chernobyl," 21-22.

[25]Paul Brodeur, "The hazards of eletromagnetic fields (I) (II) and (III)."

[26]J.A. Mort, "Return of the sweatshop: Déjà vu in the garment industry."

[27]C.J. Hogue, et al., "Class, race and infant mortality in the United States."

[28]R.M. Politzer, et al., "Primary care physician supply and the medically underserved."

[29]*Ibid.*

[30]*Ibid.*

[31]Robert Pear, "Elderly patients may get a break on medical costs: Medicare changes likely," New York *Times*, July 21, 1997, A1.

[32]G. Kowalcyk, M.S. Freeland, and K.R. Levit, "Using marginal analysis to evaluate health care trends."

[33]F.P. Albritton, *Health Care Insurance Reform in the United States: A Market Approach with Application from the Federal Republic of Germany.*

[34]"Normal science" usually looks for regularities rather than for discontinuities in system behavior. Consequently a system's *structure* often is taken as a given. To address the question of how *qualitative* change occurs, however, one has to proceed differently, rethinking concepts of structure, system, and process. These are fundamental conceptual problems for several fields, though they are not often addressed in the literature. An interdisciplinary group of scholars, ranging from organic chemists through molecular biologists to economists, psychologists, and social scientists from several disciplines, have begun to ask the following questions: (1) How do organizing principles that define a system emerge? and (2) How does the structure of relationships within a system change as a result of the interactions that make up its activity? To make this abstract, interdisciplinary, analytic approach more useable for social analysis, this book focuses attention on uniquely *social* aspects of system processes.

To understand how social transformation occurs it is useful to study interactions that develop between different levels of social organization. How do voluntary organizations and ongoing institutions respond to developments occurring at a national and international level? How do these more local responses, in turn, begin to affect what happens at higher system levels? For each time period addressed, various chapters of this book begin with a brief reminder of major changes occurring internationally which had consequences for the national political economy. These changing developments set the parameters in which health care innovation of that time period occurred, defining the issues that needed to be addressed and setting limits on how problems could be approached.

Studying social transformation from this perspective requires one to deal conceptually with what might be called *agency/structure* issues affecting transformation and its routinization: When are deliberate efforts to create social changes effective? How do structural conditions affect these efforts? When do innovations last?

Working from an *agency* perspective, this book's analysis directs attention to action choices that affected processes of change at particular moments in time. It notes how *option framing* occurred, how that affected immediate choices that were being made, and how all this in turn affected parameters that influenced choice thereafter. This account examines, as well, the role that moral communities played in framing these options. From the vantage point of *structure*, this book directs attention to the question of how *structuring* occurs—how new practices emerge at moments of social disequilibrium, when many people imitate a novel way to address a common problem. Innovations thus reinforce one another's impact, in contradiction to what "the law of large numbers" would lead us to expect. Sequences of collective innovation then become institutionalized, as the qualitative changes that are occurring at macro levels of a social system affect choices at other levels.

When structure is approached as a set of interacting processes, social influence cannot be seen as unidirectional. Therefore the analysis in this book frequently notes how more micro level responses to broader social developments also created a change of circumstance which affected the kinds of "agency" decisions that also were being made at other, more macro levels of the social system. It describes how particular structures of relationships and strategies for problem-solving arise out of earlier innovation, and notes how this creates a cumulative impact which changes the parameters shaping innovative response at later moments in time.

As its title makes clear, much of *Rethinking Health Care*'s contribution to knowledge is conceptual. The first six chapters reframe our understanding of contemporary developments previously studied by a wide range of scholars from several disciplines. These chapters make visible a larger pattern of institutional development; they identify the role of entrepreneurial innovation in structural transformations and the social dynamics which affected the impact of attempted innovations. Those chapters, thus, represent a contemporary application of the *verstehen* tradition of sociological analysis. They are intended to set the context for a different level of dialogue about health care policy. The next four chapters present information and analysis not available elsewhere, drawing lessons for health care policy from contemporary developments in medical and environmental research and from the experience of health care reform movements. The final chapters then reapproach policy discussions of health care cost containment and access to care, attempting to open a new level of health policy dialogue.

Chapter 1
Understanding How We Got Here:
Creating a Health Care Industry

[1]Useful accounts of the period of American history between 1865 and 1900 include the following: Burton J. Bledstein, *The Culture of Professionalism: The Middle Class and the Development of Higher Education in America*; Claude Bowers, *The Tragic Era*; L.D. Brandeis, *Other People's Money and How the Bankers Used It*; Andrew Carnegie, *Autobiography*; Alfred D. Chandler, *The Visible Hand: The Managerial Revolution in American Business*; Lewis Corey, *The House of Morgan*; J.T. Flynn, *God's Gold: John D. Rockefeller and His Times*; L.M. Hacker and B.B. Kendrick, *The United States Since 1865*; Murat Halstead and J.F. Beale, *Life of Jay Gould: How He Made His Fortune*; Lewis Haney, *A Congressional History of Railways in the United States*; B.J. Hendrick, *The Age of Big Business*; Carl Hovey, *The Life Story of J.P. Morgan*; Matthew Josephson, *The Robber Barons: The Great American Capitalists, 1861-1901*; S.P. Orth, *The Boss and the Machine*; J.D. Rockefeller, *Random Reminiscences of Men and Events*; D.C. Seitz, *The Dreadful Decade...1869-1879*; Ida Tarbell, *History of the Standard Oil Company*.

[2]D. Coulter, *Divided Legacy: A History of the Schism in Medical Thought*, chapter one; Martin K., *Homeopathy in America: The Rise and Fall of a Medical Heresy*; O.W. Holmes, "Homeopathy and its kindred delusions," *Medical Essays: 1842-1882*; C. Rosenberg, *The Cholera Years*, chapters two and seven. P.H. De Kruif, *The Microbe Hunters*; E. Duclaux, *Pasteur: The History of a Mind*; I.I. Mechnikov, *The Founders of Modern Medicine: Pasteur, Koch, Lister*.

[3]C. Rosenberg, *The Cholera Years*, chapters two and seven.

[4]M.J. Rosenan-Maxcy, *Preventive Medicine and Public Health*.

[5]I.I. Mechnikov, *The Founders of Modern Medicine*.

[6]See P. Starr, *The Social Transformation of American Medicine (hereafter called STAM)*, chapter one, "Medicine in a democratic culture."

[7]E.R. Brown, *Rockefeller Medicine Men: Medicine and Capitalism in America*, devotes considerable attention to relations between the Progressive Movement, the AMA, and the agendas of the Carnegie and Rockefeller Foundations.

[8]U.S. Department of Commerce, Bureau of the Census, *Historical Statistics of the United States, Part I: Colonial Times to 1970*, 76, 78; J.M. Toner, *Transactions of the American Medical Association*, 314-44.

[9]The establishment of the hegemony of medical science at the beginning of the twentieth century has been described from a variety of perspectives. See, for example, the AMA Press' *Nostrums and Quackery: Articles on the Nostrum Evil and Quackery Reprinted from the Journal of the American Medical Association*; O. Garceau, *The Political Life of the American Medical Association*; D.R. Hyde, et al., *The American Medical Association: Power, Purpose and Politics in Organized Medicine*; J.G. Burrow, *Organized Medicine in the Progressive Era: The Move Toward Monopoly*; E.R. Brown, *Rockefeller Medicine Men: Medicine and Capitalism in America*; and G. Rosen, *The Structure of American Medical Practice: 1875-1941*.

[10]A number of historians have written about the Progressive Era from several vantage points. See, for example, S.P. Hays, *Conservation and the Gospel of Efficiency: The Progressive Conservation Movement, 1890-1920*; R.J. Lustig, *Corporate Liberalism: The Origin of Modern American Political Theory, 1890-1920*; D.F. Nobel, *America by*

Design: Science, Technology and The Rise of Corporate Capitalism; M. Sklar, *The Corporate Reconstruction of American Capitalism, 1890-1916: The Market, Law and Politics.*

[11]Compare, for example, P. Starr's account of these developments, *STAM*, 116-28, with that of E.R. Brown *Rockefeller Medicine Men*, 142-59.

[12]See E.R. Brown, *Ibid.*, 156-91.

[13]P. Starr, *STAM*, 252-54.

[14]I.S. Falk, C.R. Rorem, and M.D. Ring, *The Cost of Medical Care*; Committee on the Costs of Medical Care, *Medical Care for the American People.*

[15]P. Starr, *STAM*, 266.

[16]"A statistical analysis of 2,717 hospitals," 68. See also P. Starr, *STAM*, 295.

[17]C.R. Rorem, *Blue Cross Hospital Service Plans*, 7.

[18]M.M. Davis, *The Crisis in Hospital Finance and Other Studies in Hospital Economics*, 3.

[19]O.W. Anderson, *Blue Cross Since 1929: Accountability and the Public Trust*, 40.

[20]A.R. Somers and H.N. Somers, *Doctors, Patients and Health Insurance*, 548.

[21]See F.B. Freidel, *Franklin Roosevelt: Launching the New Deal.*

[22]Respected accounts of the New Deal include the following: F.B. Freidel, *ibid.*; E. Hawley, *The New Deal and the Problem of Monopoly*; W.E. Leuctenberg, *New Deal and Global War, 1933-1945*; and A.M. Schlessinger, *The Age of Roosevelt.*

[23]See W.E. Leuctenberg, *In the Shadow of FDR: From Harry Truman to Ronald Reagan.*

[24]P. Starr, *STAM*, 340.

[25]P.H. De Kruif, *Kaiser Wakes Up the Doctors*, 20-35.

[26]For accounts of these activities see the Henry J. Kaiser Family Foundation *Annual Reports.*

[27]See D.C. Carson, *Satellite HMO Development of a Prepaid Nonprofit HMO Group Medical Practice in a Small City*; H. Berman, "Insuring the uninsured: Operational issues."

[28]The National Labor Relations Act (The Wagner Act), passed the same year as Social Security, required employers to bargain with unions that won organizing elections in their plants. Considerable ill will had resulted from the successful organizing drives in the coal, steel, and auto industries.

[29]R.C. Hill, "At the crossroads: The political economy of postwar Detroit."

[30]P. Starr, *STAM*, 311.

[31]J.L. Penick, et al., eds., *The Politics of American Science: 1939 to the Present*, 8-11.

[32]A.N. Richards, "The impact of the war on medicine," 578.

[33]Organization of Economic Cooperation and Development, *Reviews of National Science Policy: United States (1968).*

[34]J.L. Penick, et al., *The Politics of American Science.*

[35]*Stat. Abstracts*, "National health care expenditures, 1945-1970," Table 82, 62.

[36]See R.M. Freeland, *The Truman Doctrine and the Origins of McCarthyism: Foreign Policy, Domestic Politics and International Security, 1946-48*; W. Leuctenberg, *In the Shadow of FDR*; and L.C. Purifoy, *Harry Truman's China Policy: McCarthyism and the Diplomacy of Hysteria.*

[37]See E.F. Denison, *Accounting for United States Economic Growth, 1929-1969*, 102-123, and especially Table 8.5.

[38]See George Perry and William C. Brainard, eds., *Brookings Papers in Economic Activity 1.*

[39]See Samuel Bowles, David M. Gordon, and Thomas E. Weisskopf, *After the Wasteland: A Democratic Economics for the Year 2000.*

[40]Defense production's share of total American manufacturing was calculated for this period from data prepared by the U.S. Department of Commerce, Bureau of Economic Analysis, "General business indicators: Capital goods industries manufacturing sales and inventories," 14.

[41]U.S. Department of Commerce, Bureau of Economic Analysis, "General business indicators," 14 ff.

[42]W. Leonhard, *Eurocommunism: Challenge for East and West*, 49-52.

[43]See R.M. Freeland, *The Truman Doctrine.*

[44]E. Stein, *American Enterprise in the European Common Market: A Legal Profile.*

[45]U.S. Bureau of the Census, *Historical Statistics*, Series C 25-75, Estimated Net Intercensal Migration of Total, Native White, Foreign-Born White, and Negro Population by States: 1879-1970, 95.

[46]See J.M. Guttentag and S.M. Wachter, *Redlining and Public Policy*; K.T. Jackson, "Race, ethnicity, and real estate appraisal"; C. Bradford and D.M. Bradford, *Redlining and Disinvestment as a Discriminatory Practice in Residential Mortgage Loans.*

[47]See C.W. Mills, *The Power Elite.*

[48]This warning was given in Dwight Eisenhower's farewell address as President of the United States, in January of 1960.

[49]T. Marmor and A. Marmor, *The Politics of Medicare*, 24.

[50]*Ibid.*, 9-28.

[51]For a 25-year record of Hill-Burton expenditures, see U.S. Department of Health Education and Welfare, Health Services and Mental Health Administration, Health Care Facilities Service, Office of Program Planning and Analysis, *The Hill-Burton Progress Report*, 13.

[52]*Ibid.*

[53]P. Starr, *STAM*, 352-363.

[54]*Stat. Abstracts*, National Health Care Expenditures, 1945-1970, Table 82, 62.

[55]P. Starr, *STAM*, 355-56.

[56]For information about distribution in medical specialties, see M. Gonzales, D.W. Emmons, and D. Pieniozek, *Socioeconomic Characteristics of Medical Practice.*

[57]J.Z. Bowers and E.F. Purcell, *Schools of Public Health: Present and Future.*

[58]See J.J. Hanlon and G.E. Pickett, *Public Health: Administration and Practice.*

[59]For accounts of Mary Lasker's remarkable influence on congressional health budgets, see New York *Times*, 1986; and S. Siwolop and J. Brazda, "The fairy godmother of medical research."

[60]For information about pharmaceutical industry growth and profits, see *Standard & Poor's Industry Surveys*, December 17, 1959, D20-22.

[61]R. Munts, *Bargaining for Health*, 7-12.

[62]J.W. Garbarino, *Health Plans and Collective Bargaining*, 19-20.

[63]See New York *Times*, May 26, 1948, I1. May 24, 1950, I3, 43.

[64]New York *Times*, June 3, 1948, I1.

[65]New York *Times*, May 24, 1950, I3, 43.

[66]See discussions of the velocity of money in W. Baumol and A. Blinder, *Economic Principles and Policies*, or D. Fusfeld, *Economics: Principles of Political Economy.*

[67]See note 49 above.

[68]*Standard and Poor's Industry Surveys*, July 19, 1973, H19.

⁶⁹P. Starr, *STAM*, 350.

⁷⁰See G. Bush, ed., *Campaign Speeches of American Presidential Candidates 1948-1984*, 104-122.

⁷¹The Supreme Court's most important ruling on health care segregation was its 1963 ruling that hospitals which discriminate against persons on the basis of race were not eligible for Hill-Burton funds. (See P. Starr, *STAM*, 350. See also A.M. Bickel, *Politics and the Warren Court*; L.B. Bozell, *Politics, the Constitution, and the Warren Court*.)

⁷²The declining influence of the AMA as the "voice of medicine" was increasingly apparent as time went on. By 1971, less than half of American physicians were members of the AMA. (P. Starr, *STAM*, 398.)

⁷³See note 71 above.

⁷⁴H. Brownell, "Eisenhower's civil rights program"; M.S. Mayes, "With much deliberation and some speed: Eisenhower and the Brown Decision."

⁷⁵C. Stone, *Black Political Power in America*, 48-54.

⁷⁶See M. Heirich and S. Kaplan, "Yesterday's discord."

⁷⁷P. Starr, *STAM*, 366-370.

⁷⁸T. Marmor and A. Marmor, *The Politics of Medicare*, 15-21.

⁷⁹*Ibid., The Politics of Medicare*, 59-93; P. Starr, *STAM*, 368-370; R. Stevens and R. Stevens, *Welfare Medicine in America: A Case Study of Medicaid*.

⁸⁰P. Starr, *STAM*, 376; J.M. Feder, *Medicare: The Politics of Federal Hospital Insurance*.

⁸¹These figures come from the American Hospital Administration, *Survey of Sources of Hospital Construction, 1982, Capital Finance Survey, 1984*, and *Panel Survey, 1988*, with additional interpretation by David Hellman of the AHA Office on Capital Financing, in an interview conducted February 8, 1989.

⁸²An excellent review of changes in court decisions regarding hospital liability for malpractice appears in M.M. Bertlet, ed., *Hospital Liability: Law and Practice*. Beginning in the 1940s and 1950s, then with increasing frequency in the 1960s and 1970s, state and federal courts ended malpractice exemption for non-profit hospitals. The doctrine of corporate negligence, applying to hospitals, was formulated in a series of decisions citing a hospital's responsibility to provide equipment and services and to maintain them, to adapt its rules and procedures as new discoveries emerge, and to take responsibility for the selection and retention of a competent medical staff.

⁸³American Medical Association, *Physician Liability: Survey Report*.

⁸⁴See American Hospital Association, *Hospital Statistics, 1986*, 14; "Hospital employees and salaries," 67.

Chapter 2
First Efforts at Cost Control

¹National health care cost figures come from the Health Care Financing Administration, Office of the Actuary: Data from the Office of National Cost Estimates, 1988, and from Department of Health, Education, and Welfare, Social Security Administration, *Social Security Bulletin*, December, 1970.

²A. Campbell, *Guerillas*.

³See F.J. Al-Chalabi, *OPEC at the Crossroads*; A.L. Danielson, *The Evolution of OPEC*; S.M. Ghanem, *OPEC: the Rise and Fall of an Exclusive Club*; F.P. Wyant, *The United States, OPEC, and Multinational Oil*.

⁴See R. Gilpin, *U.S. Power and the Multinational Corporation: The Political Economy of Foreign Direct Investment*, 202-203.

⁵See U.S. Department of State, Bureau of Public Affairs, *Foreign Direct Investment in a Global Economy* or Table 5 in the Appendix.

⁶See M. Blomstrom, *Transnational Corporations and Manufacturing Exports from Developing Countries*; T.G. Gunn, *Manufacturing for Competitive Advantage: Becoming a World Class Manufacturer*; M. Kotabe, *Global Sourcing Strategy*.

⁷See L. Kaboolian, *Shifting Gears: Auto Workers Assess the Transformation of Their Industry*.

⁸See R. Herring, *National Monetary Policies and International Financial Markets*.

⁹Tables for this book which trace the changing profit picture for American manufacturing and other corporations are based on data provided in Table B-88, Corporate Profits by Industry, U.S. Government, *Economic Report of the President*, 350.

¹⁰E.F. Denison, *Why Growth Rates Differ: Postwar Experience in Nine Western Countries*, 23, 46-47, 51, 116.

¹¹See Table 4.1, "The productivity slowdown," in S. Bowles, D. Gordon, T. Weisskopf, *After the Wasteland*.

¹²See, for example, D. M. Gordon, "A statistical series on production worker compensation," 220.

¹³Resistance to the war in Vietnam was chronicled in T. Hayden's *Vietnam: The Struggle for Peace, 1972-73*; G.L. Heath, *Mutiny Does Not Happen Here: The Literature of the American Resistance to the Vietnam War*; and F. Halstead, *Out Now: A Participant's Account of the American Movement Against the Vietnam War*.

¹⁴J.A. Geschwender, ed., *The Black Revolt: The Civil Rights Movement, Ghetto Uprisings, and Separatism*; L. Gordon, *A City in Racial Crisis: The Case of Detroit Pre- and Post- the 1967 Riot*; P.H. Rossi, ed., *Ghetto Revolts*.

¹⁵Peter Kihss, "100,000 addicts reported in city," New York *Times*, December 14, 1967, 52.

¹⁶A.W. McCoy, *Politics of Heroin in Southeast Asia*.

¹⁷For a picture of changing employment trends by industry, see *Stat. Abstracts*, Table 631, 380.

¹⁸P. Moynihan memo in "Civil rights progress report," 23-24.

¹⁹D. Bell, *The Coming of Post-Industrial Society*.

²⁰The proportion of federal budget allocated for military use was figured from data provided in table 352 (1968), 252, and table 508 (1988), 314, *Stat. Abstracts*.

²¹See the following tables in U.S. Bureau of the Census, *Stat. Abstracts* (88th and 109th editions). Washington, D.C., 1968, 1989. Table 84: National Health Expenditures, 1940 to 1965 (1968), 68; Table 136: National Health Expenditures, by Type, 1970 to 1986 (1989), 136; Table 352: Federal Administrative Budget Expenditures for National Defense Functions and Veterans Benefits and Services (1968), 252; and Table 508: National Defense Outlays and Veterans Benefits, 1960 to 1987 (1988), 314.

²²During the eight year period from 1973 to 1980 the U.S. federal government ran up a deficit of $265.4 billion. However, if business tax revenues had continued at the 1966 level of proportionate contribution, with tax contributions from the other

revenue sources increasing at the level they actually did, there would have been a net surplus of $99.6 billion. (The comparisons become even more striking for the 1980s.) See Table 7 of the Appendix.

[23]The wage formula decisions that led to the inclusion of Cost of Living Adjustments (COLA) to wages, are discussed in Chapter 2. The exact formula for COLA figures varies from contract to contract across the industries, and health care's cost increases vary from year to year. However, by 1990 federal figures showed that health care price increases over the preceding year accounted for 12.2 percent of the overall increase in the consumer price index.

[24]Economic Report of the President, 1979, p 145. See also S. Bowles, D. Gordon, T. Weisskopf, "Long swings of the non-reproductive cycle." I appreciate James Hardy's help in sorting through studies of how investment of OPEC profits affected the American economy, countering efforts to tighten the money supply during the rapid inflation of the 1970s. See P. Ferris, *The Master Banks: Controlling the World's Finances*, and P. Hoffman, *The Deal Makers: Inside the World of Investment Banking*.

[25]See Table 738, "Consumer price indexes by major groups, 1950-86," *Stat. Abstracts*, 450.

[26]See G.L. Bach, *The New Inflation: Causes, Effects, Cures*; Economic Forum, *Inflation in the United States: Causes and Consequences*; G. Haberler, *Stagflation*; G.W. Wilson, *Inflation—Causes, Consequences and Cures*; and Milbank Memorial Fund, *Health, a Victim or Cause of Inflation?*.

[27]See K. Levit, et al., "Health spending and ability to pay," *Health Care Financing Review*, 3.

[28]Ibid.

[29]Professional Standards Review Organizations (PSROs) were set up by law in 1972 to monitor hospital performance of doctors. The legislation was amended in 1984 Peer Review Organizations (PROs). See R. Egdahl and P.M. Gertman, *Quality Assurance in Health Care*; J. Blum, P. Gertman, and J. Rabinow's *PSRO and the Law*; P.Y. Ertel and M.G. Aldridge, *Medical Peer Review: Theory and Practice*. See also P. Starr, *STAM*, 402.

[30]For a description of Nixon's wage freeze and other inflation-control attempts of 1971, see *Facts on File* XXXI(1607), August 12-18, 1971, 621. 2

[31]Interview with David Hellman of the American Hospital Association Office on Capital Financing, February 8, 1989. See also American Hospital Association, *Survey of Sources of Hospital Construction, 1982; Capital Finance Survey, 1985*; and its on-going AHA panel survey.

[32]See P. Starr, *STAM*, 398-405.

[33]In 1972 the United States ranked sixteenth among nations reporting to the United Nations World Health Organization in terms of life expectancy for its male population. In 1973 it ranked fifteenth in infant mortality. United Nations, *Demographic Yearbook* and U.S. National Center for Health Statistics, *Facts of Life and Death*.

[34]A 1972 NBC television special examined the American health care crisis under the title "What Price Health?" Also see R. Tunley, *The American Health Scandal*; D. Schorr, *Don't Get Sick in America*; S. Lewin, ed., *The Nation's Health*; A. Ribicoff, with P. Danaceau, *The American Medical Machine*; E. Ginzberg, *The Limits of Health Reform: The Search for Realism*; D.E. Rogers, *American Medicine: Challenge for the 1980s*; P. Menzel, *Medical Costs, Medical Choices: A Philosophy of Health Care Economics in*

America; V. Sidel and R. Sidel, *Reforming Medicine: Lessons of the Last Quarter Century*; S. Wohl, *The Medical Industrial Complex*; J.A. Califano, *America's Health Revolution: Who Lives? Who Dies? Who Pays?*; or V.R. Fuchs, *The Health Economy*. See also R.J. Carlson, *The End of Medicine*, R.J. Carlson and R. Cunningham, *Future Directions in Health Care: A New Public Policy*, and I. Illich, *Medical Nemesis: The Expropriation of Health*.

[35]I. Illich, *Medical Nemesis*.

[36]V. Navarro, *Medical Care in the U.S.: A Critical Analysis*.

[37]The perspective of the health planning establishment is well captured in J. Knowles, ed., *Doing Better and Feeling Worse: Health Care in the U.S.*

[38]See, for example, L.M. Carter, *Toward an Educated Health Consumer: Mass Communication and Quality in Medical Care*.

[39]This information was obtained in an interview with Lawrence W. Green, May 17, 1989.

[40]*Ibid.*

[41]For discussions of Nixon's policy of détente, see: C. Bown and P.J. Mooney, *Cold War to Détente*; E. Friedland, P. Seabury, and A. Wildavsky, *The Great Détente Disaster: Oil and the Decline of American Foreign Policy*; C. Gati and T. Trister Gati, *The Debate Over Détente*; R. Litwak, *Détente and the Nixon Doctrine: Foreign Policy and the Pursuit of Stability, 1969-1976*.

[42]The New York *Times* gave prominent coverage to columnist James Reston's appendicitis attack and the use of acupuncture for surgery anesthesia while he was accompanying President Richard Nixon as the American president toured China to establish a new foreign policy during the week of July 20, 1971. A year later the *Times* was reporting on the visits of American medical delegations to observe use of acupuncture in China.

[43]The John E. Fogarty International Center for Advanced Study in the Health Sciences, *The Barefoot Doctor's Manual: The American Translation of the Chinese Paramedical Manual*.

[44]See M. Rosenthal, *Health Care in the People's Republic of China*.

[45]David McQueen, "China's impact on American medicine in the seventies," 931-936; P.R. Wolpe, "The maintenance of professional authority? Acupuncture and the American physician."

[46]For participation rates in new health care professions, see the American Nursing Association's Nursing Information Bureau, *Facts About Nursing, 1984-85*; U.S. Department of Health and Human Services Administration's Bureau of Health Professions' *Report to the President and the Congress on the Status of Health Personnel in the United States*; and a survey of physicians' assistants conducted by the American Academy of Physicians' Assistants, 1982.

[47]National Health Service Corps (U.S.), "National Health Service Corps Scholarship Program: A Report of the Secretary of Health, Education and Welfare to Congress, 1978-1979."

[48]See J.L. Falkson, *HMOs and the Politics of Health System Reform*.

[49]P. Starr, *STAM*, 400-401, discusses the passing of legislation which set up HMOs.

[50]See David E. Kenty and Martin Wald, eds., *ERISA: A Comprehensive Guide*.

[51]Kathleen A. Lewis, *Private Sector Investment in HMOs, 1974-1980*. Excelsior, MN: InterStudy, 1981; Leslie Scism, "Travelers Inc. and Met Life to form HMO; Met

Life plans to purchase some Travelers assets to fund joint venture," The *Wall Street Journal*, June 14, 1994, A3.

[52]P. Starr, *STAM*, 402, 403, 415, 416, 419, 444.

[53]P. Starr, *STAM*, 404-405.

[54]See J.K. Inglehart, "Consensus forms for national insurance plan, proposals vary widely in scope," "National insurance plan tops Ways and Means agenda," and "The rising costs of health care—Something must be done, but what?"

[55]G. Kowalcyk, M.S. Freeland, and K.R. Levit, "Using marginal analysis to evaluate health care trends."

[56]See M. Gonzales, D.W. Emmons, and D. Pieniozek, *Socioeconomic Characteristics of Medical Practice* (1986) and the AMA's SMS Surveys of nonfederal, patient-care physicians excluding residents, that were conducted between 1983 and 1985.

[57]See D. Kotelchuck, ed., *Prognosis Negative: Crisis in the Health Care System.* In 1970 there were five times as many physicians per 100,000 persons in the population for metropolitan areas with populations over five million as in non-metropolitan areas with less than 10,000 persons, with distribution of physicians stair-stepped in between for cities of varying sizes.

[58]Information about physicians can be found in a series of publications by the American Medical Association's Center for Health Policy Research.

[59]See K. Davis and R. Reynolds, "The impact of Medicare and Medicaid on access to medical care"; and K. Davis and C. Schoen, *Health and the War on Poverty*.

[60]See Table 9 in the Appendix, "Changes in federal expenditures for personal health care costs."

[61]See U. S. General Accounting Office, *Medical Malpractice: No Agreement on the Problems or Solutions* and *Medical Malpractice: Insurance Costs Increased but Varied Among Physicians and Hospitals*; L.S. Pocincki, S.J. Dogger, and B. Schwartz, "The incidence of iatrogenic injuries"; M. Kendall and J. Haldi, "The medical malpractice insurance market"; W. R. Pabst, "An American Hospital Association professional liability study"; American Medical Association, *Report of the Special Task Force on Professional Liability and Insurance*.

Chapter 3
Health Care Innovation in a
Rapidly Changing World Economy

[1]Balance of trade figures come from the *World Almanac and Book of Facts*, 132-133.

[2]A. Skidmore, "U.S. sinks deeper in world debt holes," New York *Times*, July 1, 1993, D2.

[3]U.S. Department of Labor, Bureau of Labor Statistics, "Current Labor Statistics," 83.

[4]Employee Benefit Research Institute (EBRI), "Sources of Health Insurance and Characteristics of the Uninsured."

[5]See Table B-77, U.S. Government, *Economic Report of the President*, 338-339, and reports released by the Greenhouse Crisis Foundation and the World Watch Institute and put together in a dispatch from The Washington *Post*, January 10, 1991, A3.

[6]F. Kempe, *Divorcing the Dictator: America's Bungled Affair with Noriega.* "U.S. and other nation's agency involvement in drug trafficking continues to get media attention. See Linda Robinson and Brian Duffy, "At play in the field of the spies: a primer: How not to fight the drug war," *U.S. News and World Report* 115 (21), November 29, 1993, 37.

[7]L.D. Johnston, P.M. O'Malley, and J.G. Bachman, *National Trends in Drug Use Among High School Students and Young Adults.*

[8]See B. Eklof, *Soviet Briefing: Gorbachov and the Reform*; H.-H. Hohmann, *Soviet Reform Policy Under Gorbachev*; M. Lewin, *The Gorbachev Phenomenon: A Historical Interpretation.*

[9]R. Evans and R. Novak, *The Reagan Revolution.*

[10]See *Stat. Abstracts*, Table 497, 373.

[11]For explanations and assessments of the Reagan presidency see D. Boaz, *Assessing the Reagan Years*; M.J. Boskin, *Reagan and the Economy: The Successes, Failures and Unfinished Agenda*; H. Carter, *The Reagan Years*; R. Dallek, *Ronald Reagan, The Politics of Symbolism.*

[12]The National Safe Workplace Institute, Chicago, Illinois, "Unmet Needs," September 4, 1989, commended Secretary of Labor, Elizabeth Dole for helping the Occupational Safety and Health Administration begin recovering from the acute political neglect that it experienced in the early 1980s when the agency's budget was severely cut, cited by Bob Baker, Los Angeles *Times*, September 3, 1989, 132.

In testimony to Congress through the summer and fall of 1989, HUD staff testimony made it clear that HUD had not simply down-graded priorities for housing for low income groups but had accepted major budget cuts in these programs while also diverting other funds to pay for inappropriate private projects of political favorites.

[13]See *Tax Reform Bill of 1986: Senate Finance Committee Report on HR 3838*; Commer Clearing House, 1986.

[14]Information about corporate mergers comes from the *World Almanac and Book of Facts*, 140-ff.

[15]Information about the number of bank failures, over time, comes from the *Federal Reserve Bulletin* 75(3), March 1989, 124. In 1989, by a vote of 201-175, the U.S. House of Representatives approved a Savings and Loan Bail-Out bill which, with interest, would cost at least $159 billion between 1989 and 1999, and seemed sure to cost at least $285 billion over a period of 30 years, because the rescue effort would be financed in part through sale of thirty-year bonds.

[16]See D. Bell, *The Coming of Post-Industrial Society: A Venture in Social Forecasting.*

[17]See Table 554: Social Welfare Expenditures Under Public Programs as Percent of GNP and Total Government Outlays: 1960-1985, *Stat. Abstracts*, 1989, 336.

[18]*Ibid.*

[19]For descriptions of DRG policy and providers' strategies for dealing with this, see U.S. Congress Office of Technology Assessment, *Diagnostically Related Groups (DRGs) and the Medicare Program: Implications for Medical Technology*; D.L. Zimmerman, *DRGs and the Medicaid Program*; R.J. Fitzgibbon and B.E. Statland, *DRG Survival Manual for the Clinical Lab*; Commission of Professional and Hospital Activities, *Length of Stay by Diagnosis Related Groups, July 1984-July 1985 discharges.*

[20]D.G. Whiteis and J.W. Salmon, "The proletarization of health care and the underdevelopment of the public sector" (hereafter called "The proletarization"), 126.

[21]See E. Taylor, *Data Book on Multihospital Systems, 1980-1985*, and American Hospital Association, *Directory of Multihospital Systems*.

[22]D.G. Whiteis and J.W. Salmon, "The proletarization," 125.

[23]H.S. Berliner and C. Regan, "Multi-national operations of U.S. for-profit hospital chains: Trends and implications," 155-156.

[24]For a look at health care's participation in the movement toward corporate mergers, see the *World Almanac and Book of Facts*, 1989, 140. See also, *Health Facts*, 21(204) May 16, 1996, 2.

[25]M. Gonzales, D.W. Emmons, and D. Pieniozek, *Socioeconomic Characteristics of Medical Practice*.

[26]The January/February, 1985 issue of *Business and Health* includes the following reports: M. Schlessinger, "The rise of proprietary health care" (7-12); A. Masso, "HMOs in transition: What the future holds" (21-24); P.C. Roeder and J.H. Moxley III, "Promoting quality care in cost-effective settings" (30-31). See also description of business health coalition strategies in B. Longest, "Pittsburgh embraces HMO development," and J. Stein, "How HMOs adapt: A perspective from the inside," (an interview with Fred Wasserman of the Maxicare HMO chain).

[27]See David E. Kenty and Martin Wald, eds., *ERISA: A Comprehensive Guide*.

[28]M. Gonzales, D.W. Emmons, and D. Pieniozek, *Socioeconomic Characteristics of Medical Practice*.

[29]See A.L. Hillman, "Special report: Financial incentives for physicians in HMOs—Is there a conflict of interest?"

[30]See "Majority of hospitals consider DRG-104 to be a money-maker." See the Health Care Financing Administration's Bureau of Data Management and Strategy and Office of Research and Demonstrations' data on hospital usage by Medicare. These data show a sizeable drop in hospital admissions and in length of stay for persons admitted to the hospital after the DRG policy was implemented in 1983. See Tables 2, 3, and 10, pages 3, 4, and 7, *Health Care Financing Review* 10(1), Fall, 1988.

[31]Information about HMO cost trends was obtained in a July, 1989, interview with John Gable, a researcher for the Health Insurance Association of America. See J. Gable, "The changing world of group insurance" and J. Gable, et al., "Employer-sponsored health insurance."

[32]See note 61 in Chapter 2.

[33]U. S. General Accounting Office, *Medical Malpractice: Insurance Costs Increased but Varied Among Physicians and Hospitals*, 86-112.

[34]A larger picture of changes in rates for various kinds of operations can be seen by perusing the American College of Surgeons' *Socioeconomic Fact Book for Surgery*.

[35]On November 2, 1987, Jerry Estill of the Associated Press quoted a study written by Tanio, Manley, and Wolfe for the Public Citizen Health Research Group, Washington, D.C., noting that the national Caesarean-section rate had increased from 5.5 percent of all births in 1970 to 24 percent of all births in 1986. They estimated that in 1986 455,000 babies were delivered by Caesarean-section unnecessarily.

³⁶S.M. Rock, "Malpractice premiums and primary Caesarean section rates in New York and Illinois." In his book, *Medical Nemesis*, I. Illich draws attention to a series of studies done from the 1950s to the early 1970s, documenting how rates for various kinds of operations vary in the population, depending on the number of physicians and the kind of demand they create for their services. See for example, J.C. Doyle, "Unnecessary ovariectomies: Study based on the removal of 704 normal ovaries from 546 patients," and "Unnecessary hysterectomies: Study of 6,248 operations in thirty-five hospitals during 1948"; C.E. Lewis, "Variations in the incidence of surgery"; or E. Vayda, "A comparison of surgical rates in Canada and in England and Wales."

³⁷See M. Summer, *The Dollars and Sense of Hospital Malpractice Insurance*; H.R. Lewis and M.E. Lewis, *The Medical Offenders*; S. Rottenberg, *The Economics of Medical Malpractice*; W.B. Schwartz and N.K. Komesor, *Doctors, Damages and Deterrence: An Economic View of Medical Malpractice*; P.E. Cerlin, *Medical Malpractice Pre-Trial Screening Panels: A Review of the Evidence*, Intergovernmental Health Policy Project; F. J. Ritchey, "Medical rationalization, cultural lag, and the malpractice crisis"; and M.A. Bailey and W.I. Cikins, *The Effects of Litigation on Health Care Costs*.

³⁸American Medical Association, *Socioeconomic Monitoring System Survey, 1988*.

³⁹New York *Times*, April 12, 1989, A25. See also J.A. Califano, *America's Health Care Revolution: Who Lives? Who Dies? Who Pays?*, 485.

⁴⁰Table 147, *Stat. Abstracts of the U.S.* 109th edition, 1989.

⁴¹The tuberculosis rate among the homeless is one hundred times that of the population at large. J.D. Wright, *The Social Epidemiology of AIDS*, unpublished dissertation, University of Washington.

⁴²Congressional investigations of HUD through the summer and fall of 1989 showed that HUD staff had not simply down-graded priorities for housing for low income groups and had diverted funds to pay for inappropriate private projects of political favorites.

⁴³A. Golphin, "Homelessness," syndicated column, appearing in *Ann Arbor News*, April 15, 1989, A7.

⁴⁴L.D. Johnston, P.M. O'Malley, and J.G. Bachman, *National Trends in Drug Use Among High School Students and Young Adults*, 1987.

⁴⁵Table 130: "National Health Expenditures by Type: 1970 to 1986," *Stat. Abstracts*, 88.

⁴⁶W.L. Heyward and J.W. Curran, "The epidemiology of AIDS in the U.S."

⁴⁷P. Blaikie and T. Marnett, *AIDS in Africa: The Social and Policy Impact*; C.W. Hunt, "Migrant labor and sexually transmitted diseases: AIDS in Africa" and "Africa and AIDS: Dependent development, sexism and racism"; A. Larson, "The social epidemiology of Africa's AIDS epidemic."

⁴⁸Centers for Disease Control, "Estimates of Prevalence and Projected AIDS Cases: Summary of a Workshop, October 31-November 1, 1989."

⁴⁹Information from Centers for Disease Control poster, February, 1989.

⁵⁰C.E. Koop, *Surgeon General's Report on Acquired Immune Deficiency Syndrome*, 1987.

⁵¹For reports on the National AIDS Commission see New York *Times*, February 21, 1988, I32; February 25, 1988, I1.

[52]Study reports summarized by Mindy Fullilove, psychiatrist and AIDS researcher, at a University of Michigan conference on AIDS reported in the *Ann Arbor News*, June 28, 1989, A1.

[53]Five International Conferences on AIDS held during the 1980s were filled with reports of the HIV virus' ability to mutate rapidly, frustrating efforts to find a simple way to block its activity. Moreover, frequent use of antibiotics to control infections among the population with AIDS was producing a more rapid mutation among other organisms, making them more resistant to antibiotic formulas.

[54]Lawrence K. Altman, "AIDS deaths drop 19% in U.S., continuing a heartening trend," New York *Times*, July 15, 1997, AI.

[55]Associated Press, August 7, 1987.

[56]Centers for Disease Control, "Special Report: Treatment Rerun: Costs are High."

[57]R. Begley, "CPI airs views on trade, health care," 6.

Chapter 4
The 1990s: Efforts at More Basic Reform
in a New World Order

[1]"Senate gives final approval to close 130 military bases," New York *Times*, Sept. 21, 1993, 143, A13; "California's job losses affected base closing list," New York *Times*, March 7, 1995, 144, C18; James Bornemeier and Glenn F. Bunting, "State officials mount attack to save bases," Los Angeles *Times*, March 9, 1993, A3.

[2]E.F. Denison, *Why Growth Rates Differ: Postwar Experience in Nine Western Countries*, 23, 46-47, 51, 116.

[3]Barbara Wootton, and Laura T. Ross, "Hospital staffing patterns in urban and non-urban areas."

[4]"Trade pact anniversary — for better or worse. Is NAFTA working? One year later," *The Christian Science Monitor*, Jan. 3, 1995, 1; "How's NAFTA working? Ask the people in Avis, Pa.," *The Christian Science Monitor*, Dec. 12, 1994, 87(12):18; Bob Davis, "Two years later, the promises used to sell Nafta haven't come true, but its foes were wrong, too," The *Wall Street Journal*, Oct. 26, 1995, A24; W. von Raab, and M.F. Andy, Jr., "Will NAFTA free the drug trade? Cocaine business too will exploit open borders," The Washington *Post*, August 15, 1993, 62; J. Dillin, "NAFTA and drug threat," *The Christian Science Monitor* June 4, 1993, 3.

[5]Pauline Yoshihashi, Sarah Lubman, and Dianne Solis, "Passage of Proposition 187 sets up bitter social battle," The *Wall Street Journal*, Nov. 10, 1994, A7.

[6]Elizabeth Shogren. "Sterner penalties send U.S. prisoner count past 1 million," Los Angeles *Times*, Oct. 28, 1994, A36.

[7]See Stephen Donaldson, "Can we put an end to inmate rape?" *USA Today*, May 1995, 40-2; Tom Cahill, "Rape behind bars"; H. Pickering and G.V. Stimson, "Syringe sharing in prison," *Lancet* (North American edition) 342:621-22, Sept. 4, 1993; R.J. Kochleer, "HIV infection, TB and the health crisis in correction," *Public Administration Review* 54:3-5, Jan.-Feb. 1994.

[8]Dan Morgan, "Medicaid costs balloon into fiscal 'time bomb'," The Washington *Post*, Jan. 30, 1994, A1.; Henry A. Waxman, "My record on Medicaid," The Washington *Post*, March 6, 117, C6.

[9]Keith Bradsher, "Rise in uninsured becomes an issue in Medicaid fight," New York *Times*, August 27, 1995, A1.

[10]Michael A. Morrisey, *Cost Shifting in Health Care: Separating Evidence from Rhetoric.*

[11]"World cancer rates shifting dramatically," 161; *Environmental Change and Human Health.*

[12]J.D. Rockefeller IV, "A call for action: The Pepper Commission's blueprint for health care reform"; U.S. Government, *A Call for Action: Final Report of the Pepper Commission*; National Leadership Commission on Health Care, *For the Health of a Nation: A Shared Responsibility.*

[13]U. S. Government, *The President's Comprehensive Health Reform Program*; P. Cotton, "Preexisting Conditions 'Hold Americans Hostage'."

[14]Healthcare Information Center, *Reforming the System: Containing Health Care Costs in an Area of Universal Coverage*; C.J. Schramm, *Health Care Financing for All Americans.*

[15]Kaiser Commission on the Future of Medicaid, *The Medicaid Cost Explosion: Causes and Consequences*; K. Davis, "Expanding Medicare and employer plans to achieve universal health insurance"; K.N. Lohr and S.A. Schroeder, "Special Report: A Strategy for Quality Assurance in Medicare."

[16]Interagency Committee on Immunization (U.S.), *Action Plan to Improve Access to Immunization Services: Report of the Interagency Committee on Immunization*; M.P. Beachler, "Improving health care for underserved infants, children, and adolescents: The Robert Wood Johnson Foundation's experience."

[17]J. Rovner, "Bush Medicare premium plan is greeted warily on Hill."

[18]*Ibid.*

[19]J.D. Rockefeller IV, "A call for action: The Pepper Commission's blueprint for health care reform."

[20]*Ibid.*

[21]E. Friedman, "The uninsured"; F. Cerne, "Rate decrease unlikely despite health insurers' healthy profits."

[22]R.J. Blendon, R. Leitman, I. Morrison, and K. Donelan, "Satisfaction with health systems in ten nations"; V. Navarro, "Why some countries have national health insurance, others have national services, and the U.S. has neither"; V.R. Fuchs, "The health sector's share of gross national product."

[23]P. Starr, *STAM*, 252-54.

[24]Healthcare Information Center, *System in Crisis: The Case for Health Reform*; M. Pfaff, "Differences in health care spending across countries: Statistical evidence."

[25]F.P. Albritton, *Health Care Insurance Reform in the United States: A Market Approach with Application from the Federal Republic of Germany*; L.K. Bradford, "Health insurance values and implementation in the Netherlands and the Federal Republic of Germany: An alternative path to universal coverage."

[26]Japan's health care costs were 6.7 percent of the GNP in 1986, compared to 10.5 percent in the U.S. M. Powell, *Health Care in Japan.*

[27]Canada's health care costs were 8.7 percent of the GNP in 1988 compared to 11.5 percent in the U.S. V.R. Fuchs, "How does Canada do it? A comparison of expenditures for physician's services in the United States and Canada" (hereafter referred to as "How does Canada do it?"); J.K. Inglehart, "The United States looks at Canadian health care"; A.J. Culyer, *Health Care Expenditures in Canada: Myth and*

Reality, Past and Future; Health Insurance Association, *Canadian Health Care: The Implications of Public Health Insurance.*

[28]M. Powell, *Health Care in Japan.*

[29]F.P. Albritton, *Health Care Insurance Reform in the United States: A Market Approach with Application from the Federal Republic of Germany.*

[30] V.R. Fuchs, "How does Canada do it?"

[31]J.D. Rockefeller IV, "A call for action: The Pepper Commission's blueprint for health care reform."

[32]*Ibid.*

[33]*Ibid.*

[34]Edwin Chen, "'Jackson Hole Group' helps to shape Bush health plan; a small circle of doctors, academics and executives exerts a strong influence on the White House," Los Angeles *Times*, January 17, 1992, A22; Michael M. Weinstein, "Is it Jackson Hole-compatible? After 25 years of work, a health care standard," New York *Times*, April 25, 1992.

[35]U.S. Congressional Budget Office, *Managed Competition and Its Potential to Reduce Health Spending*; A.C. Enthoven, *Health Plan* and *Theory and Practice of Managed Competition in Health Care Finance.*

[36]White House Domestic Policy Council, *The President's Health Security Plan: The Clinton Blueprint.* See also Dan M. Peterson, and H. Jeffrey Brownawell. "A review of Health Security Act of 1993."

[37]Sallyanne Payton, "The politics of comprehensive national health care reform: Watching the 103rd and 104th Congresses at work," in Marilynn M. Rosenthal and Max Heirich (eds.), *Health Care Policy: Understanding Our Choices from National Reform to Market Force.*

[38]These developments were chronicled fully and regularly in the New York *Times* throughout this time period. Washington insiders with whom I conversed reported that the *Times* reporters had excellent informants and that their day to day reports were quite accurate.

[39]Sallyanne Payton, "The politics of comprehensive national health care reform".

[40]The health purchasing alliances would prefer to work with a few large health insurance companies, the small insurance association believed. This would lure the large insurance companies, who had withdrawn from health insurance after the large corporations had self-insured, back into competition with the smaller insurance companies. Since these large insurance companies also owned several of the largest managed care plans, the threat of their domination of the health care market became very real. The ads were filmed as if conversations between a husband and wife, Harry and Louise, expressing "average Americans'" growing worries about health care reform.) See Susan Dentzer, "Harry, Louise, and health alliances."

[41]Charles Krauthammer, "The watershed election of 1996," The Washington *Post*, March 31, 1995, A3; "Why many Democratic stars fell in 1994; and why GOP landslide left several liberal icons untouched in angry war," *The Christian Science Monitor*, Nov. 10, 1984, 3.

[42]*Ibid.*

[43]Edmund Faltermayer, "Health care: More Americans are switching to HMOs"; "Enrollment in HMOs spurted almost 10% in 1993, report says," The *Wall Street Journal*, Dec. 10, 1993, A2; Leslie Scism, "Managed care thrives as smaller insurers

'rent' HMOs; cost-conscious employers are forcing changes as Washington deliber-ates," The *Wall Street Journal,* April 28, 1994, B4; Ron Winslow, "Big health concerns agree to develop data system to gauge quality of care," The *Wall Street Journal,* Jan. 15, 1993, B2.

⁴⁴"Not a cure," The *Washington Post,* June 29, 1995, 118, A20; Suzie A. Blevins, "Antidote for health care costs," *The Christian Science Monitor,* June 29, 1995, 20.

⁴⁵Felicia Paik, "HMO competition heats up as states pick managed care to save on Medicaid" (Pennsylvania Contracts with Health Maintenance Organizations, Health Care Reform), The *Wall Street Journal,* June 13, 1994, B4.

⁴⁶Judith Havemann, "President signs insurance portability bill into law," The Washington *Post,* August 22, 1996, A9; Jane Bryant Quinn, "Insurance safety net still has gaps, "The Washington *Post,* August 25, 1996, H2; Philip R. Lee and James Scanlon, "The data standardization remedy in Kassebaum-Kennedy."

⁴⁷Adam Clymer, "White House and GOP announce deal to balance budget and trim taxes," New York *Times,* July 29, 2997, A1.

⁴⁸Edwin Chen, "Hawaii's health plan offers lessons for the future," Los Ange-les *Times,* July 8, 1994, A18; Adam Clymer, "Hawaii is a health care lab as employ-ers buy insurance," New York *Times,* May 6, 1994, 143, A1; Emily Friedman, "Health insurance in Hawaii: Paradise lost or found?"

⁴⁹M.A. Strosberg, J.M. Wiener, R.C. Fein, and I.A. Fein, eds., *Rationing America's Medical Care: The Oregon Plan and Beyond;* H.D. Klevit, et al., "Prioritization of Health Care Services: A Progress Report by the Oregon Health Services Commission."

⁵⁰Milt Freudenheim, "Health costs for workers in U.S. rose last year, reversing '94 drop," New York *Times,* Jan. 30, 1996, A1.

⁵¹R.J. Carlson, *The End of Medicine.*

Chapter 5
Contending Strategies for Reform: Underlying Principles, Unanticipated Consequences, and Unmet Problems

¹The maldistribution of physicians is not even mentioned by David U. Himmelstein and Steffie Woolhandler, major academic advocates for a single payer system, in their popularly written "Source Guide for Advocates" of a national, single payer system, which describes problems with the current American health care system and suggests how a Canadian-style, single payer plan would improve health care. Himmelstein and Woolhandler, *The National Health Program Book.*

²V.R. Fuchs, "How does Canada do it?"

³My thanks to Jeff deGraff, University of Michigan School of Business Admin-istration, for this observation.

⁴The expanding role of American business in cost containment efforts and health care policy has been described in Chapters 3 and 4. The role of American busi-nesses in sponsoring innovative prevention and health promotion programs is dis-cussed in Chapter 8.

⁵Sallyanne Payton, "Why alliances? A simpler path to health care reform through reinsurance."

⁶See A.L. Hillman, "Special Report: Financial Incentives for Physicians in HMOs—Is There A Conflict of Interest?"

[7]R.H. Brook, *The Effect of Co-insurance on the Health of Adults: Results from the Rand Health Experiment*; J.P. Newhouse, *Free for All? Lessons from the Rand Health Insurance Experiment*.

[8]Jack Maurer, PFL Life Insurance Company, reanalysis using Tillinghast's 1992 Major Medical Claims Cost Studies, reported by the Council for Affordable Health Insurance; National Center for Policy Analysis, *Controlling Health Care Costs with Medical Savings Accounts*, Report #168, January 1992.

[9]Three bills introduced into the 104th Congress House of Representatives would authorize the creation of Health Savings Accounts: HR 323, IRA Code 1986 Amendment (David M. McIntosh, R-Ind.); HR 539, IRA Code 1986 Amendment (Mike Porter, D-Miss.); and HR1818, Medical Savings Account and Investment Act (Bill Archer, R-Texas).

[10]Len Nichols, Wellesley College economist, reported Wellesley College's experience with optional health savings accounts (personal communication, Nov. 17, 1994).

[11]"Medicare Catastrophic Coverage Act of 1988;" P.J. Ferrara, "The catastrophic health care fiasco."

[12]Information from D. William Ruoff, Michigan Employee Benefits Services, interviewed July 11, 1995.

[13]Purchasing alliances would have been forbidden to dictate prices, however, because the Clinton Plan hoped to preserve market competition.

[14]Employers could choose the three plans with the most attractive combination of services and cost.

[15]My thanks to Sallyanne Payton for this analogy.

[16]Thomas S. Kuhn, *The Structure of Scientific Revolutions*.

Chapter 6
Origins of New Health-Care Perspectives

[1]J. Griffith, et al., "Cancer mortality in U.S. counties with hazardous waste sites and ground water pollution."

[2]H. Selye, *The Stress of Life*.

[3]D.A. Strickland, *Scientists in Politics: The Atomic Scientists Movement, 1945-1946*; F. Barnaby and G. Thomas *The Nuclear Arms Race, Control or Catastrophe? Proceedings of the General Section of the British Association for the Advancement of Science*; P.P. Craig, *Nuclear Arms Race: Technology and Society*.

[4]Scientists and Engineers for Social and Political Action Newsletter *Science for People*; Physician's Role Periodicals (PRS) *A Journal of Medicine and Global Survival*.

[5]C.G. Hempel, "The logic of functional analysis."

[6]A.W. Gouldner, *The Coming Crisis of Western Sociology*.

[7]P. Goodman, *Growing Up Absurd: Problems of Youth in the Organized Society*; H. Marcuse, *One Dimensional Man*; T. Roszak, *The Dissenting Academy, The Making of a Counter Culture: Reflections on the Technocratic Society and Its Youthful Opposition* and *Where the Wasteland Ends*.

[8]See, for example, discussions of students' relation to class interest in M. Rudd, et al., "What is to be done?"; T. Thomas, "The student revolt: An analysis."

[9]R.L. Blumberg, *Civil Rights: The 1960s Freedom Struggle*, 126.

[10]The Peace and Freedom movement, which brought together civil rights and anti-war efforts, is recorded in R.M. Fisher's *Rhetoric and American Democracy: Black Protest Through Vietnam Dissent*. See also D.J. Westby, *The Clouded Vision: The Student Movement in the United States in the 1960s*.

[11]See K. Mannheim's discussion of social "generations," *Essays on the Sociology of Knowledge*, R. Wuthnow's application to the 'sixties generation, *Experimentation in American Religion: The New Mysticisms and Their Implications for the Churches*; S. Allen, "Class, culture and generation"; T.A. Lambert, "Generations and change: Toward a theory of generations as a force in the historical process."

[12]P.W. Lunneborg, *Abortion: A Positive Decision*; D.M. Sloan, *Abortion: A Doctor's Perspective/A Woman's Dilemma*.

[13]S. Monteith, *AIDS: The Unnecessary Epidemic: America Under Siege*; D. Sadownick, "ACT UP makes a dpectacle of AIDS."

[14]National Institute on Alcohol Abuse and Alcoholism, *Alcohol and Alcoholism: Programs and Progress*; R. Baggot, *Alcohol, Politics and Social Policy*; R.L. Akers, *Drugs, Alcohol, and Society: Social Structure, Process, and Policy*.

[15]D.J. Denuyl, "Smoking, human rights, and civil liberties."

[16]C.G. Benello, *The Case for Participatory Democracy: Some Prospects for a Radical Society*; D.C. Kramer, *Participatory Democracy: Developing Ideals of the Political Left*.

[17]See R. Kanter, *Teaching Elephants to Dance* and *When Giants Learn to Dance: Mastering the Challenge of Strategies, Management and Career in the 1990s*.

[18]Insider accounts of the New Left include C. Oglesby's *The New Left Reader*, M. Teodori's *The New Left: A Documentary History*, and M. Friedman's *The New Left of the Sixties*. See also E.J. Bacciocco, Jr., *The New Left in America: Reform to Revolution, 1956 to 1970*.

[19]See V. Hines and L. Gerlach, *People, Power, Change: Movements of Social Transformation* and *Lifeway Leap: The Dynamics Change in America*. Gerlach also wrote "Movements of social change: Some structural characteristics." Hines first described SPIN in an article titled "The basic paradigm of a future socio-cultural system."

[20]Jan Smuts, a South African general who became influential in the British cabinet and later was architect of the plan to set up a League of Nations (the predecessor of the United Nations), also was a philosopher who looked for ways to counter *reductionist* tendencies of scientific thinking. He called his philosophic stance *Holism*. See J. Smuts, *Holism and Evolution*.

[21]B. Blauner, *Racial Oppression in America*.

[22]NATO Advanced Study Institute Paleorift *Tectonics and Geophysics of Continental Rifts*; C. Olliver, *Tectonics and Landforms*; J.M. Bird, *Plate Tectonics: Selected Papers from Publications of the American Geophysical Union*.

[23]S.M. Lipset, *Revolution and Counter Revolution*. Insider accounts of the American New Left or hippie Counter Culture include N. Von Hoffman's *We Are the People Our Parents Warned Us Against*; T. Wolfe's *The Electric Kool-Aid Acid Test*; and J. Rubin's *We Are Everywhere*.

[24]Black Power is chronicled in J. Haskins' *Profiles in Black Power*, in G.L. Jackson's *Blood in My Eye*, and in S. Carmichael and C.V. Hamilton's *Black Power: The Politics of Liberation in America*. See also L. Killian, *The Impossible Revolution, Phase II: Black Power and the American Dream*.

[25]See P. Matthiessen's *In the Spirit of Crazy Horse*, and R. Weyler's *Blood of the Land: The Government and Corporate War Against the American Indian Movement*.

²⁶The Chicano struggle, and especially that of migratory farm laborers, is chronicled by J.G. Dume in *Delano, The Story of the California Grape Strike*. See also M. Day's *Forty Acres: Cesar Chavez and the Farm Workers*, J.E. Levy's *Cesar Estrada Chavez: Autobiography of La Causa*, and R. De Toledano's *Little Cesar*.

²⁷See H.L. Perretz, *The Gray Panther Manual*; L.N. Bailis, *Bread or Justice: Grassroots Organizing in the Welfare Rights Movement*; F.F. Piven and R.A. Cloward, *Poor People's Movements: Why They Succeed, How They Fail*; A.D. Heskin, *Tenants and the American Dream: Ideology and the Tenant Movement*.

²⁸See B. Friedan's *The Feminine Mystique*; G. Steinem, *Outrageous Acts and Everyday Rebellion*; M.L. Carden, *Feminism in the Mid 1970s*; S. Stambler, *Women's Liberation: Blueprint for the Future*. Gay Liberation is examined in K. Jay and A. Young's *Out of the Closets: Voices of Gay Liberation*; L. Richmond and G. Nogura's *The Gay Liberation Book*; and D. Altman's, *Homosexual Oppression and Liberation*.

²⁹Women's Movement innovations in health care are discussed in R. Simmons, B.J. Kay and C. Regan's article, "Women's health groups: Alternatives to the health care system." See also Judith Bruce, "Women-oriented health care: New Hampshire feminist center."

³⁰J. Neihardt, *Black Elk Speaks: The Life Story of a Holy Man of the Ogalala Sioux*.

³¹For a history of gay medical clinics see D.G. Ostrow, "Homosexualities." Issues regarding care of the mentally ill are discussed in F.D. Chu, *The Madness Establishment: Ralph Nader's Study Group Report on the National Institute of Mental Health*, 3.

³²P.A.B. Clarke, *AIDS: Medicine, Politics, Society*; R. Shilts, *And the Band Played On: Politics, People, and the AIDS Epidemic*; National Institutes of Health, *The AIDS Research of the National Institutes of Health: Report of a Study*.

³³H.C. Schulberg, *The Mental Hospital and Human Services*; C.A. Kiesler, *Mental Hospitalization: Myths and Facts about a National Crisis*.

³⁴See R. Nader, *Unsafe At Any Speed: The Designed-in Dangers of the American Automobile*; *Corporate Power in America*, with M. Green; *The Consumer and Corporate Accountability*, with J. Carper.

³⁵M. McComas, G. Fookes, and G. Taucher, *The Dilemma of Third World Nutrition: Nestle and the Role of Infant Formula*.

³⁶See also R. Mills, *Young Outsiders: A Study in Alternative Communities*; B.H. Wolfe, *The Hippies*; W. Hedgepeth, *The Alternative: Communal Life in New America*; or F. Davis, *On Youth Subcultures: The Hippie Variant*.

³⁷See D.E. Smith, D.J. Bentel, and J.L. Schwartz, *The Free Clinic: A Community Approach to Health Care and Drug Abuse* and D.E. Smith and J. Luce, *Love Needs Care: A History of San Francisco's Haight-Ashbury Free Medical Clinic and Its Pioneer Role in Treating Drug-Abuse Problems*.

³⁸R. Ravich, "Patient advocacy."

³⁹T. Leary, *LSD, the Consciousness Expanding Drug* and *Politics of Ecstacy*.

⁴⁰Ram Dass, *Be Here Now*.

⁴¹Popular "New Age" authors include Marilyn Ferguson, Fritjof Capra, W. Brough Joy, M.D., Richard Moss, George Leonard, Mark Satin, David Spengler, and Ken Wilber.

⁴²Critics included C. Lasch, *The Culture of Narcissism and American Life in an Age of Diminishing Expectations* and M. Rossman, *New Age Blues and the Politics of Consciousness*.

[43]R. Crawford, "Healthism and the medicalization of everyday life (politics of delf-care)."

[44]See R. Crawford, "You are dangerous to your health: The ideology and politics of victim blaming," or "Healthism and the medicalization of everyday life (politics of self-care)." These criticisms related holistic attempts to encourage people to take responsibility for their own health to earlier social criticism about tendencies to blame victims for the problems which they are facing because of larger social policies. The best known exponent of this broader social critique is W. Ryan, *Blaming the Victim*.

[45]See, for example, S. Guttmacher, "The individual, the social context, and health policy: Whole in body, mind & spirit—Holistic health and the limits of medicine."

[46]These demonstration projects are discussed in Chapter 7.

[47]See H.R. Jones, *John Muir and the Sierra Club: The Battle for Yosemite*; F. Turner, *Rediscovering America: John Muir in His Time and Ours*; J. Muir, *Our National Parks*.

[48]S. Wexler, *The Vietnam War: An Eyewitness History*; N. Sheehan, *The Pentagon Papers, as Published by the New York Times Based on Investigative Report*; F. Halstead, *Out Now! A Participant's Account of the American Movement Against the Vietnam War*; N.L. Zaroulis, *Who Spoke? American Protest Against the War in Vietnam, 1963-1975*.

[49]H. Mitgang, *America at Random, from the New York Times' Oldest Editorial Feature, "Topics of the Times," a Century of Comments on America and Americans*; M. McLuhan, *The Global Village: Transformations in World Life and Media in the 21st Century*.

[50]F.P. Longford, *Nixon, a Study of Extremes of Fortune*; M.A. Genovese, *The Nixon Presidency: Power and Politics in Turbulent Times*; D.E. Casper, *Richard Nixon: A Bibliographic Exploration*; J. Schell, *Observing the Nixon Years: "Notes and Comments" from the New Yorker on the Vietnam War and the Watergate Crisis, 1969-1975*.

[51]U.S. Environmental Protection Agency, *EPA Reports Bibliography: A Listing of EPA Reports Available from the National Technical Information Service as of April 1, 1973*; D.F. Paulsen, *Pollution and Public Policy: A Book of Readings*; U. S. Government, *The President's 1971 Environmental Program*.

[52]D. Adamson, *Defending the World: The Politics and Diplomacy of the Environment* (hereafter called *Defending*).

[53]See C. Spratnik and F. Capra, *Green Politics*.

[54]E.J.J. Leeuw, *The Sane Revolution: Health Promotion, Backgrounds, Scope, Prospects*; Physicians for Social Responsibility, *The PSR Quarterly: A Journal of Medicine and Global Survival*.

[55]J. May, *The Greenpeace Book of the Nuclear Age: The Hidden History, the Human Cost*; Greenpeace U.S.A., *The Greenpeace Guide to Anti-Environmental Organizations*; E. Papadakis, *The Green Movement in West Germany*.

[56]A. Alekseev, *Stockholm Conference*; A.B. Lovins, *World Energy Strategies: Facts, Issues, and Options*; A. Rosencranz and J.E. Carroll, *International Environmental Diplomacy: The Management and Resolution of Transfrontier Environmental Problems*.

[57]Conference on Acid Rain (1984: Washington, DC), *Acid Rain: Economic Assessment*.

[58]D. Adamson, *Defending*, 113-116, 131.

[59]D. Adamson, *Defending*, 111-112.

Chapter 7
Holistic Health

[1]Insurance companies paying for some alternative treatments include Aetna, American Western Life, Blue Shield of California, and Mutual of Omaha.

[2]See A.G. Hasting, J. Fadiman, and J.S. Gordon, *Health for the Whole Person* or J.S. Gordon, *Holistic Medicine*.

[3]Note, for example, the fourth principle enunciated by the national Coalition of Holistic Health Organizations in 1984, which will be presented shortly.

[4]Christopher Peacocke develops these ideas more generally, *Holistic Explanation: Action, Space, Interpretation*.

[5]To get a sense of the variety of treatment approaches pursued within the holistic health movement see the Berkeley Holistic Health Center publication, *Holistic Health Lifebook: A Guide to Personal and Planetary Well-Being*.

[6]R. Dubos, *Mirage of Health: Utopias, Progress and Biological Change*.

[7]H. Benson and M.D. Epstein, "The placebo effect: A neglected asset in the care of patients."

[8]See, for example, Rick J. Carlson, *The End of Medicine*.

[9]The work of Herbert Benson and his colleagues at Harvard Medical School stands out particularly in this regard. Along with Benson's technical medical research publications are several books oriented toward the general public, including *The Relaxation Response, The Mind/Body Effect: How Behavioral Medicine Can Show You the Way to Better Health, Beyond the Relaxation Response*, and a book coauthored with W. Doyle Gentry and Charles A. Wolff, *Work, Stress and Health*.

[10]The Coalition of Holistic Health Organizations was organized in Washington, D.C., on March 3, 1984, when persons active in 30 holistic health organizations across the United States and Canada created a new organization to coordinate holistic health efforts on a national level.

[11]The statements which follow are slight paraphrases of admonitions and advice given widely in medical training in the United States. I have stated each "conventional" admonition in language that makes obvious its parallel to the eight principles of holistic health, as drawn up by the Coalition of Holistic Health Organizations (CHHO), and then cite sources for the advice in the next eight notes, whose citation numbers are placed in the text with each admonitional statement. Terrence Davies, M.D., a professor at the University of Michigan Medical School, recommended classic texts spelling out the orthodox medical perspective on appropriate stances for doctors and patients to take in approaching problems of health and disease. The wording of these admonitions, as stated in the text, is my own.

[12]Claude Bernard, *Introduction to the Study of Experimental Medicine*.

[13]Alvin R. Feinstein, *Clinical Judgment*; Philip A. Tumulty, *The Effective Clinician*.

[14]Kerr L. White, *The Task of Medicine: Dialogue at Wickenburg*. I cite Kerr White because he has stated this perspective so clearly in this volume, even though he then goes on to personally question the perspective.

[15]L. Thomas, *Medusa and the Snail* and *The Lives of a Cell: Notes of a Biology Watcher*.

[16]*The Aphorisms of Hippocrates*.

[17]M.R. Werbach, *Third Line Medicine: Modern Treatment of Persistent Symptoms*. Like Kerr White, cited in note 12, Werbach in this volume describes carefully the doctrine of specific etiology that leads to specialization in medicine in order to attack it, arguing instead for a more ecological perspective on health and disease.

[18]Kenneth M. Ludmerer, *Learning to Heal: The Development of American Medical Education*.

[19]Harold Bursctaju, Richard Feinbloom, Robert M. Hamm, and Archie Brodsky, *Medical Choices, Medical Chances: How Patients, Families and Physicians Can Cope with Uncertainty*. In their opening chapter, "A case of uncertainty," the authors state the conventional medical wisdom clearly, then use a case study to draw it into question.

[20]See, for example, Donald P. Ardsell, *High Level Wellness*.

[21]A number of American critics looked at New Age developments with considerable distrust. See, for example, Michael Rossman—one of the leaders of Berkeley, California's Free Speech Movement in the 1960s—describing the *New Age Blues: On the Politics of Consciousness*, or Christopher Lasch, *The Culture of Narcissism: American Life in an Age of Diminishing Expectations*.

[22]A larger picture of contemporary home birth practices is contained in a publication by Mary Conklin and Ruth Simmons, titled *Planned Home Childbirths: Parental Perspectives*, available as Health Monograph no. 2 from the Michigan Department of Public Health, Lansing, Michigan, 1979. They include a bibliography of relevant journal articles, as well. See also Constance J. Adams, ed., *Nurse-Midwifery: Health Care for Women and Newborns*; Barbara Katz Rothman, *[In Labor] Giving Birth: Alternatives in Childbirth*; Judy Barrett Litoff, *American Midwives: 1860 to the Present* or William Ray Arney, *Power and the Profession of Obstetrics*. For information about the hospice movement see Parker Rossman, *Hospice: Creating New Models of Care for the Terminally Ill*; Theodore H. Koff, *Hospice: A Caring Community*; Ann Munley, *The Hospice Alternative: A New Context for Death and Dying*; or Charles A. and Donna M. Corr, eds., *Hospice Care: Principles and Practices*. For a critical perspective on this movement, see Emily K. Abel, "The hospice movement: Institutionalizing innovation."

[23]These observations were developed more completely in my presentation to the American Sociological Association, "Androgyny in New Age movements," Detroit, Michigan, August 1983.

[24]Steven Finando, the founding president of the national Coalition of Holistic Health Organizations, first drew my attention to this characteristic of holistic health organizations more generally.

[25]This chapter's description of holistic health themes and public interest in them as seen in new magazines and changes in subscription rates is based on data listed yearly in *Ulrich's International Periodicals Directory* from 1960 through 1985.

[26]Information about Mandala and the American Holistic Health Association comes from notes I made at the organizing meeting for the Coalition of Holistic Health Organizations, held in Washington, D.C., March 3, 1984.

[27]*Ulrich's International Periodicals Directory*.

[28]This information comes from interviews conducted with Rick J. Carlson on March 14 and 15, 1980.

[29]The description of health care policy entrepreneurship presented here is based on a series of interviews conducted in March of 1981 and June of 1986 with the

following informants: Rick J. Carlson, Effie P. Y. Chow, Annie Collins, Jane Fullerton, Fred Heydrich, Judith LaRosa, and Alice M. McGill, as well as on field notes I made in 1978 during the Washington, D.C., conference titled, "Holistic health: A public policy?" which is described in this chapter. Additional information came from an interview with Lawrence W. Green in May of 1989.

³⁰For more information on participants in the Arlie House and first Waldorf-Astoria conferences, see note 2 in the Introduction.

³¹Key publications inspired by Rick J. Carlson's policy work in the mid-1970s include his *The End of Medicine* and *Future Directions in Health Care: A New Public Policy*, written with Robert Cunningham, reporting on the second Waldorf-Astoria conference (described in this chapter), Ivan Illich's *Medical Nemesis: The Expropriation of Health* and John Knowles' edited volume, *Doing Better and Feeling Worse: Health Care in the U.S.*

³²See note 29 above.

³³*Ibid.*

³⁴Interview with Rick J. Carlson conducted on March 14 and 15, 1980.

³⁵Blue Shield of California published a report on the subsequent experimental study done in cooperation with the Hartford Insurance Company, the Bank of America and the Siskiyou County School District in California, and researchers at Stanford University. See H.G. Pearce, "The health incentive plan evaluation: Final report to the John A. Hartford Foundation, November, 1986," prepared for C.L. Paracell, Blue Shield of California vice-president and project director.

³⁶See Robert Crawford, "You are dangerous to your health: The ideology and politics of victim blaming."

³⁷Robert Crawford, "Healthism and the medicalization of everyday life (politics of self-care)."

³⁸See Howard S. Berliner and J. Warren Salmon, "The holistic alternative to scientific medicine: History and analysis." This article is one of the few critiques of holistic health which presents a genuinely balanced appraisal of problems and benefits inherent in the movement, discussing challenges to the hegemony of medical science and social gains and problems that result from this.

³⁹See, for example, Sally Guttmacher, "The individual, the social context, and health policy: Whole in body, mind & spirit—Holistic health and the limits of medicine."

⁴⁰See Howard S. Berliner and J. Warren Salmon, "The holistic alternative to scientific medicine: History and analysis."

⁴¹A number of holistic health advocates have tried to clarify what "taking responsibility for your health" means to responsible members of this movement. See, for example, James S. Gordon, *Holistic Medicine*.

⁴²*Ibid.*

⁴³See the discussion of Type I and Type II errors in W. Allen Wallis and Harry V. Robert, *Statistics: A New Approach*, 387-396.

⁴⁴Interview with Fred Wiewel and James S. Gordon, Washington, D.C., September, 1992.

⁴⁵*Ibid.*

⁴⁶A Report to NIH, by James S. Gordon, et al., on the Status of Alternative Medicine (in process) provides the basis of this description. On June 14, 1993, the National Institutes of Health Revitalization Act of 1993 (now known as Public Law

103–43) permanently established within the Office of the Director of NIH an office to be known as the Office of Alternative Medicine, whose director is appointed by the director of NIH.

[47]This information comes from notes I made during the 1992 NIH Conference.

[48]Information from the Office of Alternative Medicine, National Institutes of Health, October 1995. In 1995, the following people and institutions received OAM grants to establish Alternative Medicine Research Centers, with responsibility for coordinating investigation of particular topic areas: Leanna Standish at Bastyr University (a naturopathic medical college in Seattle, Washington), alternative approaches to the treatment of HIV/AIDS; Thomas Kiresuk at the Minneapolis Medical Research Center, use of acupuncture for treating drug addiction; Ann Gill Taylor at the University of Virginia School of Nursing and Brian M. Berman at the University of Maryland School of Medicine, alternative approaches to pain control; Guy S. Parcel at the University of Texas Health Center at Houston, alternative approaches to cancer; Samuel Shifflett at the Kessler Institute for Rehabilitation, West Orange, New Jersey, and the University of Medicine and Dentistry, Newark, New Jersey, alternative approaches to stroke and neurological conditions; William L. Haskell at Stanford, alternative approaches to aging; M. Eric Gershwin and Judith Stern, University of California, Davis, asthma, allergy and immunology; Fredi Kronenberg, Columbia University College of Physicians and Surgeons, women's health; David N. Eisenberg, Beth Israel Hospital and Harvard Medical School, general medical conditions.

[49]David Eisenberg, "Unconventional medical practice in the United States: Prevalence, costs and patterns of use."

[50]Insurance companies paying for some alternative treatments include Aetna, American Western Life, Blue Shield of California, and Mutual of Omaha.

[51]The Oxford Health Plan, in Connecticutt, was among the first to integrate alternative medicine within an HMO context.

Chapter 8
Prevention and Health Promotion: Industry,
the Government, and Foundations Innovate

[1]Charles-Everett A. Winslow, *The Evolution and Significance of the Modern Public Health Campaign*, 57-58.

[2]"Report to the Rockefeller Foundation of William Henry Welch and Wickliffe Rose," is reprinted as Appendix C in John Z. Bowers and Elizabeth F. Purcell, *Schools of Public Health: Present and Future.*

[3]In addition to Paul Starr's account of the development of public health programs in America, *The Social Transformation of American Medicine* (STAM), I found the following to be helpful: S.P.W. Chave, "The origins and development of public health"; and Committee for the Study of the Future of Public Health, Division of Health Care Services, Institute of Medicine, "A history of the public health system," 56-72.

[4]John J. Hanlon and George E. Pickett, "Development and organization of public health in the United States."

⁵Committee for the Study of the Future of Public Health, *The Future of Public Health*.

⁶The Fogarty Center's monograph series publications on the Teaching of Preventive Medicine include a preface which describes the Center's origins, mandate, and program emphases. See, for example, L.M. Carter, *Toward an Educated Health Consumer: Mass Communication and Quality in Medical Care*.

⁷This information was obtained in an interview with Lawrence W. Green, May 17, 1989.

⁸See L.H. Kulles, K.H. Svendsen, and J.K. Ockens, "The relationship of smoking cessation to coronary heart disease and lung cancer in the Multiple Risk Factor Intervention Trial (MRFIT)."

⁹This information comes from interviews with Rick J. Carlson, June 15, 1986, and with Lawrence W. Green, May 17, 1989.

¹⁰*Ibid*.

¹¹Information about action networks within the federal government has come from a number of informants within various health bureaucracies, in other government agencies, and in private health care organizations in Washington and elsewhere around the country.

¹²See note 26 in Chapter 3.

¹³Joint National Committee on Detection, Evaluation, and Treatment of High Blood Pressure, *Hypertension Prevalence and the Status of Awareness, Treatment, and Control in the United States: Final Report of the Subcommittee on Definition and Prevalence*; The National Cholesterol Education Project, Heart Lung and Blood Institute, *Adult Treatment Guidelines*; William B. Kannell, M.D. and Thomas J. Thom, "Declining cardiovascular mortality"; David Zinnman, "Mystery of heart disease death rates."

¹⁴See, for example, David Gelman, "Fitness, corporate style: Companies are racing to invest in employee 'wellness'"; Penelope C. Roeder and John H. Moxley III, "Promoting quality care in cost-effective settings."

¹⁵Jonathan Fielding, for the Office of Disease Prevention and Health Promotion, *National Survey of Worksite Health Promotion Activities: A Summary, 1987*.

¹⁶See, for example, Steven N. Blair, Philip V. Piserchia, Curtis S. Wilbur, and James H. Crowder, "A public health intervention model for work-site health promotion: Impact on exercise and physical fitness in a health promotion plan after 24 months"; Jonathan Fielding, "Smoking: Health effects and control."

¹⁷Laura C. Leviton, "The yield from worksite cardiovascular risk reduction."

¹⁸J.C. Erfurt, A. Foote, and M.A. Heirich, "Worksite wellness programs: Incremental comparison of screening and referral alone, health education, follow-up counseling, and plant organization."

¹⁹*Ibid*.

²⁰Interview with the late Andrea Foote, October 20, 1992.

²¹J.C. Erfurt and K. Holtyn, "Health promotion in small business: What works and what doesn't work."

²²These cost estimates came from the late Jack Erfurt, based on experience working with this kind of health promotion program for General Motors, Ford, and University of Michigan employees.

²³Interview with Hank Gardner, *Options and Choices*, June 15, 1993.

[24] *Ibid.*

[25] J.C. Erfurt, A. Foote, M.A. Heirich, and B.M. Brock, *The Wellness Outreach at Work Program: A Step-by-Step Guide.*

[26] "A pat on the back says you've done the right thing: Support for Healthy People 2000 Program," *Safety & Health* 147: 62, March 1993; "Vested interests: Welcoa's Annual Well Workplace Award Winners," *Hospitals and Health Networker* 68: 44, Nov. 20, 1994.

[27] Originated in the White House, The Health Project (THP) is a public/private organization involving leading U.S. corporations, the labor movement, the academic community, public groups and government agencies. Carson Beadle, Managing Director of William M. Mercer, Inc., is its president. THP gives annual C. Everett Koop National Health Awards to effective health care innovations, named for the former U.S. Surgeon General who co-founded The Health Project.

[28] Merck and Bristol-Myers Squibb pharmaceutical companies.

[29] J.C. Erfurt and A. Foote, "Maintenance of blood pressure treatment and control after discontinuation of work site follow-up."

[30] William R. Whitmer, "Worksite health promotion and health care reform: An update," and correspondence.

[31] *Ibid.*

[32] *Ibid.*

[33] The description of philanthropic foundation preventive health programs which follow in the text were taken from the foundations' annual reports.

[34] See Alvin R. Tarlov, Barbara H. Kehrer, Donna P. Hall, Sarah E. Samuels, Gwendolyn S. Grown, Michael R.J. Felix, and Jane A. Ross, "Foundation work: The Health Promotion Program of the Henry J. Kaiser Foundation," the Henry J. Kaiser Family Foundation Annual Reports, and interview with Lawrence W. Green, May 28, 1989.

[35] These included the Benedum Foundation of Pittsburgh, Pennsylvania, the Carnegie Corporation of New York, the Denver-based Colorado Trust, the J.M. Foundation of New York, the Robert Wood Johnson Foundation, based in Princeton, New Jersey, the Ruth Mott Fund of Flint, Michigan, the Pew Charitable Trusts of Philadelphia, Pennsylvania, the Dorothy Rider Pool Health Care Trust of Allentown, Pennsylvania, the San Diego Community Foundation, the San Francisco Foundation, the Stuart Foundations (also of San Francisco) and the Wesley Foundation in Wichita, Kansas.

[36] Telephone interview with Lawrence W. Green, October 21, 1992.

[37] NCCDPHP mission statement from NCCDPHP Home Page, Internet, updated 7/95, http://www.cdc.gov/nccdphp/vision.htm.

[38] U.S. Department of Health and Human Services, Public Health Service, *Healthy People 2000: National Health Promotion and Disease Prevention Objectives.*

[39] CDC Funding Opportunities, from CDC webpage, Internet: http://www.cdcd.gov/funding.htm.

[40] Prevention Training Centers History, Internet, http://129.137.232.101/stdptc/Network/PtcHistory.html.

[41] "Effective heart health programs at the worksite," conference jointly sponsored by the Ohio Department of Health and Bristol-Myers Squibb Pharmaceutical Company, in Columbus, Ohio, April 23, 1997.

⁴²Source: "Cost-effectiveness of prevention," http://www.cdc.gov/nccdphp/costeff.htm.

⁴³Jane E. Brody, "Why bad habits drive out good ones: Lack of progress in reaching *Healthy People 2000* goals established by surgeon general in 1990," New York *Times*, February 1, 1995, C9.

⁴⁴Sheryl Gay Stolberg, "Beleaguered tobacco foe holds key to talks," New York *Times*, June 4, 1997, A1.

⁴⁵John Schwartz, "FDA chief discloses high-nicotine leaf: Cigarettes manipulated, Kessler testifies," The Washington *Post*, June 22, 1994, A1; Marlise Simons, "FDA chief calls nicotine addiction a 'pediatric disease'," Los Angeles *Times*, March 9, 1995, A15; Marlise Simons, "FDA sees 'carding' as key deterrent to teen smoking," Los Angeles *Times*, Aug. 11, 1995, A27; Laurie McGinley and Timothy Noah, "Lighting a fire: Long FDA campaign and a bit of serendipity led to tobacco move: Firm's climate; why Kessler took action," *The Wall Street Journal*, Aug. 22, 1995, A1; Jeffrey Goldberg, "Next target: Nicotine," *The New York Times Magazine*, Aug. 4, 1996, 22.

⁴⁶Stolberg, "Beleaguered tobacco foe holds key to talks."

⁴⁷Art Buchwald, "One man's sauce (Satire on Bob Dole and the tobacco issue), The Washington *Post*, July 9, 1996, C1; George F. Will, "Dole's tobacco debacle; Presidential candidate Bob Dole lost credibility and perhaps votes after he suggested that tobaccco might not be addictive," The Washington *Post*, July 7, 1996, C7.

⁴⁸Stolberg, "Beleaguered tobacco foe holds key to talks."

⁴⁹Source: Internet, http://cdc.gov/nccdphp.riskf.htm.

⁵⁰John M. Broder, "FTC charges 'Joe Camel' ad illegally takes aim at minors," New York *Times*, May 29, 1997, A1.

⁵¹John M. Broder, "2 top cigarette makers seek settlement," New York *Times*, April 17, 1997, A1; Barry Meier, "Tobacco deal still stalled over nicotine civil damages," New York *Times*, A16; and Barry Meier, "Tobacco's price tag," New York *Times*, July 15, 1997, A8.

⁵²"An open letter to the American public: Tobacco deals—will they protect our children? Or is it about money?" American Cancer Society, May 1997.

⁵³Barry Meier, "Tobacco's price tag," New York *Times*, July 15, 1997, A8.

⁵⁴Sheryl Gay Stolberg, "4 groups see urgency for accord on tobacco," New York *Times*, June 13, 1997, A10; Barry Meier, "White House: It may be willing to help resolve tobacco dispute," New York *Times*, A8; Barry Meier, "Tobacco deal still stalled," New York *Times*, A16; Barry Meier, "Tobacco's price tag," New York *Times*, July 15, 1997, A8; Adam Clymer, "White House and GOP announce deal to balance budget and trim taxes," New York *Times*, July 29, 1997, A1.

⁵⁵Lifestyle change trends reported in Chapter 7 come from several sources. The Gallup Poll data come from *Gallup Poll Monthly Report* 226 (July 1984): 9-11, from information in *Gallup Poll Surveys 989-P* and *990-P*, and from a comparison of Gallup Polls conducted in 1961 and 1985 as reported by Sarah Van Allen of the Gallup Poll organization.

⁵⁶M.A. Heirich, A. Foote, J.C. Erfurt, and B. Konopka, "Worksite physical fitness programs: Comparing the impact of different program designs on cardiovascular risks."

⁵⁷Centers for Disease Control, Division of Education, *Promoting Physical Activity Among Adults*.

[58]Information about changes in food consumption patterns and in smoking behavior comes from comparing data found in various editions of *Stat. Abstracts of the United States* published between 1970 and 1987.

[59]Centers for Disease Control, Division of Education, *Effectiveness in Disease and Injury Prevention: Public Focus Activity and the Prevention of Coronary Heart Disease*; K.E. Warner, "Effects of the anti-smoking campaign: An update." J.H. Price, R.A. Krol, and S.M. Desmond, "Comparison of three antismoking interventions among pregnant women in an urban setting: A randomized trial".

[60]U.S. Public Health Service, *Strategies to Control Tobacco Use in the U.S.: A Blueprint for Public Health Action in the 1990s*; K.E. Warner, "Television and health education: Stay tuned."

[61]Frank Riessman, "New dimensions in self-help."

[62]Thomas J. Powell, *Self-Help Organizations and Professional Practice.*

[63]See Table 1-37: Live Births by Place of Delivery, Attendant, and Race of Child: United States, Specified Years 1940-60 and Each Year 1965-86, U.S. Public Health Service, *Vital Statistics of the U.S., 1986, Volume I, Natality.*

[64]*Guide to the Nation's Hospices, Annual, 1984.*

[65]See note 41 in Chapter 6.

[66]See note 44 in Chapter 6.

[67]Lawrence W. Green interview, May 28, 1989.

[68]K.E. Warner, "Smoking and health: A 25-year perspective" and "Smoking and health implications of a change in the federal cigarette excise tax."

[69]*Ibid.*

[70]See Henry J. Kaiser Family Foundation Annual Report 1989.

[71]David R. Williams, "Macrosocial influences on African-American health," American Psychological Association meetings, Washington, D.C., 1992.

[72]J.C. Erfurt, A. Foote, M.A. Heirich, and B.M. Brock, *The Wellness at Work Program: A Step-By-Step Guide.*

[73]Robert Crawford, "You are dangerous to your health."

[74]J.C. Erfurt, A. Foote, and M.A. Heirich, "Saving lives and dollars through comprehensive preventive health care."

[75]M.A. Heirich, J.C. Erfurt, and A. Foote, "The core technology of worksite wellness."

[76]Max Heirich, Carolyn Holmes, et al., "Integrating prevention and primary care services: A proposal from the University of Michigan," February 1993, submitted to Clinton Health Reform Task Force, at the request of Joycelyn Elders, Surgeon General.

[77]J.C. Erfurt, "What can we do next to encourage worksite health promotion?" Fetzer Institute, Kalamazoo, Michigan, March 13, 1992.

[78]L.G. Coleman, "Geriatric boomers expected to strain health care system"; C. Farrell, "The age wave and how to ride it: Middle-aged baby boomers and senior-seniors mean more spending on entertainment and health care"; R.G. Schwartz, "Commentary: Investment for an aging population."

[79]Gay Luce, "S.A.G.E., a health program for senior citizens," report to the Holmes Center for Research in Holistic Healing, annual research symposium, Los Angeles, California, March 1991.

Chapter 9
Understanding the Ecology of Health and Disease

[1]M. Lappe, *Broken Code*, 13-21.

[2]U.S. OTA, *Mapping Our Genes—The Genome Projects: How Big, How Fast?*, 3-6, 13-14, 21, 116-117; M. Lappe, *Broken Code*, 101-115; S.J. Aje and J. Mori, "Birth defects: From here to eternity"; T.H. Fraser, "The future of recombinant DNA technology in medicine," 395-426, 469-482; T.F. Lee, *The Human Genome Project*, 209-234; J. Davis, *Mapping the Code*, 135-140, 159-160; "The Genome Project: Life after Watson."

[3]G. Montgomery, "Shooting the messenger," ; W.A. Haseltine and F. Wong-Staal, "The molecular biology of the AIDS virus"; J.N. Weber and R.A. Weiss, "HIV infection: The cellular picture."

[4]W.A. Haseltine and F. Wong-Staal, "The molecular biology of the AIDS virus."

[5]L. Thomas, *The Lives of a Cell*, 3-5.

[6]"The human body has 10 to the 12th number of cells and 10 to the 13th number of micro-organisms." Jon Sangeorzan, M.D., University of Michigan Medical School, lecture on infectious disease, University AIDS course, February 12, 1992.

[7]C.R. Miro and J.E. Cox, "EPA Science Board concludes passive smoke causes cancer"; "Legislation needed to protect nonsmokers"; P. Weiss, "Passive risk: EPA loads anti-smoking gun"; "Passive smokers tied to cancer risk in study," New York *Times*, October 7, 1992, C13.

[8]Kenneth A. Perkins and Leonard H. Epstein, "Smoking, stress, and coronary heart disease."

[9]"The legal implications of dietary fats: Risks of cardiovascular disease and the duty of food manufacturers"; R.A. Harmon, "American experience with nutrition and cardiovascular risk".

[10]*Nutrition, Toxicity, and Cancer; Nutrition and Cancer Prevention*; M.M. Jacobs, "Diet, nutrition, and cancer: An overview".

[11]J.N. Weber and R.A. Weiss, "HIV infection: The cellular picture."

[12]N.R. Hall and A.D. Goldstein, "Thinking well: The chemical links between emotions and health"; D.N. Khansari, A.J. Murgo, and R.E. Faith, "Effects of stress on the immune system."

[13]*Stress Neuropeptides and Systemic Disease*; "Chemical switchboard of the brain."

[14]N.M. Amin, "Antibiotic-associated pseudomembranous colitis"; M. Amdrejak et al., "The clinical significance of antibiotic-associated pseudomembranous colitis in the 1990s".

[15]M.C. Lakshmanan, et al., "Hospital admissions caused by iatrogenic disease"; H.G. Colt and A.P. Shapiro, "Drug-related illnesses as a cause for admission to a community hospital"; A.P. Jonville et al., "Characteristics of medication errors in pediatrics."

[16]H.G. Caldwell, *Mosquitos, Malaria and Man: A History of the Hostilities Since 1880*, 232-263; R.S. Desowitz, *The Malaria Capers*, 211-220.

[17]Lawrence K. Altman, "Wake-up call on threats of disease," New York *Times*, October 16, 1992, A31; Michael Specter, "Neglected for years, TB is back with strains that are deadlier," New York *Times*, October 11, 1992, A1.

[18]H. Bartsch, et al., "Carcinogen metabolism and DNA adducts in human lung tissues as affected by tobacco smoking or metabolic phenotype"; F.F. Kadlubar, "Detection of human DNA-carcinogen adducts"; F. Perera, et al., "DNA adducts and other biological markers in risk assessment for environmental carcinogens"; D.H. Phillips, et al., "Monitoring occupational exposure to carcinogens"; R.M. Santella, et al., "Immunological methods for the detection of carcinogen adducts in humans"; P. Vinels, et al., "Genetically-based a-acetyltranferese metabolic polymorphism and low-level environmental exposure to carcinogens".

[19]S. Blakeslee, "Genes tell story of why some get cancer and others don't", New York *Times*, May 17, 1994, B6.

[20]F.M. Waldman, et al., "Centromeric copy number of chromosome 7 is strongly correlated with tumor grade and labeling index in human bladder cancer"; A. Blair and S.H. Zahm, "Herbicides and cancer."

[21]S. Blakeslee, "Genes tell story of why some get cancer while others don't," New York *Times*, May 17, 1994, C3.

[22]WHO, "Update on AIDS," *Weekly Epidemiological Record*, November 29, 1991; Philip Shenon, "After years of denial, Asia faces scourge of AIDS," New York *Times*, November 8, 1992, A1; "HIV statistics and strategies".

[23]Incidence reports summarized by Mindy Fullilove, psychiatrist and AIDS researcher, at a University of Michigan conference on AIDS reported in the *Ann Arbor News*, June 28, 1989, A1.

[24]David A. Kessler, Food Drug Administration (FDA), asked Congress to give FDA rights to control tobacco manufacture and sales, as a drug, *The Washington Post*, March 26, 1994, A3; Kessler cites tobacco company use of recombinant DNA to create tobacco plants with a stronger nicotene content and their cultivation in Latin American tobacco plantations. New York *Times*, June 22, 1994, A1.

[25]T. Weiner and T. Golden, "Free-trade treaty may widen traffic in drugs" New York *Times*, May 24, 1993, 142, A1.

[26]D. Adamson, *Defending*, 9; R. Benedick, *Ozone Diplomacy*, 114-115; James Brooke, "President, in Rio, defends his stand on environment," New York *Times*, June 13, 1992, A1.

[27]D. Adamson, *Defending*, 111-112.

[28]Murray Feshback and Alfred Friendly, *Ecocide in the U.S.S.R.*, 11-12, 174-175.

[29]See, for example, O. Sursis and A. Puchalsky, "Detroit Edison fire shuts down plant," The *Wall Street Journal*, December 29, 1993, B7; P. Hadfield, "Accidents cast shadow over Japan's nuclear strategy," *New Scientist* 129:15, March 9, 1991; M. Fitzgerald, "Three Mile Island and cancer," *The Fourth Estate*, 122:32, April 22, 1989; "Cover-up after accident cited by Whistleblower (Georgia), *ENR* 225: 13-14, October 4, 1990; "Disaster on tap at French reactor," *New Scientist* 139:7, July 17, 1993.

[30]Murray Feshback and Alfred Friendly, *Ecocide in the USSR*, 11-12; David Budiansky, "The dim glow of history," 74 ff.

[31]"World cancer rates shifting dramatically," 161; *Environmental Change and Human Health*.

[32]Linda Rothstein, "PSR pinpoints problems," *Bulletin of the Atomic Scientists* 49:10, Jan-Feb, 1993.

[33]Alicia Hills Moore, "The other worry: Atomic wastes," *Fortune* 118: 114, August 1, 1988; "Further study needed," *Bul. Atomic Scientists*, 46:4, July-Aug., 1990; "Catch-22", *Bul. Atomic Scientists*, 46:6, Sept. 1990.

[34]Allen Springer, "United States environmental policy and international Law: Stockholm Principle Twenty-One revisited," 47-48; Lynton K. Caldwell, *International Environmental Policy*, 105.

[35]D. Adamson, *Defending*, 54.

[36]*Critical Condition: human health and the environment.*

[37]D. Adamson, *Defending*, 107.

[38]U.S. Environmental Protection Agency (EPA), "Executive summary on the scientific assessment of stratospheric ozone," 15099; D.J. Hofmann, et al., "Observation and possible causes of new ozone depletion in Antarctica in 1991," 283-287.

[39]"Pinatubo fails to deepen the ozone hole," 395.

[40]Fred S. Singer, *Global Climate Change*, 125.

[41]Michael Weiskopf, "First summer thinning found in U.S. ozone layer," *Congressional Record* 137(154), Oct. 24, 1991, 15098.

[42]Warren E. Leaky, "Ozone-harming agents reach a record," New York *Times*, February 4, 1992, C4.

[43]EPA, *Effects of Changes in Stratospheric Ozone and Global Climate*, 3-6.

[44]D. Adamson, *Defending*, 106. Richard E. Benedick, *Ozone Diplomacy*, 14-15.

[45]OTA, *Changing By Degrees*, 61-62.

[46]William K. Stevens, "Compromise offered at U.N. on greenhouse emissions," New York *Times*, May 2, 1992, A3; W.K. Stevens, "Accord on limits on gas emissions said to be near," New York *Times*, May 8, 1992, A1; W.K. Stevens, "143 lands adopt treaty to cut emissions of gases," New York *Times*, May 10, 1992, A14; Paul Lewis, "U.N. seeks third world ecology aid," New York *Times*, March 2, 1992, A3.

[47]Michael Weiskopf, "First summer thinning found in U.S. ozone layer," *Congressional Record* 137(154), Oct. 24, 1991, 15098.

[48]U.S. Office of Technology Assessment (OTA), *Changing by Degrees: Steps to Reduce Greenhouse Gasses, Summary*.

[49]D. Adamson, *Defending*, 106.

[50]"Toxic Wasteland," 40-43; Marlise Simons, "Massive ozone and smog defile Atlantic skies," New York *Times*, October 12, 1992, A1.

[51]EPA, *Effects of Changes in Stratospheric Ozone and Global Climate*, 3. Jeremy Leggett, "Running down to Rio," 38-42.

[52]D. Adamson, *Defending*.

[53]"Researcher discounts global warming," *Geotimes* 38:6, Sept. 1993; W. Beckerman and J. Malkin, "How much does global warming matter?" *The Public Interest* 114:3-16, Winter 1994; Suzanne Tainter, "Improving global change models: Going after better data," in special issue: *Detecting signals of global change*, University of Michigan *Research News*, 46(2):6-13,1995.

[54]IPOC, *Climate Change: The IPOC Scientific Assessment*, Executive Summary XC.

[55]D. Adamson, *Defending*, 111-112.

[56]J. Griffith, et al., "Cancer mortality in U.S. counties with hazardous waste sites and ground water pollution," 69-74; K. Baverstock, et al., "Thyroid cancer after Chernobyl," 21-22.

[57]J.E. Davies and R. Doon, "Human health effects of pesticides," 113-124; J. Stanley, *Broad Scan Analysis of Human Adipose Tissue, Executive Summary*; R. Dougherty, et al., "Negative chemical ionization studies of human and food chain contamination with xenobiotic chemicals," 103-118; C. Travis and H. Hattemer-Fray, "Global chemical pollution."

[58]L.K. Caldwell, *International Environmental Policy*, 41-42; A.L. Springer, "United States environmental policy and international law," 46.

[59]D. Adamson, *Defending*, 35.

[60]L.K. Caldwell, *International Environmental Policy*, 51.

[61]D. Adamson, *Defending*, 35.

[62]L.K. Caldwell, *International Environmental Policy*, 53-67.

[63]A. Rosencranz and J.E. Carroll, *International Environmental Diplomacy: The Management and Resolution of Transfrontier Environmental Problems*, 173-184.

[64]D. Adamson, *Defending*, 57.

[65]R. Benedick, *Ozone Diplomacy*, 46, 265; D. Adamson, *Defending*, 109-115.

[66]World Commission on Environment and Development, *Our Common Future*, 43-66; M. Jacobs, *The Green Economy*, 58-61.

[67]"Risking global disaster, Japan continues to attack the Earth's ozone layer," ad in New York *Times*, June 13, 1995, A23.

[68]R. Benedick, *Ozone Diplomacy*, 114; D. Adamson, *Defending*, 19, 152-153.

[69]D. Adamson, *Defending*, 185.

[70]D. Adamson, *Defending*, 186.

[71]D. Adamson, *Defending*, 187-189.

[72]Netherlands Ministerie van Welzijn, Volkgezondheim en Cultuur. Stuurgroep Toekwustscenario's Gezondheidzorg, *AIDS up to the year 2000: Epidemiological, sociocultural,and economic scenario analysis for the Netherlands*; Daniel M. Perrine, "The view from Platform Zero: How Holland handles its drug problem," *America* 171: 9-12, October 15, 1994.

[73]U.S. Dept. of Health and Human Services, *Health Status of the Disadvantaged Chartbook*.

[74]William K. Stevens, "Washington may change its position on climate," New York *Times*, February 18, 1992, C1; John B. Oakes, "An Environmentalist? Bush? Forget It," New York *Times*, May 8, 1992, A31; Keith Schneider, "U.S. environmental negotiator in Rio walks a tightrope in administration," New York *Times*, June 2, 1992, A11; R. Benedick, *Ozone Diplomacy*, 51-67.

[75]A.L. Springer, *Ibid.*, 52-55; L.K. Caldwell, *International Environmental Policy*, 278-279; H. Patricia Hynes, *The Recurring Silent Spring*, 140-179.

[76]"Trees aren't a magic answer," New York *Times*, June 7, 1992, A20.

[77]B. Knickerbocker, "World leaders gather at Rio for earth summit," *The Christian Science Monitor* 84:131, June 2, 1992, 12.

[78]James Brooke, "U.S. has starring role at Rio summit as villain," New York *Times*, June 2, 1992, A27.

[79]EPA, "Executive summary on the scientific assessment of stratospheric ozone"; "Ozone in northern hemisphere at lowest level in fourteen years" (Report from NASA and the National Oceanic and Atmospheric Administration) New York *Times*, April 23, 1993, A14.

[80]Paul Lewis, "U.S. informally offers to cut rise in climate-warming gases," New York *Times*, April 29, 1992, A10; William K. Stevens, "143 lands adopt treaty to cut emissions of gases," New York *Times*, May 10, 1992, A14; Keith Schneider, "White House snubs U.S. envoy's plea to sign Rio treaty" New York *Times*, June 5, 1992, A1; W.K. Stevens, "U.S., trying to buff its image, defends forests," New York *Times*, June 7, 1992, A20.

81William K. Stevens, "Lessons of Rio: A new preeminence and an effective blandness," New York *Times*, June 14, 1992, A10; Steven Greenhouse, "Ecology, the economy, and Bush," New York *Times*, June 14, 1992, D1.

82James Brooke, "U.N. chief closes summit with an appeal for action," New York *Times*, June 14, 1992, A8; William K. Stevens, "With climate treaty signal, all say they'll do even more," New York *Times*, June 13, 1992, A1.

83James Brooke, "Britain and Japan split with U.S. on species pact," New York *Times*, June 6, 1992, A1.

84"Bush plan to save forests is blocked by poor countries," New York *Times*, June 9, 1992, A7; "Earth Summit races clock to resolve differences on forest treaty," New York *Times*, June 10, 1992, A8. William K. Stevens, "U.S. at Earth Summit: Isolated and challenged," New York *Times*, June 10, 1992, A8.

85"Pinatubo fails to deepen the ozone hole."

86Charles Hanley, "Global warming: Action in '97?" Associated Press, in Ann Arbor *News*, September 28, 1997, A3.

87A. Gore, *Earth in the Balance: Ecology and the Human Spirit*; Charles J. Hanley, "Administration backs off stance on global warming," *Associated Press*, June 16, 1997; John H. Cushman, Jr., "Senate urges U.S. to pursue new strategy on emissions," New York *Times*, July 26, 1997, A8.

88George W. Hinman, Thomas C. Lowinger, and Russell J. Fuller, "The impact of nuclear power on the systematic risk and market value of electric utility common stock"; Charles R. Moyer and Raymond E. Spudeck, "A note on the stock market's reaction to the accident at Three Mile Island"; Thomas Schneeweis and Joanne Hill, "The effect of Three Mile Island on electric utility stock prices."

89R.J. Knox, "Toxic overload: The waste disposal dilemma"; J.E. Davies and R. Doon, "Human health effects of pesticides"; S.S. Sandhu, et al., "Clastogenicity evaluation of seven chemicals commonly found at hazardous industrial waste sites," AMA Council on Scientific Affairs; American Medical Association, "A permanent U.S.-Mexico border environmental health commission."

90"Manufacturers urged to make environmentalism a goal," New York *Times*, September 29, 1992, C4; "Environmental rules may spur innovation," New York *Times*, September 8, 1992, C8; Curtis Moore, "Bush's nonsense on jobs and the environment," New York *Times*, September 25, 1992, A33.

91See C-E. A. Winslow, *The Evolution and Significance of the Modern Public Health Campaign*, 57-58.

92Max Weber, "Science as a vocation."

93William K. Stevens, "Economists strive to find environment's bottom line," New York *Times*, September 8, 1992, C1.

94F.A. Sloan, *Cost, Quality, and Access in Health Care: New Roles for Health Planning in a Competitive Environment*; Institute of Medicine, *Costs of Environment-Related Health Effects: A Plan for Continuing Study*.

95W.A. Rosenbaum, *The Politics of Environmental Concern*.

96L.G. Hines, *Environmental Issues: Population, Pollution, and Economics*.

97EPA, "Executive summary on the scientific assessment of stratospheric ozone"; "Ozone in northern hemisphere at lowest level in fourteen years" (Report from NASA and the National Oceanic and Atmospheric Administration) New York *Times*, April 23, 1993, A14.

⁹⁸L.S. Gallay, "Health care, technology, and competitive environment"; Congressional Quarterly, Inc., *Environment and Health*.

⁹⁹R.R. Alford, *Health Care Politics: Ideological and Interest Groups, Barrier to Reform*.

¹⁰⁰*Canadian Aid and the Environment: The Politics and Performance of the Canadian International Development Agency*; Charles S. Pearson, *Environment, North and South: An Economic Interpretation*; Johan Galtung, *Toward Self-Reliance and Global Interdependence: Reflections on a New International Order and North-South Cooperation*.

¹⁰¹J. Schooner, "The Rio Earth Summit: What does it mean?"

Chapter 10
Reapproaching Health: Next Steps

¹R. William Whitmer, "Worksite health promotion and health care reform: An update," and correspondence.

²Information from Bruce Brock, a consultant to the Air Force for prevention planning.

³Quotations from documents circulated to MHSS2020 participants, authors not identified in the documents.

⁴*Ibid.*

⁵Jeff deGraff shared this observation of market behaviors.

⁶This information comes from notes I made while attending HERO's organizing meetings.

⁷Sallyanne Payton, "Why alliances? A simpler path to health care reform through reinsurance."

⁸The pattern of skewed health care utilization which Federal Express has documented for their employees is found much more widely, and applies to Medicare utilization as well.

⁹Ron Winslow, "Uninsured suffered higher death rate over 16-year period, researchers find," *The Wall Street Journal* (Eastern edition), Aug. 11, 1993, B3.

¹⁰The John E. Fogarty International Center for Advanced Study in the Health Sciences, *The Barefoot Doctor's Manual: The American Translation of the Chinese Paramedical Manual*, provides detail on health guidelines used for these services in China.

¹¹A larger picture of contemporary home birth practices is contained in a publication by Mary Conklin and Ruth Simmons, titled *Planned Home Childbirths: Parental Perspectives*, available as Health Monograph no. 2 from the Michigan Department of Public Health, Lansing, Michigan, 1979. They include a bibliography of relevant journal articles, as well. See also Constance J. Adams, ed., *Nurse-Midwifery: Health Care for Women and Newborns*; Barbara Katz Rothman, *[In Labor] Giving Birth: Alternatives in Childbirth*; Judy Barrett Litoff, *American Midwives: 1860 to the Present* or William Ray Arney, *Power and the Profession of Obstetrics*.

¹²Barbara Luke, Nicole Mamelle, Louis Keith, et al. "The association between occupational factors and preterm birth: A United States nurses' study."

¹³James D. Lubitz, Gerald F. Riley, "Trends in medical payments in the last year of life;" "National health care expenditures, by type."

¹⁴David R. Olmos, "AIDS activists accuse druggist of profiteering," Los Angeles *Times*, Nov. 21, 1993, 112, D1.

[15]An AIDS treatment data network has been set up with a Pfeizer grant. Laurie Lehne, Heather Branton, and Anne Bottros have collected cost data that can be used with this broader database.

[16]From literature prepared by Shanti, 1984.

[17]H. Lance Gould, Dean Ornish, and Larry Scherwitz, "Changes in myocardial perfusion abnormalities by positron emission tomography after long-term, intensive risk factor modification," *JAMA* 274: 89-901, September 20, 1995; Dean Ornish, *Clinical Cardiac Rehabilitation: A Cardiologist's Guide*, Baltimore, MD: Williams & Wilkins, 1993; Dean Ornish, *Dr. Dean Ornish's Program for Reversing Heart Disease*, NY: Random House, 1990; Dean Ornish, *Stress, Diet and Your Heart*, NY: Holt, Rinehart and Winston, 1982.

[18]Mutual of Omaha has announced its willingness to pay for the cardiac rehabilitation program developed by Dr. Dean Ornish, which relies on diet, exercise, social support, and meditation. Aetna and Blue Shield of California will do so, also. American Western Life Insurance now pays for a wider range of alternative treatments.

[19]David Eisenberg, "Unconventional medical practice in the United States: Prevalence, costs, and patterns of use."

[20]The Oxford Health Plan, in Connecticut, was among the first to integrate alternative medicine within an HMO context.

[21]George Foster, "Alternative health care takes root," Seattle *Post Intelligencer*, February 25, 1995, B1.

Chapter 11
Reapproaching Problems of Cost

[1]James D. Lubitz and Gerald F. Riley, "Trends in medical payment in the last year of life," p. 1094.

[2]Barbara Luke, Nicolle Mamelle, Louis Keith, et al., "The association between occupational factors and preterm birth: A United States nurses' study."

[3]C. Hoffman, D. Rice, and H.Y. Sung, "Persons with chronic conditions: Their prevalence and cost."

[4]Mike Cansey, "Finally some good news," (Pres. Clinton's balanced budget plan would help medically uninsured U.S. workers by requiring health plans that are part of the Federal Employees Health Benefits program to offer same coverage to employees in small firms that don't provide health insurance), The Washington *Post*, June 15, 1995, 118, D2.

[5]Jeff DeGraff suggested this possible strategy for capping public liability for hospital costs while allowing hospitals to expand their markets (personal communication, May 1993).

[6]J. Wiener, L. Illston, and R.J. Hanley, *Sharing the Burden: Strategies for Public and Private Long-Term Care Insurance*. See especially Table 2-10: "Initial individual and group premiums for two-year and four-year private long term care insurance," p 49.

[7]Marilynn Rosenthal, *Dealing with Medical Malpractice: The British and Swedish Experience*. London: Tavistock, 1987; Durham, NC: Duke Univ. Press, 1988.

[8]*Ibid.*

[9]*Benefits, Costs, and Cycles in Workers' Compensation.*

Chapter 12
New Approaches to Problems of Access

[1]Some people ask if those proposals to protect wages are enforceable. I think they could be. Employees who find their wages not increased after absorbing health benefits costs formerly paid by the employer could file complaints with IRS against their employers. Since their employer's identification number is part of those employees' W-2 forms, it would be easy to audit the tax reports of those employers, to see whether the allegations are correct.

[2]David C. Johnston, "Anti-tobacco groups push for higher cigarette taxes," New York *Times*, April 3, 1997, A1; Art Pine, "Panel Oks tax cuts, seeks levy on tobacco (Senate Finance Com.), Los Angeles *Times*, June 20, 1997, A1.

[3]Louis Uchitelle, "Not making it: We're leaner, meaner, and going nowhere faster," New York *Times*, May 12, 1996, 4, 1, *Week in Review.*

[4]Information from interviews with the Rev. Richard P. Wilson and Ms. Maggie Burton, President and chief staff person for ILC/PATCH, Inc.

[5]*Ibid.*

[6]*Ibid.*

References

Abel, Emily K. "The hospice movement: Institutionalizing innovation." *International Journal of Health Service* 16(1):71-86, 1986.

Adams, Constance J. *Nurse Mid-Wifery: Health Care for Women and Newborns.* New York: Grune & Stratton, 1983.

Adamson, David. *Defending the World: The Politics and Diplomacy of the Environment.* London: I.B. Tauris, 1990.

Aje, Samuel J. and Mori, Joseph. "Birth defects: From here to eternity." In *Genetic Perspectives in Biology and Medicine,* edited by Edward D. Garber. Chicago: University of Chicago Press, 1985.

Akers, R.L. *Drug, Alcohol, and Society: Social Structure, Process, and Policy.* Belmont, CA: Wadsworth Publ. Company, 1992.

Albritton, F.P. *Health Care Insurance Reform in the United States: A Market Approach with Application from the Federal Republic of Germany.* Lanham, MD: University Press of America, 1992.

Al-Chalabi, Fadhil J. *OPEC at the Crossroads.* Oxford and New York: Pergamon Press, 1989.

Alekseev, A. *Stockholm Conference.* Moscow: General Editorial Board for Foreign Publications, Nauka Publishers, 1986.

Alford, R.R. *Health Care Politics: Ideological and Interest Groups, Barrier to Reform.* Chicago: University of Chicago Press, 1975.

Allen, Sheila. "Class, culture and generation." *Sociological Review* 21:437-446, 1973.

Altman, Dennis. *Homosexual Oppression and Liberation.* New York: Avon, 1984.

Amdrejak, M., Schmit, J.L., and Tondriaux, A. "The clinical significance of antibiotic-associated pseudomembranous colitis in the 1990s." *Drug Safety* 6(5):339-49, Sept.-Oct. 1991.

American College of Surgeons. *Socioeconomic Fact Book for Surgery.* Chicago: ACS, 1979, 1986.

American Hospital Association. *Directory of Multihospital Systems.* Chicago: AHA, 1985.

_____. *Hospital Statistics, 1986.* Chicago: AHA, 1986.

_____. *Panel Survey, 1988.* Chicago: AHA, 1988.

_____. *Survey of Sources of Hospital Construction, 1982.* Chicago: AHA, 1982.

American Management Association. *Employee Benefit Cost Control.* New York: Am. Mgt. Assoc. Insurance Div., 1968.

American Medical Association. *Nostrums and Quackery: Articles on the Nostrum Evil and Quackery Reprinted from the Journal of the American Medical Association (JAMA).* Chicago: AMA Press, 1912.

_____. *Physician Liability: Survey Report.* Chicago: AMA, 1980.

_____. *Reference Data on Socioeconomic Issues of Health.* Chicago: AMA, 1977.

_____. *Report of the Special Task Force on Professional Liability and Insurance.* Chicago: AMA, October, 1984.

_____. *Socioeconomic Monitoring System Survey.* Chicago: AMA, 1988.

American Medical Association, Council on Scientific Affairs. "A permanent U.S.-Mexico border environmental health commission." *JAMA* 263(24):3319-3332, June 27, 1990.

American Nursing Association. *Facts About Nursing, 1984-85.* Kansas City, MO: ANA, 1985.

Amin, M. "Antibiotic-associated pseudomembranous colitis." *American Family Physician* 31:115-20, May 1985.

Anderson, Odin W. *Blue Cross Since 1929: Accountability and the Public Trust.* Cambridge, MA: Ballinger, 1975, 40.

Ardsell, Donald P. *High Level Wellness.* Berkeley, CA: Ten Speed Press, 1986.

Arney, William Ray. *Power and the Profession of Obstetrics.* Chicago: University of Chicago Press, 1982.

Bacciocco, Edward J., Jr. *The New Left in America: Reform to Revolution, 1956 to 1970.* Stanford, CA: Hoover Institute Press, 1974.

Bach, George Leland. *The New Inflation: Causes, Effects, Cures.* Providence, RI: Brown University Press, 1972.

Baggot, R. *Alcohol, Politics and Social Policy.* Aldershot: Avebury, 1990.

Bailey, May Ann, and Cikins, Warren I. (eds.). *The Effects of Litigation on Health Care Costs: Papers.* Washington, DC: Brookings Institute, 1985.

Bailis, Lawrence Neil. *Bread or Justice: Grassroots Organizing in the Welfare Rights Movement.* Lexington, MA: Lexington Press, 1974.

Barnaby, Frank, and Thomas, Geoffrey (eds.). *The Nuclear Arms Race, Control or Catastrophe? Proceedings of the General Section of the British Association for the Advancement of Science.* London: Frances Pinter, 1982.

Bartsch, H., Petruzzelli, S., De Flora, S., Hietanen, E., Camus, A.M., Castegnaro, M., Geneste D., Camoirano, A., Saracci, R., Giuntini, C., "Carcinogen metabolism and DNA adducts in human lung tissues as affected by tobacco smoking or metabolic phenotype." *Mutation Research* 250(1-2):103-14, Sept.-Oct. 1991.

Baumol, William, and Blinder, Alan. *Economic Principles and Policies.* New York: Harcourt, Brace, 1986.

Baverstock, K., Egloff, B., Pinchera, A., Ruchti, C., and Williams, D. "Thyroid cancer after Chernobyl." *Nature* 359:21-22, September 3, 1992.

Beachler, M.P. "Improving health care for underserved infants, children, and adolescents: The Robert Wood Johnson Foundation's experience." *American Journal of Diseases of Children (AJDC)* 145:565-568, 1991.

Beckerman, Wilfred and Malkin, Jesse "How much does global warming matter?" *The Public Interest* 114:3-16, Winter 1994.

Bell, Daniel. *The Coming of Post-Industrial Society: A Venture in Social Forecasting.* New York: Basic Books, 1973, 1976.

Benedick, Richard E. *Ozone Diplomacy.* Cambridge, MA: Harvard University Press, 1991.

Benefits, Costs, and Cycles in Workers' Compensation. Boston: Kluwer Academic Publishers, 1990.

Benello, C. George. *The Case for Participatory Democracy: Some Prospects for a Radical Society*. New York: Viking Press, 1972.

Benson, Herbert. *Beyond the Relaxation Response*. New York: Times Books, 1984.

_____. *The Mind/Body Effect: How Behavioral Medicine Can Show You the Way to Better Health*. New York: Simon & Schuster, 1979.

_____. *The Relaxation Response*. New York: Morrow, 1975.

Benson, Herbert and Epstein, Mark D. "The placebo effect: A neglected asset in the care of patients." Chapter 6, in *Health for the Whole Person: The Complete Guide to Holistic Medicine*, edited by Hastings, Arthur C., Fadiman, James, and Gordon, James S. New York: Bantam Books, 1981: 184-190.

Benson, Herbert, Gentry, W. Doyle, and Wolff, Charles A. *Work, Stress and Health*. Boston: Kluever, 1985.

Berkeley Holistic Health Center. *Holistic Health Lifebook: A Guide to Personal and Planetary Well-Being*. E. Rutherford, NJ: Greene, 1984.

Berliner, Howard S., and Regan, Carol. "Multi-national operations of U.S. for-profit hospital chains: Trends and implications." In *The Corporate Transformation of Health Care: Issues & Directions*, edited by Salmon, J. Warren. Amityville, NY: Baywood Publishing Company, Inc., 1990, 155-156.

Berliner, Howard S. and Salmon, J. Warren. "The holistic alternative to scientific medicine: History and analysis." *Journal of International Health Services* 10(1):133-148, 1974.

Berman, Henry. "Insuring the uninsured: Operational issues." *Proceedings of the 1990 Group Health Institute* 21-35, 1990.

Bernard, Claude. *Introduction to the Study of Experimental Medicine*. Paris, 1865. Classics in Medicine Series. New York: Macmillan, 1927.

Bertlet, Mary M. (ed.). *Hospital Liability: Law and Practice*. 5th ed. New York: Practicing Law Institute, 1987.

Bickell, Alexander M. *Politics and the Warren Court*. New York: Harper and Row, 1965.

Bien, Sandra. *Women's Liberation: An Historical View*. Independence, KY: Feminist Publications, 1971.

Bird, J.M. *Plate Tectonics: Selected Papers from Publications of the American Geophysical Union*. 2nd ed. Washington, DC: AGU, 1980.

Birenbaum, A. *Putting Health Care on the National Agenda*. Westport, CT: Praeger, 1993.

Blaikie, Piers, and Barnett, Tony. *AIDS in Africa: The Social and Policy Impact*. Lewiston: Edwin Meller Press, 1988.

Blair, A. and Zahm, S.H. "Herbicides and cancer: A review and discussion of methodological issues." *Recent Results Cancer Research* 120:132-95, 1990.

Blair, Steven N., Piserchia, Philip V., Wilbur, Curtis S., and Crowder, James H. "A public health intervention model for work-site Health promotion: Impact on exercise and physical fitness in a health promotion plan after 24 months." *JAMA* 255(7):921-926, February 21, 1986.

Blauner, Bob. *Racial Oppression in America*. New York: Harper and Row, 1972.

Bledstein, Burton J. *The Culture of Professionalism: The Middle Class and the Development of Higher Education in America*. New York: W.W. Norton, 1976.

Blendon, R.J., Leitman, R., Morrison, I., and Donelan, K. "Satisfaction with health systems in ten nations." *Health Affairs* 9:185-192, 1990.

Blendon, R.J., and Tracey, S.H. (eds.). *Reforming the System: Containing Health Care Costs in an Era of Universal Coverage*. New York: Faulkner and Gray, 1992.

Blomstrom, Magnus. *Transnational Corporations and Manufacturing Exports from Developing Countries*. New York: UN, 1990.

Blum, B.B. "Children's services in an era of budget deficits." *AJDC* 145:575-578, 1991.

Blum, John, Gertman, Paul, and Rabinow, Jean. *PSRO and the Law*. Germantown, MD: Aspen Press, 1977.

Blumberg, Rhoda Lois *Civil Rights: The 1960s Freedom Struggle*. Boston: Twayne Publishers, 1984: 126.

Boaz, David. *Assessing the Reagan Years*. Washington, DC: Cato Institute, 1988.

Borysenko, Joan, with Rothstein, Larry. *Minding the Body, Healing the Mind*. Reading, MA: Addison-Wesley, 1987.

Boskin, Michael J. *Reagan and the Economy: The Successes, Failures and Unfinished Agenda*. San Francisco: Institute for Contemporary Studies, 1987.

Boston Women's Health Collective. *Our Bodies/Ourselves: A Book by and for Women*. New York: Simon & Schuster, 1976, revised, 1984.

Bowers, Claude. *The Tragic Era*. Boston: Houghton Mifflin Company, 1929.

Bowers, John Z., and Purcell, Elizabeth F. *Schools of Public Health: Present and Future*. New York: Josiah Macy, Jr., Foundation, 1974.

Bowles, Samuel, Gordon, David M., and Weisskopf, Thomas E. "Long swings and the non-reproductive cycle." *Americian Economic Review* 152-157, May 1983.

_____. *After the Waste Land: A Democratic Economics for the Year 2000*. Armonk, NY: M.E. Sharpe, Inc., 1990.

Bown, Colin, and Mooney, Peter J. *Cold War to Détente*. London: Heinemann Education, 1976.

Bozell, L. Brent. *The Warren Revolution: Reflections on the Consensus Society*. New York: Arlington House, 1966.

Bradford, Calvin, and Bradford, Dennis Marinol. *Redlining and Disinvestment as a Discriminatory Practice in Residential Mortgage Loans*. Washington, DC: U.S. Department of Housing and Urban Development, U.S. Government Printing Office, 1977.

Bradford, L.K. "Health insurance values and implementation in the Netherlands and the Federal Republic of Germany: An alternative path to universal coverage." *JAMA* 265:2496-2502, 1991.

Brandeis, L.D. *Other People's Money and How the Bankers Used It*. New York: Frederick A. Stokes Company, 1932.

Broadus, J., Milliman, J., Edwards, S., Aubrey, D., and Gable, F. "Rising sea level and damming of rivers: Possible effects in Egypt and Bangladesh." In U.S. Environmental Protection Agency, *Effects of Changes in Stratospheric Ozone and Global Climate*, James G. Titus (ed.), vol. 4. Washington, DC: U.S. EPA and UNEP. August, 1989.

Brodeur, Paul. "The hazards of electromagnetic fields (I)." *The New Yorker*, 65:51-2, June 12, 1989.

_____. "The hazards of electromagnetic fields (II)." *The New Yorker*, 65:47-9, June 19, 1989.

_____. "The hazards of electromagnetic fields (III)." *The New Yorker*, 65:39-42, June 26, 1989.

Brook, Robert H. *The Effect of Co-insurance on the Health of Adults: Results from the Rand Health Experiment.* Santa Monica, CA: Rand Corporation, 1984.

Brown, E. Richard. *Rockefeller Medicine Men: Medicine and Capitalism in America.* Berkeley: University of California Press, 1979.

Brownell, Herbert. "Eisenhower's civil rights program: A personal assessment." *Presidential Studies Quarterly* 21:234-42, Spring 1991.

Bruce, Judith. "Women-oriented health care: New Hampshire feminist center." *Studies in Family Planning* 12:331-340, 1981.

Brun, Per. "Worldwide impact of sea level rise on shorelines." In U.S. Environmental Protection Agency, *Effects of Changes in Stratospheric Ozone and Global Climate,* James G. Titus (ed.), vol. 4, 19. Washington, DC: U.S. EPA and UNEP. August, 1989.

Budiansky, David. "The dim glow of history." *U.S. News and World Report,* April 18, 1994, 74 ff.

Burghardt, Stephen. *Tenants and the Urban Housing Crisis.* Dexter, MI: New Press, 1972.

Burrow, James G. *AMA: Voice of American Medicine.* Baltimore: Johns Hopkins Press, 1963.

_____. *Organized Medicine in the Progressive Era: The Move Toward Monopoly.* Baltimore: Johns Hopkins Press, 1977.

Bursctaju, Harold, Feinbloom, Richard, Hamm, Robert M., and Brodsky, Archie. *Medical Choices, Medical Changes: How Patients, Families and Physicians Can Cope with Uncertainty.* New York: Delacorte Press, 1981.

Bush, Gregory (ed.). *Campaign Speeches of American Presidential Candidates 1948-1984.* New York: Frederick Ungar Publishing Co., 1985, 104-122.

Cahill, Tom. "Rape behind bars." *The Progressive* 49:32-4, November 1985.

Caldwell, Harrison Gordon. *Mosquitos, Malaria and Man: A History of the Hostilities Since 1880.* New York: Dutton, 1978.

Caldwell, Lynton K. *International Environmental Policy.* Durham, NC: Duke University Press, 1984.

Califano, Joseph A., Jr. *America's Health Care Revolution: Who Lives? Who Dies? Who Pays?* New York: Random House, 1986.

Callan, John P. "Holistic health or holistic hoax?" *JAMA* 241(11):1156, March 16, 1979.

Campbell, Arthur. *Guerillas.* London: C. Tinling and Co., 1967.

Canadian Aid and the Environment: The Politics and Performance of the Canadian International Development Agency. Ottawa: North-South Institute, 1981.

Capra, Fritjof. *The Tao of Physics.* New York: Science Library and Boulder, CO: Shambhala Publications, 1975.

_____. *The Turning Point: Science, Society, and the Rising Culture.* New York: Simon & Schuster, 1982, Bantam, 1987.

Carden, Mary Lockwood. *Feminism in the Mid 1970s: The Non-Establishment, the Establishment and the Future.* New York: Ford Foundation, 1977.

Carlson, Rick J. *The End of Medicine.* New York: Wiley, 1975.

Carlson, Rick J., and Cunningham, Robert (eds.). *Future Directions in Health Care: A Public Policy.* Cambridge: Ballantine Press, 1978.

Carmichael, Stokely and Hamilton, Charles V. *Black Power: The Politics of Liberation in America.* New York: Random House, 1967.

Carnegie, Andrew. *Autobiography*. Boston: Houghton Mifflin Company, 1920.

Carson, Clayborne. *In Struggle: SNCC and the Black Awakening of the 1960s*. Cambridge, MA: Harvard University Press, 1981.

Carson, David C. *Satellite HMO Development of a Prepaid Nonprofit HMO Group Medical Practice in a Small City*. Seattle: Group Health Cooperative of Puget Sound, 1972.

Carson, Rachel. *The Silent Spring*. Greenwich, CT: Fawcett, 1962.

Carter, Hodding. *The Reagan Years*. New York: George Braziller, 1988.

Carter, L. Marshall, *Toward an Educated Health Consumer: Mass Communication and Quality in Medical Care*. Vol. 7, John E. Fogarty International Center for Advanced Studies in the Health Sciences, monograph series on the Teaching of Preventive Medicine. Washington, DC: U.S. Government Printing Office, DHEW Publication No. (NIH) 77-881, 1977.

Casper, D.E. *Richard Nixon: A Bibliographic Exploration*. New York: Garland Publishers, 1988.

"Catch 22." *Bulletin of the Atomic Scientists* 46:6, Sept. 1990.

Centers for Disease Control. "Estimates of prevalence and projected AIDS cases: Summary of a workshop, October 31-November 1, 1989." *Morbidity, Mortality, Weekly Report* (3)7:110-119, February 23, 1990.

———. "Special report: Treatment rerun: Costs are high." *HIV-AIDS Prevention*, February 19, 1991.

Centers for Disease Control, Division of Education. *Effectiveness in Disease and Injury Prevention: Public Focus Activity and the Prevention of Coronary Heart Disease*. Rockville, MD: U.S. Department of Health and Human Services, 1993.

———. *Promoting Physical Activity Among Adults*. Rockville, MD: U.S. Department of Health and Human Services, 1988.

Cerlin, Peter E. *Medical Malpractice Pre-Trial Screening Panels: A Review of the Evidence, Intergovernmental Health Policy Project*. Washington, DC: George Washington University Press, 1980.

Cerne, F. "Rate decrease unlikely despite health insurers' healthy profits." *American Hospital Association News* 26:8, November 5, 1990.

Chandler, Alfred D. *The Visible Hand: The Managerial Revolution in American Business*. Cambridge, MA: Belknap Press of Harvard University, 1977.

Charlton, John R.H., and Velez, Ramon. "Some international comparisons of mortality amenable to medical intervention." *British Medical Journal* 292:295-301, February 1, 1986.

Chave, S.P.W. "The origins and development of public health." In *Oxford Textbook of Public Health*, Vol. 1: History, Determinants, Scope and Strategy, edited by Holland, Walter W., Detels, Roger, and Knox, George. Oxford and New York: Oxford University Press, 1984.

"Chemical switchboard of the brain." *The Economist* 291:74-75, June 30, 1984.

Chollet, D., and Mages, Foley J. *Uninsured in the United States: The Nonelderly Population without Health Insurance, 1988*. Washington, DC: Employee Benefit Research Institute, 1990.

Chu, Franklin D. *The Madness Establishment: Ralph Nader's Study Group Report on the National Institute of Mental Health*. New York: Grossman Publishers, 1974, 3.

Clarke, P.A.B. *AIDS: Medicine, Politics, Society*. London: Lester Cook Academic Publishers, 1988.

Clayton, Edward (ed.). *The SCLC Story*. Atlanta: Southern Christian Leadership Conference, 1964.

Clayton, R.R., and Ritter, C. "The epidemiology of alcohol and drug abuse among adolescents." *Adv. Alcohol and Substance Abuse* 4(3-4):69-97, Spring-Summer 1985.

Cleveland, W.W. "Redoing the health care quilt: Patches or whole cloth?" *JAMA* 265:499-504, 1991.

Clinton, B., and Gore, Al. *Putting People First: How We Can All Change America*. New York: Times Books, 1992.

Cohen, Richard E. "Into the swamp." *National Journal* 642-654, March 19, 1994.

Coleman, L.G. "Geriatric boomers expected to strain health care system." *Marketing News* 25:17, May 13, 1991.

Colt, H.G., and Shapiro, A.P. "Drug-related illnesses as a cause for admission to a community hospital." *Journal of the American Geriatric Society* 37(4):279, April 1989.

Commission on Professional and Hospital Activities. *Length of Stay by Diagnosis Related Groups, July 1984-July 1985 Discharges*. Ann Arbor, MI: CPHA Probe Series, 1986.

Committee for the Study of the Future of Public Health, Division of Health Care Services, Institute of Medicine. *The Future of Public Health*. Washington, DC: National Academy Press, 1988.

_____. "A history of the public health system." In *The Future of Public Health*. Washington, DC: National Academy Press, 1988, 56-72.

Committee on the Costs of Medical Care. *Medical Care for the American People*. Chicago: University of Chicago Press, 1932.

Conference on Acid Rain (1984: Washington, DC). *Acid Rain: Economic Assessment*. New York: Plenum Press, 1985.

Congressional Quarterly, Inc. *Environment and Health*. Washington, DC: 1981.

Conklin, Mary, and Simmons, Ruth. *Planned Home Childbirths: Parental Perspectives*. Lansing: Michigan Department of Public Health, 1979.

Corey, Lewis. *The House of Morgan*. New York: G. Howard Watt, 1930.

Corr, Charles A., and Corr, Donna M. (eds.). *Hospice Care: Principles and Practices*. New York: Springer Publications, 1983.

Cotton, Paul "Pre-existing conditions 'hold Americans hostage' to employers and insurance." *JAMA* 265(19):2451-2454, May 15, 1991.

Coulter, David. *Divided Legacy: A History of the Schism in Medical Thought*. Washington, DC: McGrath Publishing, 1973.

Craig, P.P. *Nuclear Arms Race: Technology and Society*. New York: McGraw-Hill, 1986.

Cranston, Alan. "AIDS update." *American Family Physician* 44:682, August 1991.

Crawford, Robert. "Healthism and the medicalization of everyday life (politics of self-care)." *International Journal of Health Services* 10(3):365-388, 1980.

_____. "You are dangerous to your health: The ideology and politics of victim-blaming." *International Journal of Health Services* 7(4):663-688, 1977.

Critical Condition: Human Health and the Environment. Cambridge, Mass.: MIT Press, 1993.

Culyer, A.J. *Health Care Expenditures in Canada: Myth and Reality, Past and Future*. Toronto: Canadian Tax Foundation, 1988.

Dallek, Robert. *Ronald Reagan, The Politics of Symbolism.* Cambridge, MA: Harvard University Press, 1984.

Danielson, Albert L. *The Evolution of OPEC.* New York: Harcourt, Brace, Jovanovich, 1982.

Davies, J.E. and Doon, R. "Human health effects of pesticides." In *Silent Spring Revisited,* edited by Gino J. Marco, Robert M. Hollingworth, and William Durham. Washington, DC: American Chemical Society, 1987, 121-122.

Davis, Fred. *On Youth Subcultures: The Hippie Variant.* New York: General Learning Press, 1971.

Davis, Joel. *Mapping the Code.* New York: Wiley, 1990.

Davis, K. "Expanding Medicare and employer plans to achieve universal health insurance." *JAMA* 265:2525-2528, 1991.

Davis, Karen, and Reynolds, Roger. "The impact of Medicare and Medicaid on access to medical care." In *The Role of Health Insurance in the Health Service Sector,* edited by E. Rossett. New York: National Bureau of Economic Research, 1976.

Davis, Karen, and Schoen, Cathy. *Health and the War on Poverty.* Washington, DC: The Brookings Institute, 1978.

Davis, Michael Marks. *The Crisis in Hospital Finance and Other Studies in Hospital Economics.* Chicago: University of Chicago Press, 1932.

Day, Mark. *Forty Acres: Cesar Chavez and the Farm Workers.* New York: Praeger, 1971.

DeGrasse, Robert W., Jr., *Military Expansion Economic Decline: the Impact of Military Spending on U.S. Economic Performance.* Armonk, NY: M.E. Sharpe, Inc., 1983.

De Kruif, Paul Henry. *Kaiser Wakes the Doctors.* New York: Harcourt-Brace, 1943.

_____. *The Microbe Hunters.* New York: Harcourt, Brace and Company, 1926.

De Toledano, Ralph. *Little Cesar.* Washington. DC: Anthem Books, 1971.

Denison, Edward F. *Accounting for United States Economic Growth, 1929-1969.* Washington, DC: The Brookings Institute, 1974.

_____. *The Sources of Economic Growth in the United States and the Alternatives Before Us, a Supplementary Paper for the Committee for Economic Development.* New York: Committee for Economic Development, 1962.

_____. *Why Growth Rates Differ: Postwar Experience in Nine Western Countries.* Washington, DC: The Brookings Institute, 1967.

Dentzer, Susan. "Harry, Louise, and health alliances." *U.S. News and World Report* 116:62, March 7, 1994.

Denuyl, Douglass J. "Smoking, human rights, and civil liberties." In *Smoking and Society,* edited by Robert D. Tollison. Lexington: Lexington Books, 1986.

Desowitz, Robert S. *The Malaria Capers.* New York: Norton, 1991.

Dougherty, R., Whitaker, M., Smith, L, Stalling, D., and Kuehl, D. "Negative chemical ionization studies of human and food chain contamination with xenobiotic chemicals, *Archives of Environmental Health Perspectives* 36:103-118, 1980.

Doyle, James C. "Unnecessary hysterectomies: Study of 6,248 operations in thirty-five hospitals during 1948." *JAMA* 151:360-365, 1953.

_____. "Unnecessary ovariectomies: Study based on the removal of 704 normal ovaries from 546 patients." *JAMA* 148:1105-1111, 1952.

Dubos, Rene. *Mirage of Health: Utopias, Progress and Biological Change.* New York: Harper and Row, 1971.

Duclaux, Emile. *Pasteur: The History of a Mind.* Translated by Erwin F. Smith and Florence Hedges. Metuchen, NJ: Scarecrow Reprint Corporation, 1973.

Dume, John Gregory. *Delano: The Story of the California Grape Strike*. New York: Farrar, Strauss and Giroux, 1967.

Economic Forum. *Inflation in the United States, Causes and Consequences, Proceedings*. New York: Conference Board, 1974.

Egdahl, Richard, and Gertman, Paul M. *Quality Assurance in Health Care*. Germantown, MD: Aspen Systems Corporation, 1976.

Eisenberg, David "Unconventional medical practice in the United States: Prevalence, costs and patterns of use." *New England Journal of Medicine (hereafter NEJM)* 328:246-56, Jan. 28, 1993.

Eklof, Ben. *Soviet Briefing: Gorbachev and the Reform Period*. Boulder, CO: Westview Press, 1989.

Employee Benefit Research Institute (EBRI). "Sources of health insurance and characteristics of the uninsured." #123. Washington, DC: EBRI, 1992.

Enthoven, A.C. *Health Plan*. Reading, MA: Addison-Wesley Publishing Co., 1980.

_____. "The history and principles of managed competition." *Health Affairs* 12(Supplement):24-48, March 1993.

_____. *Theory and Practice of Managed Competition in Health Care Finance*. Amsterdam and New York: Elsevier Science Publishing Company, 1988.

Enthoven, A.C., and Kronick, R. "A consumer-choice health plan for the 1990s: Universal health insurance in a system designed to promote quality and economy." *NEJM* 320:29-37, 94-101, 1989.

Environmental Change and Human Health. Chilchester, NY: J. Wiley and Sons, 1993.

Erfurt, J.C. "What can we do next to encourage worksite health promotion?" Fetzer Institute, Kalamazoo, MI, March 13, 1992.

Erfurt, J.C., and Foote, A. "Maintenance of blood pressure treatment and control after discontinuation of work site follow-up." *Journal of Occupational Medicine (hereafter JOM)* 32(6):513-520, 1990.

Erfurt, J.C., Foote, A., and Heirich, M.A. "Worksite wellness programs: Incremental comparison of screening and referral alone, health education, follow-up counseling, and plant organization." *American Journal of Health Promotion (hereafter Am. J. Health Promo.)* 5(6):438-448, 1991.

Erfurt, J.C., Foote, A., Heirich, M.A., and Brock, B.M. *The Wellness Outreach at Work Program: A Step-by-Step Guide*. Rockville, MD: National, Heart, Lung and Blood Institute, publ. #95-3043, 1995.

Erfurt, J.C., Foote, A., Heirich, M.A., and Holtyn, K. "Saving lives and dollars through comprehensive preventive health care." *Family Business Review* 6(2):163-172, Summer 1993.

Erfurt, John C. and Holtyn, Kenneth, M.S. "Health promotion in small business: What works and what doesn't work." *JOM* 33(1):66-73, January 1991.

Ertel, Paul Y., and Aldridge, M. Gene. *Medical Peer Review: Theory and Practice*. St. Louis: C.V. Mosby, 1977.

Evans, Rowland, and Novak, Robert. *The Reagan Revolution*. New York: Dutton, 1981.

Falk, I.S., Rorem, C. Rufus, and Ring, Martha D. *The Cost of Medical Care*. Chicago: University of Chicago Press, 1933.

Falkson, Joseph L. *HMOs and the Politics of Health System Reform*. Chicago: American Hospital Association, 1986.

Faltermayer, Edmund. "Health care: More Americans are switching to HMOs." *Fortune* 129:14, Jan. 10, 1994.

Farrell, C. "The age wave and how to ride it: Middle-aged baby boomers and senior-seniors mean more spending on entertainment and health care." *Business Week*, October 16, 1989, 112.

Feinstein, Alvin R. *Clinical Judgment*. Baltimore: Williams and Wilkins Co., 1967.

Feldstein, Paul J. *Health Associations and the Demand for Legislation: The Political Economy of Health*. Cambridge, MA: Ballinger Publishing Company, 1977.

_____. *The Politics of Health Legislation: An Economic Perspective*. Ann Arbor, MI: Health Administration Press, 1988, 5-38.

Ferguson, Marilyn. *The Aquarian Conspiracy: Personal and Social Transformation in the 1980s*. Los Angeles: J.P. Tarcher, 1980.

_____. *The Brain Revolution: The Frontiers of Mind Research*. New York: Taplinger, 1973.

_____. *The Brain/Mind Bulletin*. Box 42211, Los Angeles, CA, 90042.

_____. *Leading Edge: A Bulletin of Social Transformation*. Box 42247, Los Angeles, California 90042.

Ferrara, Peter J. "The catastrophic health care fiasco," *Consumer Research Magazine* 73:28-29, February 1990.

Ferris, Paul. *The Master Banks: Controlling the World's Finances*. New York: Wm. Morrow and Co., Inc., 1984.

Feshback, Murray and Friendly, Alfred. *Ecocide in the USSR*. New York: Basic Books, 1992.

Fielding, Jonathan. *National Survey of Worksite Health Promotion Activities: A Summary, 1987*. Silver Springs, MD: USDHHS, Public Health Service, National Technical Information Service, Summer 1987.

_____. "Smoking: Health effects and control." *NEJM* 313(9):555-561, 1986.

Fisher, Randall. *Rhetoric and Democracy: Black Protest through Vietnam Dissent*. Lanham, MD: University Press of America, 1985.

Fitzgibbon, Robert J., and Statland, Bernard E. *DRG Survival Manual for the Clinical Lab*. Oradell, NJ: Medical Economics Books, 1985.

Flynn, J.T. *God's Gold: John D. Rockefeller and His Times*. New York: Harcourt Brace and Company, 1932.

Foote, A., and Erfurt, J.C. "Hypertension control at the worksite: Comparison of screening and referral alone, referral and follow-up, and on-site treatment." *NEJM* 308:809-813, April 7, 1983.

Foote, A., Erfurt, J.C., Strauch, P.A., and Guzzardo, T.L. *Cost-Effectiveness of Occupational Employee Assistance Programs: Test of an Evaluation Method*. Ann Arbor: University of Michigan Institute of Labor & Industrial Relations, 1978.

Fowles, Jinnet, Gibbs, James O., Ina, Vickie, Larsen, Arne, and Pearce, H.G. "The Health Incentive Plan Evaluation: Final Report to the John A. Hartford Foundation, November, 1986." San Francisco: Blue Shield of California, 1986.

Fraser, Thomas H. "The future of recombinant DNA technology in medicine." In *Genetic Perspectives in Biology and Medicine*, edited by Edward D. Garber. Chicago: University of Chicago Press, 1985.

Freeland, Richard M. *The Truman Doctrine and the Origins of McCarthyism: Foreign Policy, Domestic Politics and International Security, 1946-48*. New York: Knopf, 1972.

Freidel, Frank Burt. *Franklin Roosevelt: Launching the New Deal.* Boston: Little, Brown, 1973.

Friedan, Betty. *The Feminine Mystique.* New York: Norton, 1963.

_____. *It Changed My Life: Writings on the Women's Movement.* New York: Random House, 1976.

Friedland, Edward, Seabury, Paul, and Wildavsky, Aaron. *The Great Détente Disaster: Oil and the Decline of American Foreign Policy.* New York: Basic Books, 1975.

Friedman, Emily "The uninsured: From dilemma to crisis." *JAMA* 265(19):2491-2495, May 15, 1991.

_____. "Health insurance in Hawaii: Paradise lost or found?" *Business & Health* 8:52, June 1990.

Friedman, Michael. *The New Left of the 'Sixties.* Berkeley, CA: Independent Socialist Press, 1972.

Fuchs, V.R. "The best health care system in the world." *JAMA* 268(7):916-917, 1992.

_____. *The Health Economy.* Cambridge: Harvard University Press, 1986.

_____. "The health sector's share of gross national product." *Science* 247:418-422, 1990.

_____. "How does Canada do it? A comparison of expenditures for physician's services in the United States and Canada." *NEJM* 323:884-890, 1990.

"Further study needed." *Bul. of the Atomic Scientists* 46:4, July-Aug. 1990.

Fusfeld, Daniel. *Economics: Principles of Political Economy.* Glenview, IL: Scott-Foresman, 1987.

Gable, John. "The changing world of group insurance." *Health Affairs* 7(2):48-65, Summer 1988.

Gable, J., DiCarlo, S., Sullivan, C., and Rice, T. "Employer sponsored health insurance, 1989." *Health Affairs* (Milwood) 8(2):116-128, Summer 1989.

Gallay, L.S. "Health care, technology, and competitive environment." *Journal of the American Planning Association* 59:127-128, Winter 1993.

Galtung, Johan. *Toward Self-Reliance and Global Interdependence: Reflections on a New International Order and North-South Cooperation.* Ottawa: Environment Canada: Canadian International Development Agency, 1978.

Garbarino, Joseph W. *Health Plans and Collective Bargaining.* Institute of Industrial Relations, Berkeley: University of California Press, 1960.

Garceau, Oliver. *The Political Life of the American Medical Association.* Hernden, CT: Anchor Books, 1941, 1961.

Gati, Charles, and Gati, Toby Trister. *The Debate Over Détente.* New York: Foreign Policy Association, 1977.

Gelman, David. "Fitness, corporate style: Companies are racing to invest in employee 'wellness'." *Newsweek*, November 5, 1984, 96.

"The Genome Project: Life after Watson." *Science*, May 15, 1992.

Genovese, M.A. *The Nixon Presidency: Power and Politics in Turbulent Times.* New York: Greenwood Press, 1990.

Gerlach, Luther. "Movements of social change: Some structural characteristics." *American Behavioral Scientist* 14(6):812-835, 1970.

Geschwender, James A. (ed.). *The Black Revolt: The Civil Rights Movement, Ghetto Uprisings, and Separatism.* Englewood Cliffs, NJ: Prentice-Hall, 1971.

Ghanem, Shukri Mohammed. *OPEC: The Rise and Fall of an Exclusive Club.* London: KPI, 1986.

Gibbons, Don C., Jones, Joseph F., and Backstrand, John A. "Who is in jail? An examination of the rabble hypothesis." *Crime and Delinquency* 38:219-29, April 1992.

Gilpin, Robert. *U.S. Power and the Multinational Corporation: The Political Economy of Foreign Direct Investment.* New York: Basic Books, 1975.

Ginzberg, Eli. *The Limits of Health Reform: The Search for Realism.* New York: Basic Books, Inc., 1971.

Ginzberg, Eli, and Ostow, Miriam. "Beyond universal health insurance to effective health care." *JAMA* 265(19):2559-2562, May 15, 1991.

Goldstein, J.C. "Access to care—The problem for the uninsured and underinsured." *Archives of Otolaryngology—Head and Neck Surgery* 117:490-492, 1991.

Gonzales, Martin, Emmons, David W., and Pieniozek, Don. *Socioeconomic Characteristics of Medical Practice.* Chicago: American Medical Association Center for Health Policy Research, 1986.

Goodin, Robert E. *No Smoking.* Chicago: University of Chicago Press, 1989.

Goodman, Paul. *Growing Up Absurd: Problems of Youth in an Organized Society.* New York: Random House, 1960.

Gordon, David M. "A statistical series on production worker compensation," Technical Note No. 3, in Economics Institute of the Center for Democratic Research, *What's Wrong with the Economy?* Boston: South End Press, 1982, 220.

Gordon, James S. *Holistic Medicine.* New York: Chelsea House Publishers, 1988.

Gordon, Leonard. *A City in Racial Crisis: The Case of Detroit Pre- and Post- the 1967 Riot.* Dubuque, IA: W.C. Brown Co., 1971.

Gore, A. *Earth in the Balance: Ecology and the Human Spirit.* Boston: Houghton Mifflin, 1992.

Gould, H. Lane, Ornish, Dean, and Scherwitz, Larry. "Changes in myocardial perfusion abnormalities by positron emission tomography after long-term, intensive risk factor modification." *JAMA* 274:89-901, September 20, 1995.

Gouldner, Alvin W. *The Coming Crisis of Western Sociology.* New York: Basic Books, 1970.

Greenpeace U.S.A. *The Greenpeace Guide to Anti-Environmental Organizations.* Berkeley, CA: Odonian Press, 1993.

Griffith, J., Duncan, R.C., Riggan, W.B., and Pellom, A.C. "Cancer mortality in U.S. counties with hazardous waste sites and ground water pollution." *Arch. Environ. Health* 44(2):69-74, 1989.

Guide to the Nation's Hospices, Annual, 1984. Arlington, VA: National Hospice Organization, 1984.

Gunn, Thomas G. *Manufacturing for Competitive Advantage: Becoming a World Class Manufacturer.* Cambridge, MA: Ballinger Publications, 1987.

Guttentag, Jack M., and Wachter, Susan M. *Redlining and Public Policy.* New York: New York University, Graduate School of Business Administration, Salomon Brothers Center for the Study of Financial Institutions, 1980.

Guttmacher, Sally. "The individual, the social context, and health policy: Whole in body, mind, & spirit—Holistic health and the limits of medicine." *Hastings Center Report* 9(2):15-21, April 1979.

Haberler, Gottfried. *Stagflation: An Analysis of Its Causes and Cures.* Washington, DC: American Enterprise Institute for Public Policy Research, 1977.

Hacker, L.M. and Kendrick, B.B. *The United States Since 1865.* New York: F.S. Crofts and Co., 1932.

Hall, Nicholas and Goldstein, Allan D. "Thinking well: The chemical links between emotions and health." *The Sciences* 34-39, Feb.-Mar. 1985.

Halstead, F. *Out Now! A Participant's Account of the American Movement Against the Vietnam War.* 2nd ed. New York: Monad Press, 1979.

Halstead, Murat and Beale, J.F. *Life of Jay Gould: How He Made His Fortune.* New York: Edgewood Publishing Company, 1892.

Haney, Lewis. *A Congressional History of Railways in the United States.* Madison: University of Wisconsin Economics and Political Science Series, Vol. 3, No. 2; Vol. 6, No. 1, 1908-10.

Hanlon, John J., and Pickett, George E. "Development and organization of public health in the United States." In *Public Health: Administration and Practice.* St. Louis: C.V. Mosby Co., 1950, 13-46.

Harmon, R.A. "American experience with nutrition and cardiovascular risk." *Bibl Nutr Dieta* 49:18-23, 1992.

Haseltine, William A., and Wong-Staal, Flossie. "The molecular biology of the AIDS virus." *Scientific American* 259(4):52-62, October 1988.

Haskins, James. *Profiles in Black Power.* Garden City, NY: Doubleday, 1972.

Hasting, Arthur J., Fadiman, James, and Gordon, James S. *Health for the Whole Person.* Boulder, CO: Westview Press, 1980.

Havlicek, Penny. *Medical Groups in the U.S.* Chicago: American Medical Association, 1990: 21.

Hawley, Ellis. *The New Deal and the Problem of Monopoly.* Princeton, NJ: University Press, 1966.

Hayden, Tom. *Vietnam: The Struggle for Peace, 1972-73.* Santa Monica, CA, Cambridge, MA: The Indo China Peace Campaign, 1973.

Hays, Samuel P. *Conservation and the Gospel of Efficiency: The Progressive Conservation Movement, 1890-1920.* Cambridge, MA: Harvard University Press, 1987.

Health Care Cost Containment: Challenge to Industry. NY: FERF, 1980.

Health Care Financing Administration, Office of the Actuary. *Data from the Office of National Cost Estimates,* 1991.

Health Insurance Association. *Canadian Health Care: The Implications of Public Health Insurance.* Washington, DC: Health Insurance Association, 1990.

Healthcare Information Center. *Reforming the System: Containing Health Care Costs in an Area of Universal Coverage.* New York: Faulkner and Gray, 1992.

_____. *System in Crisis: The Case for Health Reform.* New York: Faulkner and Gray, 1991.

Heath, G. Louis. *Mutiny Does Not Happen Here: The Literature of the American Resistance to the Vietnam War.* Metuchen, NJ: Scarecrow Press, 1976.

Hedgepeth, William. *The Alternative: Communal Life in New America.* New York: Macmillan, 1970.

Hedinger, F.R. *The Social Role of Blue Cross as a Device for Financing the Costs of Medical Care.* Social Research Series no. 2. Iowa City: Graduate Program in Hospital and Health Administration, University of Iowa, 1966.

Heirich, M.A. *The Spiral of Conflict: Berkeley, 1964-65.* New York: Columbia University Press, 1971.

Heirich, M.A., Erfurt, J.C., and Foote, A. "The core technology of worksite wellness." *JOM* 34(6)627-637, 1992.

Heirich, M.A., Foote, A., Erfurt, J.C., and Konopka, B. "Worksite physical fitness programs: Comparing the impact of different program designs on cardiovascular risks." *JOM* 35(5):510-517, May 1993.

Heirich, M.A., Holmes, Carolyn, et al., "Integrating prevention and primary care services: A proposal from the University of Michigan." February 1993, submitted to Clinton Health Reform Task Force, at the request of Joycelyn Elders, Surgeon General.

Heirich, M.A., and Kaplan, S. "Yesterday's discord." *California Monthly* LXXV(5):20-34, February 1965.

Hellman, S. *Medicare and Medigaps: A Guide to Retirement Health Insurance.* Newbury Park, CA: Sage Publications, 1991.

Hempel, Carl G. "The logic of functional analysis." *Aspects of Scientific Explanation.* New York: The Free Press, 1965, 297-330.

Hendrick, B.J. *The Age of Big Business.* New Haven, CT: Yale University Press, 1919.

Herring, Richard. *National Monetary Policies and International Financial Markets.* Amsterdam and New York: Elsevier/North Holland, 1977.

Heskin, Allen David. *Tenants and the American Dream: Ideology and the Tenant Movement.* New York: Praeger, 1983.

Heyward, William L. and Curran, James W. "The epidemiology of AIDS in the U.S." *The Science of AIDS: Readings from Scientific American Magazine.* New York: W. H. Freeman and Company, 1988, 1989, 39-49.

Hill, Richard C. "At the crossroads: The political economy of postwar Detroit," presented to an American Sociological Association conference on Urban Political Economy at the University of California, Santa Cruz, April 8-10, 1977.

Hillman, Alan L. "Special report: Financial incentives for physicians in HMOs—Is there a conflict of interest?" *NEJM* 317(27):1743-1748, 1987.

Himmelstein, David U. and Woolhandler, Steffie. *The National Health Program Book: A Source Guide for Advocates.* Monroe, ME: Common Courage Press, 1993.

Hines, L.G. *Environmental Issues: Population, Pollution, and Economics.* New York: W.W. Norton & Company, 1973.

Hines, Virginia. "The basic paradigm of a future socio-cultural system." *World Issues* 19-22, April-May 1977.

Hines, Virginia, and Gerlach, Luther. *Lifeway Leap: The Dynamics of Change in America.* Minneapolis: University of Minnesota Press, 1973.

_____. *People, Power, Change: Movements of Social Transformation.* Indianapolis: Bobbs-Merrill, 1970.

Hinman, A.R. "What will it take to fully protect all American children with vaccines?" *AJDC* 145(5):559-562, May 1991.

Hinman, George W., Lowinger, Thomas C., and Fuller, Russell J. "The impact of nuclear power on the systematic risk and market value of electric utility common stock." *Energy Journal* 11:117-133, April 1990.

Hippocrates. *The Aphorisms of Hippocrates.* Birmingham, AL: Classics of Medicine Library, 1982.

Hoffman, C., Rice, D., and Sung, H.Y. "Persons with chronic conditions: Their prevalence and cost." *JAMA* 276(18): 1473-1479, Nov. 13, 1996.

Hoffman, Paul. *The Deal Makers: Inside the World of Investment Banking.* New York: Doubleday, 1984.

Hofmann, D.J., Oltmans, S.J., Hams, J.M., Solomon, J., and Deshler, T. "Observation and possible causes of new ozone depletion in Antarctica in 1991." *Nature* 359:283-287, 1992.

Hogue, C.J., and Hargraves, M.A. "Class, race and infant mortality in the United States." *AJPH* 831(1):9-12, January 1993.

Hohmann, Hans-Hermann. *Soviet Reform Policy under Gorbachev: Concepts, Problems, Perspectives.* Cologne: Bundesinstitut für Ostwissenschaft und Internationale Studien, 1987.

Holahan, John, et al. "An American approach to health system reform." *JAMA* 265(19):2537-2540, May 15, 1991.

Hovey, Carl. *The Life Story of J.P. Morgan.* London: William Heinemann, 1911.

Hunt, Charles W. "Africa and AIDS: Dependent development, sexism, and racism." *Monthly Review* 39:10-22, February 1988.

_____. "Migrant labor and sexually transmitted disease: AIDS in Africa." *Journal of Health and Social Behavior* 38:533-73, December 1989.

Hyde, David R., and Wolff, Payson, with Ann Gross and Elliot Lee Hoffman. *The American Medical Association: Power, Purpose and Politics in Organized Medicine.* New Haven: Yale University Press, 1954.

Hynes, H. Patricia. *The Recurring Silent Spring.* New York: Pergamon, 1989.

Illich, Ivan. *Medical Nemesis: The Expropriation of Health.* New York: Pantheon, 1976.

Inglehart, J.K. "Consensus forms for national insurance plan, proposals vary widely in scope." *National Journal Reports* 5:1855-56, December 12, 1973.

_____. "The United States looks at Canadian health care." *NEJM* 321:1767-1772, 1989.

Institute of Medicine. *Costs of Environment-Related Health Effects: A Plan for Continuing Study.* Washington, DC: National Academy Press, 1981.

_____. *Preventing Low Birth Weight.* Washington, DC: National Academy Press, 1985.

Interagency Committee on Immunization (U.S.). *Action Plan to Improve Access to Immunization Services: Report of the Interagency Committee on Immunization.* Washington, DC: Department of Health and Human Services, Public Health Services, National Vaccine Program, 1992.

IPOC. *Climate Change: The IPOC Scientific Assessment.* Executive Summary, XC, 1991.

Jackson, George L. *Blood in My Eye.* New York: Random House, 1972.

Jackson, Kenneth T. "Race, ethnicity, and real estate appraisal." *Journal of Urban History* 6(4):419-452, August 1980.

Jackson, Larry R., and Johnson, William A. *Protest by the Poor: The Welfare Rights Movement in New York City.* Lexington, MA: Lexington Press, 1974.

Jacobs, Margo M. "Diet, nutrition, and cancer: An overview." *Nutrition Today* 28:19-25, May-June 1993.

Jacobs, Michael. *The Green Economy.* London: Pluto Press, 1991.

Jay, Karla, and Young, Alan. *Out of the Closets: Voices of Gay Liberation.* New York: Douglas Book Corporation, 1972.

The John E. Fogarty International Center for Advanced Study in the Health Sciences. *The Barefoot Doctor's Manual: The American Translation of the Chinese Paramedical Manual.* Philadelphia: Running Press, 1977.

Johnston, L.D., O'Malley, P.M., and Bachman, J.G. *National Trends in Drug Use Among High School Students and Young Adults*. U.S. Department of Health and Human Services. Washington, DC: U.S. Government Printing Office, 1984.

Joint National Committee on Detection, Evaluation, and Treatment of High Blood Pressure. *Hypertension Prevalence and the Status of Awareness, Treatment, and Control in the United States: Final Report of the Subcommittee on Definition and Prevalence*. Heart, Lung and Blood Institute of the National Institutes of Health, Bethesda, MD. Washington, DC: U.S. Government Printing Office, 1984.

Jones, Holway R. *John Muir and the Sierra Club: The Battle for Yosemite*. San Francisco: Sierra Club, 1965.

Jonville, A.P., Autret, E., Bavoux, F., Bertrand, P.P., Barbier, P., and Gauchez, A.S. "Characteristics of medication errors in pediatrics." *DICP* 25(10):1113-8, October 1991.

Josephson, Matthew. *The Robber Barons: The Great American Capitalists, 1861-1901*. New York: Harcourt, Brace, Janovich, 1934, 1962.

Joy, W. Brough, M.D. *Joy's Way: A Map for the Transformational Journey*. Los Angeles: J.P. Tarcher and New York: St. Martin's Press, 1979.

Kaboolian, Linda. *Shifting Gears: Auto Workers Assess the Transformation of Their Industry*. Unpublished dissertation. Ann Arbor: University of Michigan, 1990.

Kadlubar, F.F. "Detection of human DNA-carcinogen adducts." *Nature* 360(6400):189, Nov. 12, 1992.

Kaiser Commission on the Future of Medicaid. *The Medicaid Cost Explosion: Causes and Consequences*. Baltimore, MD: Kaiser Commission on the Future of Medicaid, 1993.

Kannell, William B., M.D., and Thom, Thomas. "Declining cardiovascular mortality." *Circulation* 331-336, September 1984.

Kanter, Rosabeth. *Teaching Elephants to Dance*. New York: Simon & Schuster, 1989.

_____. *When Giants Learn to Dance: Mastering the Challenge of Strategies, Management and Career in the 1990s*. New York: Simon & Schuster, 1990.

Kempe, Frederick. *Divorcing the Dictator: America's Bungled Affair with Noriega*. New York: G.P. Putnam's Sons, 1990.

Kendall, Mark, and Haldi, John. "The medical malpractice insurance market." In U.S. Department of Health, Education, and Welfare, *Report of the Secretary's Commission on Medical Malpractice*. Washington, DC: DHEW Publication no. 72-89, January 16, 1973.

Kenty, David E., and Wald, Martin (eds.). *ERISA: A Comprehensive Guide*. Wiley Law Publications, 1991.

Khansari, D.N., Murgo, A.J., and Faith, R.E. "Effects of stress on the immune system." *Immunology Today* 11:170-175, 1990.

Kiesler, C.A. *Mental Hospitalization: Myths and Facts about a National Crisis*. Beverly Hills, CA: Sage Publications, 1987.

Killian, Lewis. *The Impossible Revolution, Phase II: Black Power and the American Dream*. New York: Random House, 1975.

King, Martin Luther, Jr. *Stride Toward Freedom*. New York: Harper and Row, 1958.

_____. *Why We Can't Wait*. New York: American Library, 1963.

Klevit, H.D., et al. "Prioritization of health care services: A progress report by the Oregon Health Services Commission." *Archives of Internal Med.* 155:912-916, 1991.

Knowles, John (ed.). *Doing Better and Feeling Worse: Health Care in the U.S.* New York: Norton, 1977.

Knox, Robert J. "Toxic overload: The waste disposal dilemma." *Job Environmental Health* 53(8):15-17, May/June 1991.

Kochler, Richard J."HIV infection, TB, and the health crisis in corrections." *Public Administration Review* 54:3-5, Jan.-Feb. 1994.

Koff, Theodore H. *Hospice: A Caring Community*. Cambridge, MA: Winthrop Publishers, 1980.

Koop, C. Everett. *Surgeon General's Report on Acquired Immune Deficiency Syndrome*. Washington, DC: Surgeon General's Office, 1987.

Kotabe, Masoaki. *Global Sourcing Strategy: R&D, Manufacturing, and Marketing Interfaces*. New York: Quorum Books, 1992.

Kotelchuck, David (ed.). *Prognosis Negative: Crisis in the Health Care System, a Health PAK Book*. New York: Vintage Books, 1976.

Kotz, Nick, and Kotz, Mary Lynn. *A Passion for Equality: George A. Wiley and the Movement*. New York: Norton, 1977.

Kowalcyk, George, Freeland, Mark S., and Levit, Katherine R. "Using marginal analysis to evaluate health care trends." *Health Care Financing Review* 10(2):123-129, Winter 1988.

Kramer, Daniel C. *Participatory Democracy: Developing Ideals of the Political Left*. Cambridge, MA: Schenkman Pub. Co., 1972.

Kuhn, Thomas S. *The Structure of Scientific Revolutions*. Chicago: University of Chicago Press, 1970.

Kulles, Lewis H., Svendsen, Kenneth H., and Ockens, Judith K. "The relationship of smoking cessation to coronary heart disease and lung cancer in the Multiple Risk Factor Intervention Trial (MRFIT)." *AJPH* 80:954-8, August 1990.

Lakshmanan, M.C., Hershy, C.O., and Breslau, D. "Hospital admissions caused by iatrogenic disease." *American Family Physician* 35:1931-34, April 1987.

Lambert, T. Allen. "Generations and change: Toward a theory of generations as a force in the historical process." *Youth and Society* 4:21-45, 1972.

Langwell, Kathryn M. "Structure and performance of health maintenance organizations: A review." *Health Care Financing Review* 12(1):71-9, 1990.

Lappe, Marc. *Broken Code*. San Francisco: Sierra Club, 1984.

Larson, Ann. "The social epidemiology of Africa's AIDS epidemic." *African Affairs* 89:5-25, 1990.

Lasch, Christopher. *The Culture of Narcissism and American Life in an Age of Diminishing Expectations*. New York: Norton, 1978.

Law, Sylvia. *Blue Cross: What Went Wrong? A Health Law Project of the University of Pennsylvania*. New Haven: Yale University Press, 1976.

Leary, Timothy. *LSD, the Consciousness Expanding Drug*. New York: G.P. Putnam's Sons, 1964.

_____. *Politics of Ecstasy*. New York: G.P. Putnam's Sons, 1968.

Lee, Philip R., and Scanlon, James. "The data standardization remedy in Kassebaum-Kennedy." *Public Health Reports*, March-April 1997, 112(2): 114.

Lee, Thomas F. *The Human Genome Project*. New York: Plenum, 1991.

Leeuw, E.J.J. *The Sane Revolution: Health Promotion, Backgrounds, Scope, Prospects*. Assen/Maastricht, The Netherlands: Van Gorcum, 1989.

LeFeve, N.M., Ashley, M.J., Pederson, L.L. and Keys, J.J. "The health risks of passive smoking: The growing case for control measures in closed environments." *Chest* 84(1):90-95, July 1983.

"The legal implications of dietary fats: Risks of cardiovascular disease and the duty of food manufacturers." *Journal of Nutrition* 121(4):578-82, April 1991.

Leggett, Jeremy. "Running down to Rio." *New Scientist* 134 (May 2, 1992):38-42.

"Legislation needed to protect nonsmokers." *New Scientist* 117:18, March 31, 1988.

Leonard, George. *The Silent Pulse: The Search for the Perfect Rhythm that Exists in Each of Us.* New York: Dutton, 1986.

———. *The Ultimate Athlete.* New York: Avon, 1977.

———. *The Transformation: A Guide to the Inevitable Changes in Mankind.* Los Angeles: J.P. Tarcher, 1987.

Leonhard, Wolfgang. *Eurocommunism: Challenge for East and West,* translated by Mark Vecchio. New York: Rinehart and Winston, 1978.

Leuctenberg, William Edward. *In the Shadow of FDR: From Harry Truman to Ronald Reagan.* Ithaca, NY: Cornell University Press, 1983.

———. *New Deal and Global War, 1933-1945.* New York: Time Life Books, 1963.

Levit, Katherine R., and Cowan, Cathy A. "Business, households, and governments: Health care costs 1990." *Health Care Financing Review* 13(2):88, Winter 1991.

Levit, Katherine R., Freeland, Mark S., and Waldo, Daniel R. "Health spending and ability to pay: Business, individual and government." *Health Care Financing Review* 10:3ff, Spring 1989.

Leviton, Laura C. "The yield from worksite cardiovascular risk reduction." *JOM* 29:931-936, December 1987.

Levy, Jacques E. *Cesar Estrada Chavez: Autobiography of La Causa.* New York: Norton, 1975.

Lewin, Moshe. *The Gorbachev Phenomenon: A Historical Interpretation.* Berkeley: University of California Press, 1991.

Lewin, Stephen (ed.). *The Nation's Health. The Reference Shelf,* Vol. 43, No. 3. New York: The H.W. Wilson Co., 1971.

Lewis, Charles E. "Variations in the incidence of surgery." *NEJM* 281:880-884, 1969.

Lewis, Howard R., and Lewis, Martha E. *The Medical Offenders.* New York: Simon & Schuster, 1970.

Lewis, Kathleen A. *Private Sector Investment in HMOs, 1974-1980.* Excelsior, MN: InterStudy, 1981.

Light, D.W. "Escaping the traps of postwar western medicine—How to maximize health and minimize expenses." *European Journal of Public Health* 3:281-289, 1993.

Lipset, S.M. *Revolution and Counter Revolution.* New Brunswick, NJ: Transaction Publications, 1967.

Litoff, Judy Barrett. *American Midwives: 1860 to the Present.* Westport, CT: Greenwood Press, 1978.

Litwak, Robert. *Détente and the Nixon Doctrine: American Foreign Policy and the Pursuit of Stability, 1969-1976.* New York: Cambridge University Press, 1984.

Lohr, K.N., and Schroeder, S.A. "Special report: A strategy for quality assurance in Medicare." *NEJM* 322:707-712, 1990.

Longest, Beaufort B., Jr. "Pittsburgh embraces HMO development." *Business and Health* 11-13, December 1985.

Longford, F.P. *Nixon, a Study of Extremes of Fortune*. London: Weidenfeld and Nicolson, 1980.

Lovins, A.B. *World Energy Strategies: Facts, Issues, and Options*. San Francisco: Friends of the Earth International, 1975.

Lubitz, James D., Riley, Gerald F. "Trends in medical payments in the last year of life." *NEJM* 328(15): 1092-1096, April 15, 1996.

Luce, Gay. "S.A.G.E., a health program for senior citizens," report to the Holmes Center for Research in Holistic Healing, annual research symposium, Los Angeles, California, March 1991.

Ludmerer, Kenneth M. *Learning to Heal: The Development of American Medical Education*. New York: Basic Books, 1985.

Luft, Harold S. "For-profit hospitals: A cost problem or a solution?" *Business and Health* 13-16, Jan./Feb. 1985.

Luke, Barbara, Nicole Mamelle, Louis Keith, et al. "The association between occupational factors and preterm birth: A United States nurses' study." *Am. J. Obstet. Gynecol.* 173:849-62, 1995.

Lunneborg, P.W. *Abortion: A Positive Decision*. New York: Bergin & Garvey, 1992.

Lustig, Robert Jeffrey. *Corporate Liberalism: The Origin of Modern American Political Theory, 1890-1920*. Berkeley: University of California Press, 1982.

MacDonald, Gordon J. *Climate Change and Acid Rain*. McLean, VA: MITRE Corp, 1985.

"Majority of hospitals consider DRG-104 to be a money-maker." *Modern Health Care* 16(4):84, Feb. 14, 1986.

Mannheim, Karl. *Essays on the Sociology of Knowledge*. New York: Oxford University Press, 1952.

Marcuse, Herbert. *One Dimensional Man: Studies in the Ideology of Advanced Industrial Society*. Boston: Beacon Press, 1964.

Marmor, Ted, and Marmor, Ann. *The Politics of Medicare*. Chicago: Aldine Publishing Co., 1970, 24.

Masso, Anthony R. "HMOs in transition: What the future holds." *Business and Health* 21-24, Jan./Feb. 1985.

Matthiesen, Peter. *In the Spirit of Crazy Horse*. New York: Viking Press, 1983.

May, J. *The Greenpeace Book of the Nuclear Age: The Hidden History, the Human Cost*. New York: Pantheon Books, 1989.

Mayes, Michael S. "With much deliberation and some speed: Eisenhower and the Brown Decision." *Journal of Southern History* 52:43-76, February 1986.

Maynard, Roberta. "The power of pooling." *Nation's Business* 83:16-22, March 1995.

McCarry, Charles. *Citizen Nader*. New York: Saturday Review Press, 1972.

McComas, Maggie, Fookes, Geoffrey, and Taucher, George. *The Dilemma of Third World Nutrition: Nestle and the Role of Infant Formula U.S.A.*: Nestle.

McCoy, Alfred W. *Politics of Heroin in Southeast Asia*. New York: Harper and Row, 1972.

McKinlay, John B., and Stoeckle, John D. "Corporatization and the social transformation of doctoring." In *The Corporate Transformation of Health Care: Issues and Directions*, edited by Salmon, J. Warren. Amityville: Baywood Publishing Co., 1990:134.

McLuhan, M. *The Global Village: Transformations in World Life and Media in the 21st Century*. New York: Oxford University Press, 1989.

McPhee, Stephen J., Showstack, Jonathan A., and Schroeder, Steven A. "Influencing physicians decisions to use medical technology." In *The Medical Cost Containment Crisis: Fears, Opinions, and Facts*, edited by McCue, Jack D. Ann Arbor, MI: Health Administration Press, 1989:194.

McQueen, David. "China's impact on American medicine in the seventies: A limited and preliminary inquiry." *Social Science and Medicine* 21(83):931-36, 1985.

Mechnikov, Ilie Ilich. *The Founders of Modern Medicine: Pasteur, Koch, Lister*. New York: Walden Publications, 1939.

"Medicare Catastrophic Coverage Act of 1988," *Health Care Financing Review* 10(3):56, Winter 1988.

Menzel, Paul. *Medical Costs, Moral Choices: A Philosophy of Health Care Economics in America*. New Haven: Yale University Press, 1983.

"Met Life, Seattle HMO market long term care." *Employee Benefit Plan Review* 41:93-94, May 1987.

Meyer, J.A., Sharon, S., and Carl, J.S. "Universal access to health care: A comprehensive tax-based approach." *Archives of Internal Medicine* 151:917-22, 1991.

Michigan Department of Public Health, *Promoting Cardiovascular Health in Michigan: Recommendations for Action. Report of the Cardiovascular Disease Subcommittee of the Chronic Disease Advisory Committee*. Lansing, MI: MDPH, December 1991.

Milbank Memorial Fund. *Health, a Victim or Cause of Inflation?* New York: Prodist, 1976.

Mills, C. Wright. *The Power Elite*. New York: Oxford University Press, 1956.

Mills, Richard. *Young Outsiders: A Study in Alternative Communities*. New York: Pantheon Books, 1973.

Miro, Charles R. and Cox, J.E. "EPA Science Board concludes passive smoke causes cancer." *ASHRAE Journal* 3:12, March 1991.

Mitgang, H. *America at Random, from the New York Times' Oldest Editorial Feature, "Topics of the Times," a Century of Comments on America and Americans*. New York: Coward-McCann, 1969.

Monteith, S. *AIDS: The Unnecessary Epidemic: America Under Siege*. Sevierville, TN: Covenant House Books, 1991.

Montgomery, Geoffrey. "Shooting the messenger." *Discover* 10:32, November 1989.

Moore, Alicia Hills. "The other worry: Atomic waste." *Fortune* 118:114, August 1, 1988.

Morrisey, Michael A. *Cost Shifting in Health Care: Separating Evidence from Rhetoric*. Washington, DC: AEI Press, 1994.

Mort, Jo Ann. "Return of the sweatshop: Déjà vu in the garment industry." *Dissent* 35:363-366, Summer 1988.

Moss, Richard. *The I That Is We: Awakening to Higher Energies Through Unconditional Love*. Millbrae, CA: Celestial Arts, 1981.

Moyer, R. Charles, and Spudeck, Raymond E. "A note on the stock market's reaction to the accident at Three Mile Island." *J. of Economics and Business* 41:235-240, August 1989.

Moynihan, Patrick. "Civil rights progress report." *Congressional Quarterly*. Washington, DC: Congressional Quarterly Inc., 23-24, 1970.

Muir, John. *Our National Parks*. Boston: Houghton Mifflin Co. 1909.

Munley, Ann. *The Hospice Alternative: A New Context for Death and Dying*. New York: Basic Books, Inc., 1983.

Munts, Raymond. *Bargaining for Health*. Madison: University of Wisconsin Press, 1960.

Nader, Ralph. *Unsafe At Any Speed: The Designed-in Dangers of the American Automobile*. New York: Grossman, 1965.

Nader, Ralph, with Carper, Jean. *The Consumer and Corporate Accountability*. New York: Harcourt, Brace and Jovanovich, 1973.

Nader, Ralph, with Green, Mark. *Corporate Power in America*. New York: Grossman, 1973.

The National Cholesterol Education Project, Heart Lung and Blood Institute, National Institutes of Health, Health Prospects. *Adult treatment guidelines*. Rockville, MD: NHLBI, 1987.

"National health care expenditures, by type." *Health Care Financing Review*, Spring 1996.

National Health Service Corps (U.S.). *National Health Service Corps Scholarship Program: A Report by the Secretary of Health, Education and Welfare to Congress, 1978-79*. Hyattsville, MD: Department of HEW, 1978-79.

National Institute of Health. *The AIDS Research of the National Institute of Health: Report of a Study*. Washington, DC: National Academy Press, 1991.

National Institute on Alcohol Abuse and Alcoholism (U.S.). *Alcohol and Alcoholism: Programs and Progress*. Washington, DC: Government Printing Office, 1972.

National Leadership Commission on Health Care. *For the Health of a Nation: A Shared Responsibility*. Ann Arbor, MI: Health Administration Press, 1990.

NATO Advanced Study Institute Paleorift. *Tectonics and Geophysics of Continental Rifts*. Dordrecht: D. Reidel Pub. Co., 1978.

Navarro, Vincente. *Medical Care in the U.S.: A Critical Analysis*. Farmingdale, NY: Heywood Publications, 1977.

————. "Why some countries have national health insurance, others have national services, and the U.S. has neither." *Soc. Sci. Med.* 30:887-898, 1989.

NBC. "What price health?" NBC Special Report, 1992.

Neihardt, John G. *Black Elk Speaks: Being the Life Story of a Holy Man of the Ogalala Sioux*. Lincoln: University of Nebraska Press, 1932, 1988.

Netherlands Ministerie van Welzijn, Volkgezondheim en Cultuur. Stuurgroep Toekwustscenario's Gezondheidzorg. *AIDS up to the year 2000: Epidemiological, sociocultural,and economic scenario analysis for the Netherlands*. Dordrecht, Boston: Kluwer Academic Publishers, 1992.

New Age Directory. Chicago: Twenty-First Century Press, (no date).

Newhouse, Joseph P. *Free for All? Lessons from the Rand Health Insurance Experiment*. Cambridge, MA: Harvard Univ. Press, 1993.

Nobel, David F. *America by Design: Science, Technology and the Rise of Corporate Capitalism*. New York: Oxford University Press, 1979.

Nutrition and Cancer Prevention: Investigating the Role of Micronutrients. New York: Dekkas, 1989.

Nutrition, Toxicity, and Cancer. Boca Raton: CRC Press, 1991.

Oglesby, Carl (ed.). *The New Left Reader*. New York: Grove Press, 1969.

Olliver, C. *Tectonics and Landforms*. London: Longman, 1981.

O'Malley, P.M., Johnston, L.D., and Bachman, J.G. *Quantitative and Qualitative Changes in Cocaine Use Among High School Seniors, College Students, and Young Adults.* Rockville, MD: NIDA Research Monograph, 1991, 110-19-43.

Organization of Economic Cooperation and Development. *Reviews of National Science Policy: United States.* Geneva: OECD, 1968.

Ornish, Dean. *Stress, Diet and Your Heart.* New York: Holt, Rinehart and Winston, 1982.

_____. *Dr. Dean Ornish's Program for Reversing Heart Disease.* New York: Random House, 1990.

_____. *Clinical Cardiac Rehabilitation: A Cardiologist's Guide.* Baltimore, MD: Williams & Wilkins, 1993.

Orth, S.P. *The Boss and the Machine.* New Haven, CT: Yale University Press, 1919.

Ostrow, D.G. "Homosexualities." Chapter Sixteen, in *Sexually Transmitted Diseases*, edited by Holmes, K., Wisener, P., and A. Mardagh, second edition, 1990.

Pabst, William R., Ph.D. "An American Hospital Association Professional Liability Study." In U.S. Department of Health, Education and Welfare, *Report of the Secretary's Commission on Medical Malpractice.* Washington, DC: DHEW Publication no. 72-89, January 16, 1973.

Papadakis, Elim. *The Green Movement in West Germany.* New York: St. Martin's Press, 1984.

Patrick, Clifford H., and Johnson, Katrina W. "Health differentials between blacks and whites: Recent trends in morbidity and mortality." *Milbank Quarterly* 65 supp. 1:129-199, 1987.

Patton, Cindy. *Sex and Germs: The Politics of AIDS.* Boston: South End Press, 1985.

Paulsen, D.F. *Pollution and Public Policy: A Book of Readings.* New York: Dodd, 1973.

Payton, Sallyanne. "Why alliances? A simpler path to health care reform through reinsurance." Conference on Paths to Health Care Reform, Duke Medical School, February 10, 1994.

_____. "The politics of comprehensive national health care reform: Watching the 103rd and 104th Congresses at work," in Rosenthal, Marilynn M. and Max Heirich, Max (eds.). *Health Care Policy: Understanding Our Choices from National Reform to Market Force.* Boulder, CO: Westview Press, 1997.

Peacocke, Christopher. *Holistic Explanation: Action Space, Interpretation.* New York: Oxford University Press, 1979.

Pearce, H.G. "The Health Incentive Plan Evaluation: Final Report to the John A. Hartford Foundation, November, 1986." Prepared for C.L. Paracell, vice-president and project director, Blue Shield of California (unpublished).

Pearson, Charles S. *Environment, North and South: An Economic Interpretation.* New York: Wiley, 1978.

Penick, James L., Pursell, Carrol W., Sherwood, Morgan B., and Swain, Donald (eds.). *The Politics of American Science: 1939 to the Present.* Cambridge: MA: The MIT Press, 1965, 1972.

Perera, F., Mayer, J., Santella, R.M., Brenner, D., Tsai, W.Y., Brandt-Rauf, P., Hemminki, K. "DNA adducts and other biological markers in risk assessment for environmental carcinogens." *Annali dell Instituto Superiore di Sanita* 227(4):615-20, 1991.

Perkins, Kenneth Al., and Epstein, Leonard H. "Smoking, stress, and coronary heart disease." *Journal of Consulting and Clinical Psychology* 56:342-9, June 1988.

Perretz, Harriet. *The Gray Panther Manual*. Philadelphia: Gray Panthers, 1978.

Perrine, Daniel M. "The view from Platform Zero: How Holland handles its drug problem," *America* 171: 9-12, October 15, 1994.

Perry, George and Brainard, William C. (eds.). *Brookings Papers in Economic Activity* 1. Brookings Institution, 1987.

Pert, Candace B. "The wisdom of the receptors: Neuropeptides, the emotions, and bodymind." *Advances, Institute for the Advancement of Health* 3(3):4-16, Summer 1986.

Peterson, Dan M., and Brownawell, H. Jeffrey. "A review of Health Security Act of 1993." *Health Care Financial Management* 48:44, January 1994.

Pfaff, M. "Differences in health care spending across countries: Statistical evidence." *J. Health Politics Policy Law* 15:1-24, 1990.

Phillips, D.H., Hemminki, K., Alhonen, A., Hewer, A., Grover P.L. "Monitoring occupational exposure to carcinogens: Detection by 32P- postlabeling of aromatic DNA adducts in white blood cells from iron foundry workers." *Mutation Research* 204:3:531-41, March 1988.

Physicians for Social Responsibility. *The PSR Quarterly: A Journal of Medicine and Global Survival*. Baltimore, MD: Williams & Wilkins, 1991.

Physician's Role Periodicals (PRS). *A Journal of Medicine and Global Survival* 1(1), March 1991.

Pickering, Helen and Stimson, Gerry V. "Syringe sharing in prison." *Lancet* (North American edition) 342:521-22, Sept. 4, 1993.

"Pinatubo fails to deepen the ozone hole." *Science* 258:395, October 16, 1992.

Pink, Louis H. *The Story of Blue Cross*. New York: Public Affairs Commission, Inc., 1945.

Piven, Francis Fox and Cloward, Richard A. *Poor People's Movements: Why They Succeed, How They Fail*. New York: Vintage, 1979.

Pocincki, Leon S., Dogger, Stuart J., and Schwartz, Barbara. "The incidence of iatrogenic injuries." In U.S. Department of Health, Education and Welfare, *Report of the Secretary's Commission on Medical Malpractice*. Washington, DC: DHEW Publication no. 72-89, January 16, 1973.

Poen, Monte M. *Harry S. Truman Versus the Medical Lobby: The Genesis of Medicare*. Columbia, MO: University of Missouri Press, 1979.

Politzer, Robert M., Harris, Dona L., Gaston, Marilyn H., and Bitzburgh, Mullan. "Primary care physician supply and the medically underserved." *JAMA* 266(1):J123-J128, July 3, 1991.

Powell, M. *Health Care in Japan*. London: Routledge, 1990.

Powell, Thomas J. *Self-Help Organizations and Professional Practice*. Silver Springs, MD: National Association of Social Workers, 1987.

Price, J.H., Krol, R.A., and Desmond, S.M. "Comparison of three antismoking interventions among pregnant women in an urban setting: A randomized trial." *Psychological Report* 68:595-604, April 1992.

Price, J.R. *National Health Insurance*. Washington, DC: American Enterprise Institute for Public Policy Research, 1992.

Purifoy, Lewis Carroll. *Harry Truman's China Policy: McCarthyism and the Diplomacy of Hysteria*. New York: New Viewpoints, 1976.

Ram Dass. *Be Here Now*. New York: Crown Publishing, 1971.

Ravich, Ruth. "Patient advocacy." In *Advocacy in Health Care: The Power of a Silent Constituency*, edited by Marks, Joan H. Clifton, NJ: Humana Press, 1986: 51-60.

Renner, Michael. "Creating substainable jobs in industrial countries." In *State of the World, 1992*, Brown, Lester (ed.). New York: Norton, 1992.

"Researcher discounts global warming." *Geotimes* 38:6, Sept. 1993.

Resnick, Rosalind. "Miami Chamber joins HMO for small firms." *Business & Health* 10:56-7, Oct. 1992.

Ribicoff, Senator Abraham, with Danaceau, Paul. *The American Medical Machine*. New York: Saturday Review Press, 1972.

Richards, A.N. "The impact of the war on medicine." *Science* 103:578, May 10, 1946.

Richmond, Len, and Nogura, Gary. *The Gay Liberation Book*. San Francisco: Ramparts Press, 1973.

Riessman, Frank. "New dimensions in self-help." *Social Policy* XV:2-4, Winter 1985.

Riley,Gerald F., Iannacchione, Vincent G., and Garfinkel, Steven A. "High-cost users of medical care," *Health Care Financing Review* 9:41-52, Summer 1988.

Ritchey, Ferris J. "Medical rationalization, cultural lag, and the malpractice crisis." *Human Organization* 40(2):97-112, Summer 1981.

Rivlin, R.S., Shils, M.D., Sherlock, P. "Nutrition and cancer." *American Journal of Medicine* 75:843-54, November 1993.

Rock, Steven M. "Malpractice premiums and primary caesarean section rates in New York and Illinois, *Public Health Reports* 103(5):459-463, Sept.-Oct. 1988.

Rockefeller, J.D. *Random Reminiscences of Men and Events*. New York: Doubleday, Page and Co., 1909.

Rockefeller, Senator John D., IV. "A call for action: The Pepper Commission's blueprint for health care reform." *JAMA* 265(19):2507-2510, May 15, 1991.

_____. "The Pepper Commission report on comprehensive health care." *NEJM* 323:1005-1007, 1990.

Roeder, Penelope C. and Moxley, John H., III. "Promoting quality care in cost-effective settings." *Business and Health* 30-31, Jan./Feb. 1985.

Rogers, David E. *American Medicine: Challenge for the 1980s*. Cambridge, MA: Ballinger Publishing Company, 1978.

Rorem, C. Rufus. *Blue Cross Hospital Service Plans*. Chicago: Hospital Service Plan Commission, 1944, 7.

_____. "Group hospitalization plans forge ahead." *Hospitals* 10:62-66, April 1936.

Rosen, George. *The Structure of American Medical Practice: 1875-1941*. Philadelphia: University of Pennsylvania Press, 1983.

Rosenan-Maxcy, Milton Joseph. *Preventive Medicine and Public Health*. Edited by Sartwell, Philip E. New York: Appleton-Century-Crofts, 1965.

Rosenbaum, W.A. *The Politics of Environmental Concern*. New York: Praeger Publishers, 1974.

Rosenberg, Charles. *The Cholera Years*. Chicago: University of Chicago Press, 1962.

Rosencranz, Armin, and Carroll, John E. (eds.). *International Environmental Diplomacy: The Management and Resolution of Transfrontier Environmental Problems*. New York: Cambridge University Press, 1988.

Rosenthal, Marilynn. *Health Care in the People's Republic of China: Moving Towards Modernization*. Boulder, CO: Westview Press, 1987.

_____. *Dealing with Medical Malpractice: The British and Swedish Experience*. London: Tavistock, 1987; Durham, NC: Duke Univ. Press, 1988.

Rosenthal, Marilynn M. and Max Heirich, Max (eds.). *Health Care Policy: Understanding Our Choices from National Reform to Market Force.* Boulder, CO: Westview Press, 1997.

Rossi, Peter H. (ed.). *Ghetto Revolts.* Chicago: Aldine Pub. Co., 1970.

Rossman, Michael. *New Age Blues: On the Politics of Consciousness.* New York: E. P. Dutton, 1979.

Rossman, Parker. *Hospice: Creating New Models of Care for the Terminally Ill.* New York: Association Press, 1977.

Roszak, Theodore. *The Dissenting Academy.* New York: Pantheon Press, 1968.

————. *The Making of a Counter Culture: Reflections on the Technocratic Society and Its Youthful Opposition.* Garden City, NY: Doubleday, 1969.

————. *Where the Wasteland Ends: Politics and Transcendance in Postindustrial Society.* Garden City, NY: Doubleday, 1972.

Rothman, Barbara Katz. *[In Labor] Giving Birth: Alternatives in Childbirth.* New York: Penguin Books, 1982, 1984.

Rothstein, Linda "PSR pinpoints problems." *Bul. of the Atomic Scientists* 49:10, Jan.-Feb. 1993.

Rottenberg, Simon (ed.). *The Economics of Medical Malpractice.* Washington, DC: American Enterprise Institute for Public Policy Research, 1978.

Rovner, Julie. "Bush Medicare premium plan is greeted warily on Hill" *Congressional Quarterly* 49(8):467-468, February 23, 1991.

Rubin, Jerry. *We Are Everywhere.* New York: Macmillan, 1970.

Rudd, Mark, Roth, Rob, Sokolow, Jeff, Cole, Lew, et al. "What is to be done?" In *The University Crisis Reader: Confrontation and Counter Attack,* edited by Immanual Wallerstein and Paul Starr. New York: Vintage Books, 1971, 201-205.

Sadownick, D. "ACT UP makes a spectacle of AIDS." *High Performance* 13:26-31, Spring 1990.

Salmon, J. Warren (ed.). *Alternative Medicines: Popular and Policy Perspectives.* New York: Tavistock Publications, 1984.

————. *The Corporate Transformation of Health Care: Issues & Directions.* Amityville, NY: Baywood Publishing Company, Inc., 1990.

Sandhu, S.S., Ma T.H., Peng, Y., and Zhou, X. "Clastogenicity evaluation of seven chemicals commonly found at hazardous industrial waste sites." *Government Reports, Announcements, and Index (1990)* issue 13.

Santella, R.M., Young, X.Y., Hsieh, L.L., Young, T.L., Lu, X.Q., Stefanidis, M., Perara, F.F. "Immunological methods for the detection of carcinogen adducts in humans." *Basic Life Science* 53:33-44, 1990.

Satin, Mark. *New Age Politics: Healing Self and Society.* New York: Dell, 1979.

Scarpa, A. "Pre-scientific medicines: Their extent and value." *Social Sciences and Medicine* 15:317-326, 1981.

Schell, J. *Observing the Nixon Years: "Notes and Comments" from the New Yorker on the Vietnam War and the Watergate Crisis, 1969-1975.* New York: Pantheon Books, 1989.

Scherer, John L. (ed.). *The U.S.S.R. Facts and Figures Annual.* Gulf Breeze, Florida: Academic International Press, 1987.

Schieber, George. *Financing and Delivering Health Care: A Comparative Analysis of OECD Countries.* Paris: Organization for Economic Co-operation and Development, 1987.

Schlessinger, Arthur M. *The Age of Roosevelt*. Boston: Houghton-Mifflin, 1957.
———. *The Bitter Heritage: Vietnam and American Democracy, 1914-1966*. Boston: Houghton-Mifflin, 1966.
Schlessinger, Mark. "The rise of proprietary health care." *Business and Health* 7-12, Jan./Feb. 1985.
Schneeweis, Thomas, and Hill, Joanne. "The effect of Three Mile Island on electric utility stock prices." *Journal of Finance* 38:1285-1292, September 1983.
Schooner, J. "The Rio Earth Summit: What does it mean?" *Environmental Science & Technology* 27:18-22, January 1993.
Schorr, A.L. "Job turnover: A problem with employer-based health care." *NEJM* 322:463-466, 1990.
Schorr, Daniel, with an introduction by Senator Ted Kennedy. *Don't Get Sick in America*. Nashville and London: Aurora Publishers, 1970.
Schramm, C.J. *Health Care Financing for All Americans: Private Market Reform and Public Responsibility*. Washington, DC: The Association, 1991.
Schroeder, S.A., and Sandy, L.G. "Specialty distribution of U.S. physicians: The invisible driver of health care costs." *NEJM* 328(13):961-963, April 1, 1993.
Schulberg, H.C. *The Mental Hospital and Human Services*. New York: Behavioral Publications, 1975.
Schwartz, R.G. "Commentary: Investment for an aging population." *Statistical Bulletin* 70:2, July-Sept. 1989.
Schwartz, William B., and Komesor, Neil K. *Doctors, Damages and Deterrence: An Economic View of Medical Malpractice*. Santa Monica, CA: Rand, 1978.
Scientists and Engineers for Social and Political Action Newsletter. *Science for the People* 2(2), August 1970-Sept. 1975.
Scitovsky, Anne A., and Rice, Dorothy P. "Estimates of the direct and indirect costs of acquired immunodeficiency syndrome in the United States, 1985, 1986, and 1991." *Public Health Reports, Journal of the Public Health Service* 102(1):5-17, Jan./Feb. 1987.
Scocpol, Theta. "Targeting within universalism." In *The Urban Underclass*, edited by Jencks, Christopher, and Peterson, Paul E. Washington, DC: Brookings Institute, 1991, 411-436.
Seidman, B. (ed.). *Curing U.S. Health Care Ills*. Washington, DC: National Planning Association, 1991.
Seitz, D.C. *The Dreadful Decade, 1869-1879*. Indianapolis: Bobbs-Merrill Company, 1926.
Selye, H. *The Stress of Life*. New York: McGraw-Hill Book Company, 1956.
Shaw, Seth H. "The compelling issue of access to capital." *Business and Health* 17-20, Jan./Feb. 1985.
Sheehan, N. *The Pentagon Papers, as Published by the New York Times, Based on Investigative Report*. New York: Bantam Books, 1971.
Shilts, R. *And the Band Played On: Politics, People, and the AIDS Epidemic*. Harrisonburg: R.R. Donnelley & Sons Co., 1988.
Short, P.F. *National Medical Expenditure Survey: Estimates of the Uninsured Population, Calendar Year 1987: Data Summary 2*. Rockville, MD: National Center for Health Services Research and Health Care Technology Assessment, 1990.
Sidel, Victor, and Sidel, Ruth (eds.). *Reforming Medicine: Lessons of the Last Quarter Century*. New York: Pantheon Books, 1984.

Simmons, Ruth, Kay, Bonnie J., and Regan, Carol. "Women's health groups: Alternatives to the health care system." *International Journal of Health Services* 14(4):619-634, 1984.

Singer, Fred S. *Global Climate Change.* New York: Paragon House, 1989.

Siwolop, Sana, and Brazda, Jerry. "The fairy godmother of medical research." *Business Week* 67, July 14, 1986.

Sklar, Martin. *The Corporate Reconstruction of American Capitalism, 1890-1916: The Market, Law and Politics.* Cambridge: Cambridge University Press, 1988.

Sloan, D.M. *Abortion: A Doctor's Perspective/A Woman's Dilemma.* New York: D.I. Fine, 1992.

Sloan, F.A. *Cost, Quality, and Access in Health Care: New Roles for Health Planning in a Competitive Environment.* San Francisco: Jossey-Bass Publishers, 1988.

Smith, D.G. *Paying for Medicare: The Politics of Reform.* New York: A. deGruyter, 1992.

Smith, David Elvin, Bentel, David J., and Schwartz, Jerome L. (eds.). *The Free Clinic: A Community Approach to Health Care and Drug Abuse—Proceedings of the First National Free Clinic Council Symposium.* Beloit, WI: Stash Press, 1971.

Smith, David Elvin and Luce, John. *Love Needs Care: A History of San Francisco's Haight-Ashbury Free Medical Clinic and Its Pioneer Role in Treating Drug-Abuse Problems.* Boston: Little Brown, 1971.

Smuts, Jan. *Holism and Evolution.* New York: Macmillan, 1926 and Delta, 1979.

Somers, Anne R., and Somers, Herbert N. *Doctors, Patients and Health Insurance.* Washington, DC: The Brookings Institute, 1961.

Sorkin, A.L. *Health Care and the Changing Economic Environment.* Lexington, MA: Lexington Books, 1986.

"South Carolina's program for aggressive outreach." *Health Advocate: Newsletter of the National Health Law Program* 169:9, Summer 1991.

Spengler, David. *Revelation, the Birth of a New Age.* San Francisco: The Rainbow Ridge, 1976.

Spratnik, Charlene, and Capra, Fritjof. *Green Politics.* Santa Fe, NM: Bear, 1986.

Springer, Allen L. "United States environmental policy and international law: Stockholm Principle Twenty-One revisited." *International Environmental Diplomacy.* John E. Carroll (ed.). Cambridge: Cambridge University Press, 1990.

Stambler, Sookie. *Women's Liberation: Blueprint for the Future.* New York: Ace Books, 1970.

Standard & Poor's. *Standard & Poor's Industry Surveys.* New York: Standard & Poor's Corp., December 17, 1959.

Stanley, J. *Broad Scan Analysis of Human Adipose Tissue, Executive Summary.* Springfield, VA: USEPA, 1986.

Starr, Paul. *The Social Transformation of American Medicine: The Rise of a Sovereign Profession and the Making of a Vast Industry.* New York: Basic Books, Inc., 1984.

Statistical Abstracts of the United States. Washington, DC: U.S. Government Printing Office, 1970-1987.

Statistical Abstracts of the United States. Work Stoppage, Major Issues and Durations, 1946-60. Washington, DC: U.S. Government Printing Office, 1946-60.

"A statistical analysis of 2,717 hospitals." *Bulletin of the American Hospital Association* 4:68, July 1930.

Stein, Eric, (ed.). *American Enterprise in the European Common Market: A Legal Profile.* Ann Arbor, MI: University of Michigan Law School, 1960.

Stein, Jane. "How HMOs adapt: A perspective from the inside." an interview with Fred Wasserman of the Maxicare HMO Chain. *Business and Health* 44-46, October 1986.

Steinberg, Earl P., Feder, Judith, and Hadley, Jack. "Comparison of uninsured and privately insured hospital patients: Condition on admission, resource use, and outcome." *JAMA* 265:374-379, Jan. 16, 1991.

Steinem, Gloria. *Outrageous Acts and Everyday Rebellion.* New York: Holt, Rinehart and Winston, 1983.

Steslicke, W.E. "Medical care security and the 'vitality of private sector' in Japan". In *Comparative Health Policy and the New Right: From Rhetoric to Reality,* edited by C. Allenstetter and S.C. Haywood. New York: St. Martin's Press, 1991, 247-282.

Stevens, Robert, and Stevens, Rosemary. *Welfare Medicine in America: A Case Study of Medicaid.* New York: Free Press, 1974.

Stone, Chuck. *Black Political Power in America.* New York: Dell Publishing Co., 1968, 48-54.

Stress, Neuropeptides and Systemic Disease. San Diego: Academic Press, 1991.

Strickland, D.A. *Scientists in Politics: The Atomic Scientists Movement, 1945-1946.* Lafayette, IN: Purdue University Studies, 1968.

Strosberg, M.A., Wiener, Joshua M., Fein, Robert C., and Fein, I. Alan (eds.). *Rationing America's Medical Care: The Oregon Plan and Beyond.* Washington, DC: Brookings Institution, 1992.

Summer, Michael T. *The Dollars and Sense of Hospital Malpractice Insurance.* Cambridge, MA: Abt Books, 1979.

Taragin, M.I., Wilczek, A.P., Karns, M.E., Trout, R., and Carson, J.L. "Physician demographics and risk of medical malpractice." *American J. of Medicine* 93(5):537-542, November 1992.

Tarbell, Ida. *History of the Standard Oil Company.* New York: MacMillan, 1904, 1925, 2 volumes.

Tarlov, Alvin R., Kehrer, Barbara H., Hall, Donna P., Samuels, Sarah E., Grown, Gwendolyn S., Felix, Michael R.J., and Ross, Jane A. "Foundation work: The Health Promotion Program of the Henry J. Kaiser Foundation." *Am. J. Health Promo.* 2(2):74-80, Fall 1987.

Taylor, Elsworth. *Data Book on Multi-Hospital Systems, 1980-1985.* Chicago: American Hospital Association, 1985.

Teodori, Massimo. *The New Left: A Documentary History.* Indianapolis: Bobbs-Merrill, 1969.

Thomas, Lewis. *The Lives of a Cell: Notes of a Biology Watcher.* New York: Viking, 1974.

_____. *Medusa and the Snail.* New York: The Viking Press, 1979.

Thomas, Robert. "Future sea level rise and its early detection by satellite remote sensing." In U.S. Environmental Protection Agency, *Effects of Changes in Stratospheric Ozone and Global Climate,* James G. Titus (ed.), vol. 4. Washington, DC: U.S. EPA and UNEP. August, 1989.

Thomas, Tony "The student revolt: An analysis." In *The University Crisis Reader: Confrontation and Counter Attack*, edited by Immanual Wallerstein and Paul Starr. New York: Vintage Books, 1971, 205-226.

Todd, J.S., et al. "Health access America—Strengthening the U.S. health care system." *JAMA* 265:2503-2506, May 15, 1991.

Toner, J.M. "Statistics of regular medical associations and hospitals of the United States." *Transactions of the American Medical Association* 24:314-344, 1973.

"Toxic wasteland." *U.S. News and World Report* 40-43, April 13, 1992.

Travis C., and Hattemer-Fray, H. "Global chemical pollution." *Environmental Science Technology* 25:814-819, 1991.

Treloar, Alan Edward, and Chill, Don. *Hill-Burton Hospital Survey and Construction Act*. Chicago: American Hospital Association, 1961.

Tunley, Roul. *The American Health Scandal*. New York: Harper and Row, 1966.

Turner, Frederick. *Rediscovering America: John Muir in His Time and Ours*. New York: Viking, 1985.

Ulrich's International Periodicals Directory. New York: Bowker, 1960-1986.

United Nations. *Demographic Yearbook*. New York: UN, 1955, 1973.

University of Hawaii (Honolulu). *Health Care Status: Selected Pacific Areas*. Springfield, VA: National Technical Information Service, U.S. Dept. of Commerce, 1973.

U.S. Congress. *Managed Competition and Its Potential to Reduce Health Spending*. Washington, DC: Congressional Budget Office, 1993.

_____. *Projections of National Health Expenditures*. Washington, DC: U.S. Congressional Budget Office, 1992.

_____. *Trends in Health Spending: An Update*. Washington, DC: U.S. Congressional Budget Office, 1993.

U.S. Congress Office of Technology Assessment. *Diagnostically Related Groups (DRGs) and the Medicare Program: Implications for Medical Technology*, OTA-TM-H-17. Washington, DC: U.S. Printing Office, 1983.

U.S. Congress Senate Committee on Finance. *Implementation of Peer Review Organization Program (PRO) Hearings, 98th Congress, Second Session*. Washington, DC: U.S. Printing Office, 1984.

U.S. Congressional Budget Office. *Managed Competition and Its Potential to Reduce Health Spending*. Washington, DC: U.S. Congress, 1993.

U.S. Department of Commerce, Bureau of the Census. *Historical Statistics of the United States, Part I: Colonial Times to 1970*. Washington, DC: U.S. Government Printing Office, 1975.

U.S. Department of Commerce, Bureau of Economic Analysis. "General business indicators: Capital goods industries manufacturing sales and inventories." *Business Statistics, 1986*. Washington, DC: U.S. Government Printing Office, 1986, 14.

U.S. Department of Health, Education and Welfare. *PRSO Fact Book*. Washington, DC: U.S. Government Printing Office, 1977.

_____. *Report of the Secretary's Commission on Medical Malpractice*, Publication no. 72-89. Washington, DC: DHEW, 1973.

_____. "The supply of health manpower: 1970 profiles and projections to 1990." In *Medical Specialists*. Washington, DC: U.S. Government Printing Office, 1974: 57.

U.S. Department of Health, Education and Welfare, Health Services and Mental Health Administration, Health Care Facilities Service, Office of Program Planning and Analysis. *The Hill-Burton Progress Report.* Rockville, MD: U.S. Government Printing Office, 1973.

U.S. Department of Health, Education and Welfare, Social Security Administration. *Social Security Bulletin.* Washington, DC: U.S Government Printing Office, December 1970.

U.S. Department of Health and Human Services Administration's Bureau of Health. *Report to the President and the Congress on the Status of Health Personnel in the United States.* Rockville, MD: May, 1984.

U.S. Department of Health and Human Services, Public Health Service. *Health United States, 1995.* Rockville, MD: Department of Health and Human Services, 1995.

_____. *Healthy People 2000: National Health Promotion and Disease Prevention Objectives.* Washington, DC: U.S. Government Printing Office, publ. no. PHS 91-50212, 1991.

_____. *Strategies to Control Tobacco Use in the U.S.: A Blueprint for Public Health Action in the 1990s.* Rockville, MD: National Institutes of Health, 1991.

_____. *Vital Statistics of the U.S., 1986, Volume 1, Natality.* Hyattsville, MD: U.S. Department of Health and Human Services, Public Health Service, Center for Disease Control, National Center for Health Statistics, 1988.

U.S. Department of Health and Human Services, Public Health Service, Health Resources and Services Administration, Bureau of Health Professions, Division of Disadvantaged Assistance. *Health Status of the Disadvantaged Chartbook.* Rockville, MD: Department of Health and Human Services, 1986.

U.S. Department of Labor, Bureau of Labor Statistics. *Bulletin 2307.*

_____. *Employment and Earnings,* monthly.

_____. "Current labor statistics." *Monthly Labor Review* 83, June 1988.

_____. *Our Changing Economy: A BLS Centennial Chartbook, Bulletin 2211.* Washington, DC: Department of Labor, 1984.

U.S. Department of State, Bureau of Public Affairs. *Foreign Direct Investment in a Global Economy.* Washington, DC: U.S. Government Printing Office, 1989.

U.S. Environmental Protection Agency. *Effects of Changes in Stratospheric Ozone and Global Climate,* James G. Titus (ed.), vol. 3. Washington, DC: U.S. EPA and UNEP. August, 1986.

_____. *EPA Reports Bibliography: A Listing of EPA Reports Available from the National Technical Information Service as of April 1, 1973.* Washington, DC: U.S. Government Printing Office, 1973.

_____. "Executive summary on the scientific assessment of stratospheric ozone." *Congressional Record* 137, October 24, 1991.

_____. *Potential Effects of Global Climate Change on the U.S.,* edited by Joel B. Smith and Dennis Tirpah. Washington, DC: EPA, December, 1989.

U.S. General Accounting Office. *Health Care Reform.* Washington, DC: U.S. Government Accounting Office, 1993.

_____. *Medical Malpractice: Insurance Costs Increased but Varied Among Physicians and Hospitals,* GAO/HRD-86-112. Washington, DC: September, 1986.

_____. *Medical Malpractice: No Agreement on the Problems or Solutions,* GAO/HRD-86-50. Washington, DC: February, 1986.

U.S. Government. *A Call for Action: Final Report of the Pepper Commission.* Washington, DC: U.S. Government Printing Office, 1990.

_____. *Economic Report of the President. Annual Report of the Council of Economic Advisers, Appendix B: Statistical Tables Relating to Income, Employment and Production.* Washington. DC: U.S. Government Printing Office, 1992.

_____. *The President's Comprehensive Health Reform Program.* Washington, DC: The President, 1992.

_____. *The President's 1971 Environmental Program.* Washington, DC: U.S. Government Printing Office, 1971.

U.S. National Center for Health Statistics. *Facts of Life and Death.* Rockville, MD: NCHS, 1974.

U.S. Office of Technology Assessment, *Energy in Developing Countries.* OTA-E-486, Washington, DC: U.S. Government Printing Office, January, 1991.

_____. *Changing By Degrees: Steps to Reduce Greenhouse Gasses,* Summary. OTA-0-483 Washington, DC: Government Printing Office, February, 1991.

_____. *Mapping Our Genes—The Genome Projects: How Big, How Fast?* OTA-BA-373. Washington, DC: USGDO. (April, 1988): 3-6.

Vayda, Eugene. "A comparison of surgical rates in Canada and in England and Wales." *NEJM* 289:1224-1229, 1973.

Vinels, Paolo, Bartsch, Helmut, Caporade, Neil, Harrington, Anita M., Kadlabor, Fred F., Landi, Maria Theresa, Malavectle, Christian, Shields, Peter G., Skipper, Paul, Talaslec, Glenn, and Tannenbaum, Steven R. "Genetically-based a-acetyltranferese metabolic polymorphism and low-level environmental exposure to carcinogens." *Nature* 369:154-56, May 12, 1994.

von Hoffman, Nicholas. *We Are the People Our Parents Warned Us Against.* Chicago: Quadrangle Books, 1968.

Waitzkin, Howard. *The Second Sickness: Contradictions of Capitalist Health Care.* New York: The Free Press, 1983.

Waldman, F.M., Carroll, P.R., Kerschmann, R., Cohen, M.B., Field, F.G., Mayall, B.H. "Centromeric copy number of chromosome 7 is strongly correlated with tumor grade and labeling index in human bladder cancer." *Cancer Research* 51(14):3807-13, July 15, 1991.

Wallis, W. Allen, and Robert, Harry V. *Statistics: A New Approach.* Glencoe, IL: The Free Press of Glencoe, 1960.

Warner, K.E. "Effects of the anti-smoking campaign: An update." *AJPH* 79:144-151, 1989.

_____. "Smoking and health: A 25-year perspective." *AJPH* 79:141-143, 1989.

_____. "Smoking and health implications of a change in the federal cigarette excise tax." *JAMA* 255:1028-1032, February 1986.

Watson, James. *The Double Helix.* New York: Norton, 1980.

Weber, Jonathan and Weiss, Robin A. "HIV infection: The cellular picture." *Scientific America* 259(4):101-9, October 1988.

Weber, Max. "Science as a vocation." In Gentle, H.H., and Mills, C. Wright, *From Max Weber: Essays in Sociology.* New York: Oxford University Press, 1958, 129-156.

Weiss, Peter. "Passive risk: EPA loads anti-smoking gun." *Science News* 138:4, July 7, 1990.

Werbach, Melvyn R. *Third Line Medicine: Modern Treatment for Persistent Symptoms.* New York: Arkana, 1986.

Westby, David J. *The Clouded Vision: The Student Movement in the United States in the 1960s.* London: Associated University Press, 1976.

Wexler, S. *The Vietnam War: An Eyewitness History.* New York: Facts on File, 1992.

Weyler, Rex. *Blood of the Land: The Government and Corporate War Against the American Indian Movement.* New York: Everett House, 1982.

White House Domestic Policy Council. *The President's Health Security Plan: The Clinton Blueprint.* Washington, DC: New York Times Books, 1993.

White, Kerr. *The Task of Medicine: Dialogue at Wickenburg.* Menlo Park, CA: Henry Kaiser Family Foundation, 1988.

Whiteis, David G., and Salmon, J. Warren. "The proletarization of health care and the underdevelopment of the public sector." In *The Corporate Transformation of Health Care: Issues & Directions,* edited by Salmon, J. Warren. Amityville, NY: Baywood Publishing Company, Inc., 1990, 117-131.

Whitmer, R. William. "Worksite health promotion and health care reform: An update." *Am. J. Health Promo.* 9(1):5-8, Sept.-Oct. 1994.

WHO. "Update on AIDS." *Weekly Epidemiological Record,* November 29, 1991.

Wiener, J., Illston, L., and Hanley, R.J. *Sharing the Burden: Strategies for Public and Private Long-Term Care Insurance.* Washington, DC: The Brookings Institute, 1994.

Wikler, Daniel. "Forming an ethical response to for-profit health care." *Business and Health* January/February 1985, 25-29.

Wilber, Ken. *The Atman Project: A Transpersonal View of Human Development.* Wheaton, IL: Theosophical Publishing House, 1980.

_____. *The Holistic Paradigm and Other Paradoxes: Exploring the Leading Edge of Science.* Boulder, CO: Shambhala, 1982.

Wilkinson, Doris Yvonne. *Black Revolt: Strategies of Protest.* Berkeley: McCutchan Pub. Corp., 1969.

Williams, David R. "Macrosocial influences on African-American health." American Psychological Association meetings, Washington, DC, 1992.

Williams, Greer. *Kaiser-Permanente Health Plan: Why It Works.* Oakland, CA: Henry J. Kaiser Foundation, 1971.

Williams, Phil. *The Living Will and the Durable Power of Attorney for Health Care.* Oak Park, IL: Gaines, 1991.

Wilson, George Wilton. *Inflation—Causes, Consequences, and Cures.* Bloomington: University of Indiana Press, 1982.

Wilson, William J. *The Truly Disadvantaged: The Inner City, the Under Class, and Public Policy.* Chicago: Chicago Univ. Press, 1987.

Winslow, Charles-Everett A. *The Evolution and Significance of the Modern Public Health Campaign.* New Haven: Yale University Press, 1923.

Wohl, Stanley, M.D. *The Medical Industrial Complex.* New York: Harmony Books, 1984.

Wolfe, Burton H. *The Hippies.* New York: New American Library, 1968.

Wolfe, Tom. *The Electric Kool-Aid Acid Test.* New York: Bantam, 1968.

Wolff, M.S., Voorhees, J.J., and Selikoff, I.J. "Cutaneous effects of exposure of polybrominated biphenyls (PBBS): The Michigan PBB incidents." *Environmental Research* 29:97-108, 1982.

Wolpe, Paul Root. "The maintenance of professional authority: acupuncture and the American physician." *Social Problems* 32:409-24, June 1985.

Wootton, Barbara, and Ross, Laura T. "Hospital staffing patterns in urban and non-urban areas," *Monthly Labor Review* 118:23-33, March 1995.

World Almanac and Book of Facts. New York: Newspaper Enterprise Association, 1992.

World Commission on Environment and Development. *Our Common Future.* Oxford: Oxford University Press, 1989.

"Worldwide cancer rates shifting dramatically." *Journal of Environmental Health* 53:16, Nov.-Dec. 1990.

Wright, James D. *The Social Epidemiology of AIDS in Africa,* unpublished dissertation, University of Washington, 1989.

Wuthnow, Robert. *Experimentation in American Religion: The New Mysticisms and Their Implications for the Churches.* Berkeley: University of California Press, 1978.

Wyant, Frank P. *The United States, OPEC and Multinational Oil.* Lexington, MA: Lexington Books, 1977.

Zaroulis, N.L. *Who Spoke? American Protest Against the War in Vietnam, 1963-1975.* 1st ed. New York: Holt, Rinehart, and Winston, 1985.

Zimmerman, Donald Lee. *DRGs and the Medicaid Program.* Washington, DC: Intergovernmental Health Project, George Washington University, 1984.

Zinn, Howard. *SNCC: The New Abolitionists.* Boston: Beacon Press, 1964.

Zinnman, David. "Mystery of heart disease death rates." *Newsday* April 28, 1987.

Index

Abortions, 88, 160
Accidents, 224
Acid rain, 176, 255, 262
Act Up, 160
Acupuncture, 69, 70, 170, 182, 193, 292, 293, 374(n42)
Adducts, 250, 259
Adolescents, 226–227, 232, 233, 252. *See also* Young people
Advertising, 234
Advertising Council, 225
Aetna Life and Casualty Insurance Company, 92
Africa, 99, 162
African Americans, 7, 18, 58, 84, 99, 100, 106, 158, 165, 329, 330. *See also* Civil rights movement
Agenda 21,
Rio, 267
Aging, 290, 291. *See also* Elderly people
Agricultural yields, 258, 271
Agriculture, southern, 33
AHA. *See* American Hospital Association
AIDS/HIV infections, 80, 83, 99–103, 106, 110, 128, 129, 160, 167, 203, 205, 223, 245, 248, 251–252, 264, 271, 276, 290–291, 293, 309, 379(n53), 400(n15)
AIDS Quarterly, 223
Air Force Office for Prevention and Health Services Assessment, 280–281
Alcohol consumption, 185, 216, 223, 224, 228, 230, 247
Alcoholics Anonymous, 238
Altered states of consciousness, 169, 184
Alternative Medicine Research Centers, 390(n48)
AMA. *See* American Medical Association
American Cancer Society, 29, 38, 233
American College of Physicians and Surgeons, 69

American Health: Fitness of Body and Mind, 190
American Heart Association, 38
American Holistic Health Association, 190
American Holistic Medical Association, 68, 190
American Hospital, 92
American Hospital Association, 22, 23, 29, 36, 65, 198, 213
American Medical Association (AMA), 16–17, 17–18, 18–19, 22, 29, 35, 36, 44, 46, 47, 49, 63, 65, 76, 108, 112, 114, 190, 210, 371(n72)
Committee on Professional Liability, 96
See also Journal of the American Medical Association
American Nursing Association, 193
American Public Health Association, 38
Analytic strategy, 12, 366(n34)
Anthropology, 156
Antibiotics, 28, 39, 249, 276, 379(n53)
Antitrust legislation, 84, 85
Antiwar movement, 57, 67, 156, 158, 161, 173
Arms race, 80, 82, 83, 154, 155, 174, 175, 253
Association for the Conservation of Energy, 263
Atmospheric issues, 164, 174, 175, 176. *See also* Global warming; Ozone layer
Australia, global warming policy, 268
Automobiles, 61, 97, 155, 263, 264, 269

Baby boom generation, 56, 57, 109, 129, 153–154, 158, 159, 243, 336. *See also* Generational perspective
Banks, 14, 21, 87
Baxter-Travenol, 92
Bedell, Berkley, 203
Bell, Daniel, 59
Benefits packages. *See under* Health care
Benson, Herbert, 365(n8), 387(n9)